T0210148

Abdominal Imaging

Case Review Series

Abdominal Imaging
Case Review Series

MANJIRI K. DIGHE, MD, FSAR, FSRU
Professor, Radiology
Medical Director of Ultrasound
Department of Radiology, University of Washington
Seattle, WA, USA

JOSEPH R. GRAJO, MD
Associate Professor of Radiology & Urology
Chief of Abdominal Imaging
Vice Chair for Research
Abdominal Imaging Fellowship Director
Department of Radiology, University of Florida
Gainesville, FL, USA

LESLIE K. LEE, MD
Assistant Division Chief, Abdominal Imaging and Intervention
Director, Abdominal MRI
Department of Radiology, Brigham and Women's Hospital
Instructor of Radiology, Harvard Medical School
Boston, MA, USA

ELSEVIER

Elsevier
1600 John F. Kennedy Blvd.
Ste 1800
Philadelphia, PA 19103-2899

ABDOMINAL IMAGING: CASE REVIEW SERIES

ISBN: 978-0-323-67984-8

Copyright © 2022 by Elsevier, Inc. All rights reserved.

No part of this publication may be reproduced or transmitted in any form or by any means, electronic or mechanical, including photocopying, recording, or any information storage and retrieval system, without permission in writing from the publisher. Details on how to seek permission, further information about the Publisher's permissions policies and our arrangements with organizations such as the Copyright Clearance Center and the Copyright Licensing Agency, can be found at our website: www.elsevier.com/permissions.

This book and the individual contributions contained in it are protected under copyright by the Publisher (other than as may be noted herein).

Notice

Practitioners and researchers must always rely on their own experience and knowledge in evaluating and using any information, methods, compounds or experiments described herein. Because of rapid advances in the medical sciences, in particular, independent verification of diagnoses and drug dosages should be made. To the fullest extent of the law, no responsibility is assumed by Elsevier, authors, editors or contributors for any injury and/or damage to persons or property as a matter of products liability, negligence or otherwise, or from any use or operation of any methods, products, instructions, or ideas contained in the material herein.

Library of Congress Control Number : 2020949633

Content Strategist: Kayla Wolfe
Content Development Specialist: Erika Ninsin
Publishing Services Manager: Shereen Jameel
Project Manager: Rukmani Krishnan
Design Direction: Amy Buxton

Printed in China

Last digit is the print number: 9 8 7 6 5 4 3 2 1

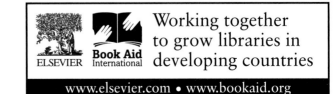

Working together to grow libraries in developing countries

www.elsevier.com • www.bookaid.org

Dedication

*To my parents, Kiran and Vaishali, for their
unwavering support, for inspiring the love of learning
in me and raising me to do my best in everything.
To my husband, Sandeep, my children, Sameer and
Myra, thank you for your love and support.
To my siblings, Anjali and Deepen, for your love,
support, and appreciation.*
—Manjiri K. Dighe, MD, FSAR, FSRU

*To my wife and best friend, Nicolette, who inspires
me and loves me unconditionally, and our daughter,
Brooklyn, who amazes me each day.
To my parents, Joseph and Ruth, who raised me to set no
limits to my potential, and my sister, Jennifer, who has
always supported and appreciated me.
To my mentors, colleagues, and trainees, who challenge
me and encourage my academic aspirations.*
—Joseph R. Grajo, MD

*To my wife, Kim, and our children, Maddy and Landon,
thank you for filling my life with love and joy.
To my parents, Sam and Christine, and my sister, Laurel,
thank you for your loving support.
To my colleagues, mentors, fellows and residents,
thank you for your friendship and inspiration.*
—Leslie K. Lee, MD

Series Foreword

Series Editor

David M. Yousem, MD, MBA
Professor of Radiology
Director of Neuroradiology
Russell H. Morgan Department of Radiology and Radiological Science
The Johns Hopkins Medical Institutions
Baltimore, Maryland

Volumes in the *Case Review* series

Series Foreword

I have been very gratified by the popularity and positive feedback that the authors of the *Case Review* series have received on the publication of their volumes. Reviews in journals and online sites as well as word-of-mouth comments have been uniformly favorable. The authors have done an outstanding job in filling the niche of an affordable, easy-to access, case-based learning tool that supplements the material in The Requisites series. I have been told by residents, fellows, and practicing radiologists that the *Case Review* series books are the ideal means for studying for rotations and clinical practice.

Although some students learn best in a non-interactive study book mode, others need the anxiety or excitement of being quizzed. The selected format for the *Case Review* series (which consists of showing a few images needed to construct a differential diagnosis and then asking a few clinical and imaging questions) was designed to simulate the board examination experience. The only difference is that the Case Review books provide the correct answer and immediate feedback. The limit and range of the reader's knowledge are tested through scaled cases ranging from relatively easy to very hard. The *Case Review* series also offers feedback on the answers, a brief discussion of each case, a link back to the pertinent Requisites volume, and up-to-date references from the literature. In addition, we have recently included labeled figures, figure legends, and supplemental figures in a new section at the end of the book, which provide the reader more information about the case and diagnosis.

We have upcoming volumes yet to be published, so stay tuned for even more Case Review favorites to come. Personally, I am very excited about the future. Join us.

David M. Yousem, MD, MBA

Foreword

I am very happy to announce the publication of the *Abdominal Imaging* edition within the *Case Review* series authored by Manjiri K. Dighe, Joseph R. Grajo, and Leslie K. Lee. This is a compilation of cases from the gastrointestinal and genitourinary systems in a volume that includes plain films, ultrasound, CT, and MRI. In a way, this is a more practical way of approaching an abdominal examination where one does not know in advance which organ system is involved. As many examinations are ordered with clinical comments of "belly pain," "nausea-vomiting," "colic," or "malignant lymphadenopathy / lung metastases—evaluation for abdominal primary tumor," having an *Abdominal Imaging* edition in the *Case Review* series is essential.

Abdominal radiology is a discipline that must address oncologic, vascular, traumatic, degenerative, iatrogenic, and infectious diseases. One must master diseases of many organ systems. I admire the abdominal imager who must keep up with so many branches of the radiology literature—I only have to know my tiny field of neuroradiology. I do very few things, very well. These authors do many things, very well. I also recognize that, in this branch of radiology, understanding the roles of multiple imaging modalities is essential.

I congratulate Drs. Dighe, Grajo, and Lee on this *Abdominal Imaging* edition of the *Case Review* series. I know that it will be influential and important in preparing trainees and practitioners for mastering this region of the body.

David M. Yousem, MD, MBA

Preface

Dear Reader,

We are pleased to present *Abdominal Imaging*, published as part of the *Case Review* series. It was wonderful to receive an invitation from Dr. Yousem to create this edition on abdominal imaging as a comprehensive collection of cases that are most commonly seen in clinical practice.

In writing this, we aimed to provide a wide range of cases encompassing gastrointestinal (GI) and genitourinary (GU) radiology, including providing CT- and MRI-rich cases with multiple images and cases encountered commonly in clinical practice, but also rare and important cases.

We directed the content and images toward radiology residents and fellows in abdominal/body imaging, and also toward new posttraining abdominal imagers.

Some of the changes compared to prior volumes in the Gastrointestinal and Genitourinary Imaging series include combining GI and GU cases in one edition, focus on CT and MR exams, and an entirely new set of images from prior editions.

We would like to thank the entire team at Elsevier for working with us in creating this book.

Manjiri K. Dighe, MD, FSAR, FSRU
Joseph R. Grajo, MD
Leslie K. Lee, MD

Contents

🌐 Online cases and supplemental figures can be accessed at
www.expertconsult.com

Abdominal Imaging

Case Review Series

Case 1

History: 74-year-old man with history of atherosclerotic disease, status postthoracoabdominal vascular bypass, presents with abdominal pain and altered mental status.

1. In the provided figures, the branching linear hypodensities in the liver represent gas in:
   A. Portal vein branches
   B. Hepatic arteries
   C. Hepatic veins
   D. Intrahepatic bile ducts
2. Which of the following is a potential etiology of the branching linear hypodensities in the liver shown in the provided figures?
   A. Colitis
   B. Diverticulitis
   C. Peptic ulcer disease
   D. Mesenteric ischemia
   E. All of these

3. From the provided figures, the most likely diagnosis is:
   A. Portal venous gas, secondary to mesenteric ischemia
   B. Pneumobilia, secondary to recent endoscopic retrograde cholangiopancreatography (ERCP)
   C. Portal venous gas, secondary to diverticular abscess
   D. Pneumobilia, secondary to gallstone ileus
4. Upon reviewing the provided figures, the next best step in the management of the patient is:
   A. ERCP
   B. Abdominal magnetic resonance imaging (MRI)/MRCP
   C. Nasogastric tube placement
   D. Surgical consultation

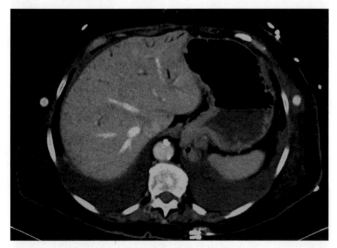

Fig. 1.1

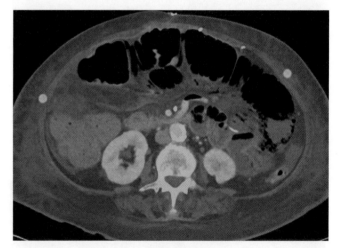

Fig. 1.2

Case 2

History: 34-year-old female with incidentally discovered liver mass.

1. What is the most likely diagnosis for the liver lesion depicted on this magnetic resonance imaging (MRI)?
   A. Hemangioma
   B. Hepatic adenoma
   C. Focal nodular hyperplasia
   D. Hepatocellular carcinoma
2. Focal nodular hyperplasia is distinguished from hepatic adenoma by which characteristic?
   A. Arterial phase hyperenhancement
   B. Hepatobiliary phase uptake
   C. Predilection for young women
   D. Association with oral contraceptives
3. Which of the following may be associated with focal nodular hyperplasia? (Choose all that apply.)
   A. Hemangiomas
   B. Arteriovenous malformation
   C. Hereditary hemorrhagic telangiectasia
   D. Fibrolamellar hepatocellular carcinoma
4. Focal nodular hyperplasia is most easily identified on which phase of dynamic contrast-enhanced imaging?
   A. Unenhanced
   B. Arterial
   C. Portal venous
   D. Equilibrium

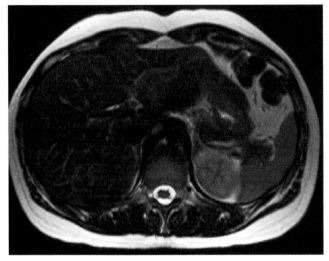

Fig. 2.1

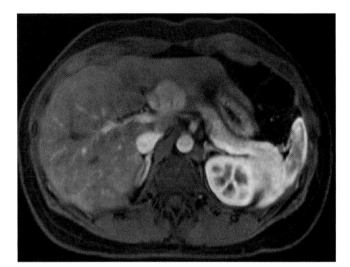

Fig. 2.2

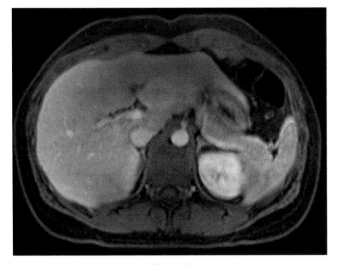

Fig. 2.3

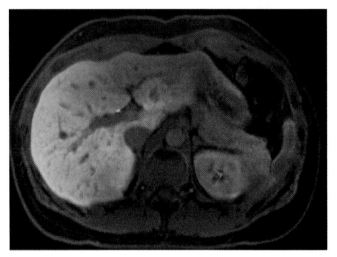

Fig. 2.4

Case 3 is online only and accessible at www.expertconsult.com.

Case 4

History: 34-year-old woman with upper abdominal pain and elevated liver function enzymes.

1. Which of the following would be included in the differential diagnosis for the imaging findings presented? (Choose all that apply.)
   A. Focal nodular hyperplasia (FNH)
   B. Adenoma
   C. Hepatocellular carcinoma
   D. Hemangioma
2. Which of the following are recognized risk factors for development of hepatic adenomas? (Choose all that apply.)
   A. Oral contraceptive (OC) use
   B. Obesity
   C. Hepatitis C infection
   D. Cirrhosis

3. Which of the following is a characteristic appearance of hepatic adenoma on magnetic resonance imaging (MRI)?
   A. Hypointense to the surrounding liver on T1 weighted in-phase images
   B. Relatively hyperintense to the liver on T1 weighted opposed phase images
   C. Hypovascular on postcontrast arterial phase
   D. Hyperintense on hepatobiliary phase during hepatocyte-specific postcontrast T1 weighted images.
4. Which of the following are recognized treatment options for hepatic adenomas?
   A. Surgery
   B. Cessation of hormone therapy
   C. Serial radiologic follow-up
   D. Serial alpha-fetoprotein measurement

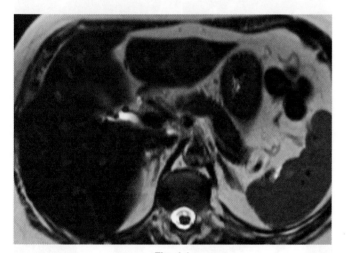

Fig. 4.1

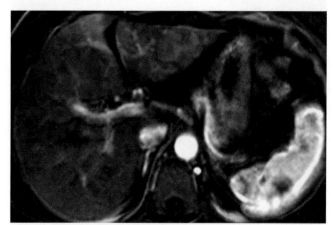

Fig. 4.2

Case 5

History: 56-year-old with abdominal pain and distension.

1. Which of the following should be included in the differential diagnosis of the imaging findings shown? (Choose all that apply.)
   A. Cirrhosis
   B. Nutmeg liver
   C. Carcinomatosis
   D. Hemochromatosis
2. What process within the liver gives rise to the appearance of the nutmeg liver?
   A. Chronic systemic venous congestion
   B. Chronic portal venous congestion
   C. Chronic arterial obstruction
   D. Chronic biliary obstruction
3. Which of the following features suggest Budd-Chiari syndrome as a cause of diffuse mottled nutmeg liver appearance?
   A. Presence of ascites
   B. Biliary duct dilation
   C. Caudate lobe enlargement
   D. Distention of the inferior vena cava
4. Which of the following would be included in the differential diagnosis of a hypervascular mass within the liver in Budd-Chiari syndrome? (Choose all that apply.)
   A. Metastasis
   B. Regenerative nodule
   C. Hepatocellular carcinoma
   D. Cyst

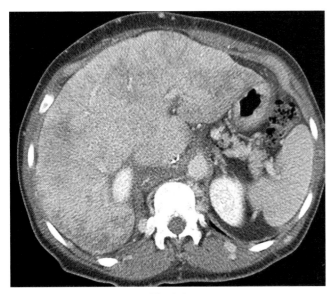

Fig. 5.1

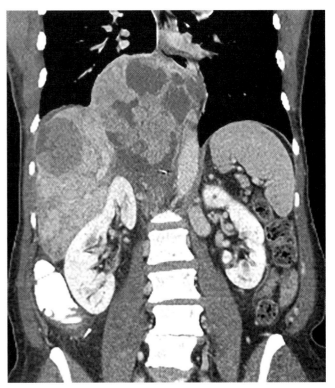

Fig. 5.2

Case 6 is online only and accessible at www.expertconsult.com.

Case 7

History: 75-year-old woman with acute right-sided abdominal pain, fever, and sepsis.

1. Which of the following would be included in the differential diagnosis for the imaging findings presented?
   A. Hepatic abscess
   B. Gallbladder perforation
   C. Hepatic cyst
   D. Dilated bowel loop
2. What is the most common type of gallbladder polyp?
   A. Adenoma
   B. Papilloma
   C. Cholesterol
   D. Hyperplastic

3. Which of the following is a description of the "sonographic-hole" sign seen on ultrasound in gallbladder perforation?
   A. Gallbladder wall thickening
   B. Pain elicited during compression of the gallbladder by the ultrasound transducer
   C. Direct visualization of the gallbladder wall defect
   D. Dirty shadowing seen in the gallbladder fossa due to air
4. Which of the following complications are seen with gallbladder perforation? (Choose all that apply.)
   A. Bile leak
   B. Peritonitis
   C. Intrahepatic abscesses
   D. Bowel obstruction

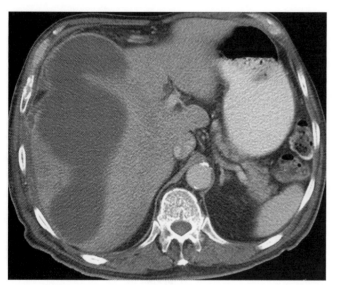

Fig. 7.1

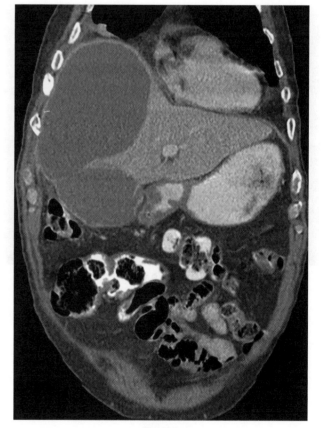

Fig. 7.2

Case 8 is online only and accessible at www.expertconsult.com.

Case 9

History: 36-year-old woman with recurrent abdominal pain.

1. Which of the following would be included in the differential diagnosis for the imaging findings presented?
   A. Polyps
   B. Adherent calculi
   C. Adenomyosis
   D. Gallbladder carcinoma
2. What is the most common type of gallbladder polyp?
   A. Adenoma
   B. Papilloma
   C. Cholesterol
   D. Hyperplastic

3. Which of the following are considered risk factors for development of gallbladder carcinoma? (Choose all that apply.)
   A. Age less than 50 years
   B. Pedunculated polyp
   C. Primary sclerosing cholangitis (PSC)
   D. Indian ethnicity
4. At what size do most guidelines recommend cholecystectomy for a gallbladder polyp?
   A. <3 mm
   B. 3 to 5 mm
   C. 6 to 10 mm
   D. >10 mm

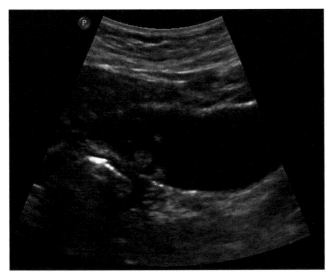

Fig. 9.1

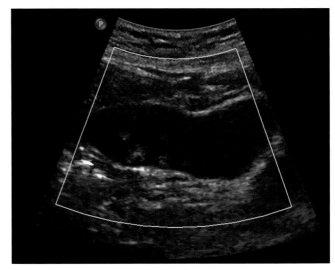

Fig. 9.2

Case 10

History: 45-year-old man presents with severe abdominal pain.

1. Which of the following are causes of acute pancreatitis? (Choose all that apply.)
   A. Alcohol
   B. Gallstones
   C. Endoscopic retrograde cholangiopancreatography (ERCP)
   D. Pancreas divisum
2. What time frame distinguishes acute peripancreatic fluid collection from pseudocyst in acute interstitial edematous pancreatitis according to the 2012 Revised Atlanta Classification?
   A. 4 hours
   B. 4 days
   C. 4 weeks
   D. 4 months
3. What is the main role of ultrasound in the evaluation of acute pancreatitis?
   A. To identify pancreatic edema
   B. To identify cholelithiasis as a potential cause
   C. To identify underlying chronic pancreatitis
   D. To identify pancreatic necrosis
4. Which laboratory marker serves as one of three major diagnostic criteria for the diagnosis of acute pancreatitis?
   A. Lipase
   B. Bilirubin
   C. International normalized ratio (INR)
   D. Aspartate aminotransferase (AST)

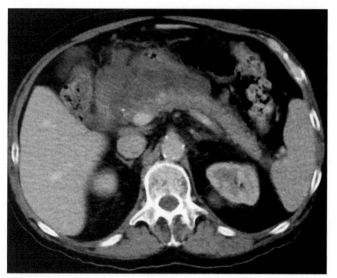

Fig. 10.1

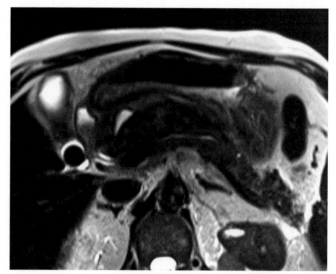

Fig. 10.2

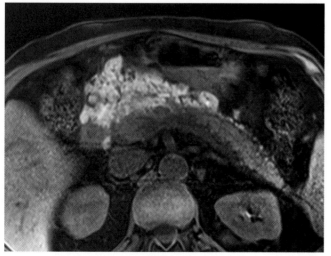

Fig. 10.3

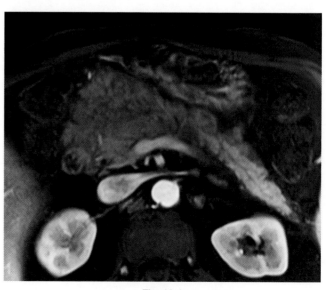

Fig. 10.4

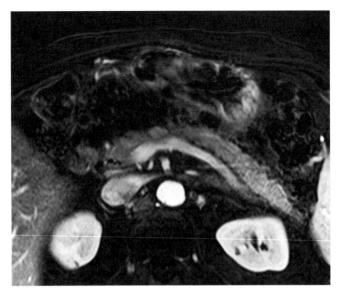

Fig. 10.5

Case 11

History: 56-year-old man with long history of alcohol use presents with chronic abdominal pain.

1. What is the most common cause of chronic pancreatitis worldwide?
   A. Alcohol
   B. Hypertriglyceridemia
   C. Gallstones
   D. Malnutrition
2. What is the most sensitive imaging modality for detecting findings of chronic pancreatitis?
   A. Ultrasound
   B. Fluoroscopy
   C. Computed tomography (CT)
   D. Magnetic resonance imaging (MRI)
3. Which imaging finding is the most specific for the diagnosis of chronic pancreatitis?
   A. Pancreatic atrophy
   B. Pancreatic enlargement
   C. Main duct dilation
   D. Intraductal stones
4. Decreased early enhancement with progressive delayed enhancement of the pancreas on dynamic contrast-enhanced imaging reflects what underlying process?
   A. Inflammation
   B. Fibrosis
   C. Acinar atrophy
   D. Ductal sclerosis

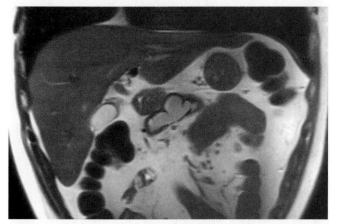

Fig. 11.1

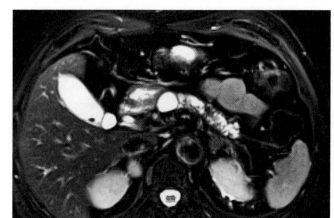

Fig. 11.2

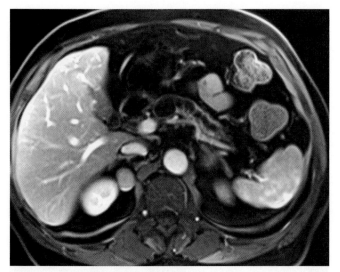

Fig. 11.3

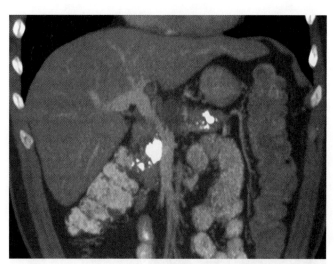

Fig. 11.4

Case 12

History: 67-year-old man presents with gradual onset of abdominal pain and jaundice.

1. Which of the following is the most common form of pancreatic malignancy?
   A. Neuroendocrine tumor
   B. Ductal adenocarcinoma
   C. Mucinous cystic neoplasm
   D. Metastatic disease
2. Which of the following represent risk factors for the development of pancreatic ductal adenocarcinoma? (Check all that apply.)
   A. Family history
   B. Cigarette smoking
   C. Chronic pancreatitis
   D. Obesity

3. What is the most common presenting symptom of pancreatic cancer?
   A. Abdominal pain
   B. Painless jaundice
   C. Early satiety
   D. Diarrhea
4. Which modality is most commonly utilized in the staging of pancreatic cancer?
   A. Ultrasound
   B. Computed tomography
   C. Magnetic resonance imaging
   D. Positron emission tomography

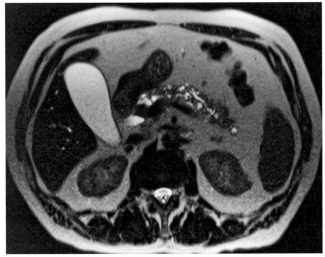

Fig. 12.1

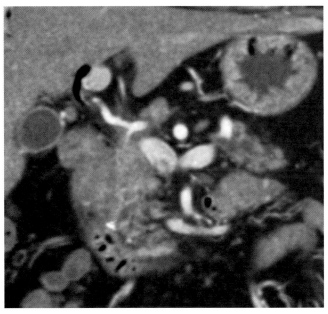

Fig. 12.2

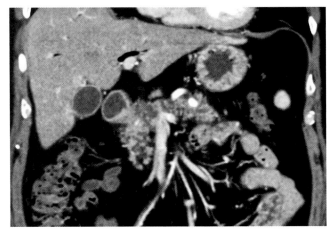

Fig. 12.3

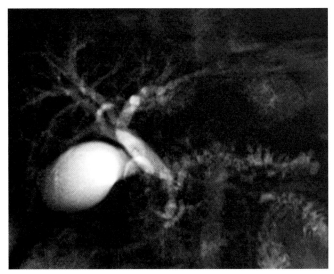

Fig. 12.4

Case 13

History: 58-year-old female with abdominal pain and fever.

1. Which of the following is a reason for the rising incidence of splenic abscess?
   A. Immunosuppression
   B. Diverticulitis
   C. Pancreatic cancer
   D. Portal hypertension
2. Which of the following imaging signs is pathognomic for splenic abscess?
   A. Peripheral enhancement
   B. Low attenuation on computed tomography (CT)
   C. Internal septations
   D. Air

3. Which source of splenic abscess most likely demonstrates a multifocal presentation?
   A. Bacterial
   B. Viral
   C. Fungal
   D. Septic emboli
4. Which of the following conditions can mimic splenic abscess on nuclear medicine gallium scan?
   A. Lymphoma
   B. Splenic infarct
   C. Splenic hemangioma
   D. Sclerosing adenomatoid nodular transformation

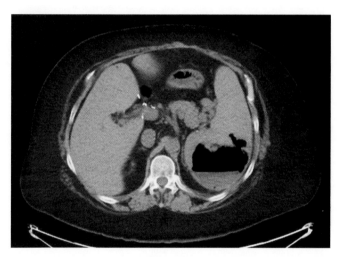

Fig. 13.1

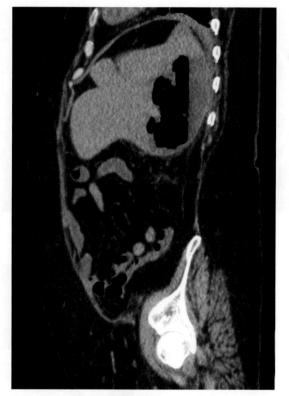

Fig. 13.2

Case 14 is online only and accessible at www.expertconsult.com.

Case 15

History: 64-year-old male with chronic hepatitis C.

1. Gamna-Gandy bodies of the spleen are most commonly seen in the setting of which condition?
   A. Paroxysmal nocturnal hemoglobinuria
   B. Portal hypertension
   C. Lymphoma
   D. Melanoma
2. What is the typical appearance of Gamna-Gandy bodies in terms of size and number?
   A. Solitary and subcentimeter
   B. Numerous and subcentimeter
   C. Solitary and large
   D. Numerous and large

3. The radiologic and pathologic appearance of Gamna-Gandy bodies is related to the deposition of which substance?
   A. Melanin
   B. Gadolinium
   C. Iodine
   D. Hemosiderin
4. Gamna-Gandy bodies are best characterized on which magnetic resonance imaging (MRI) pulse sequence?
   A. Postgadolinium T1 weighted fat suppressed images
   B. T2 weighted images
   C. In-phase and out-of-phase T1 gradient echo sequences
   D. Diffusion weighted imaging

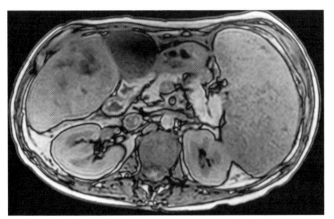

Fig. 15.1

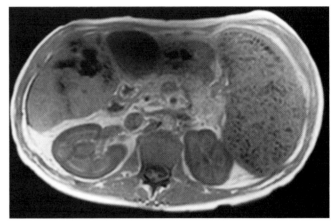

Fig. 15.2

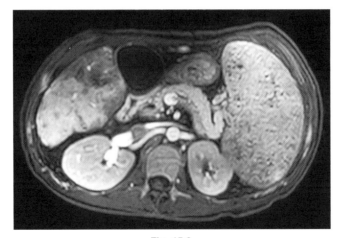

Fig. 15.3

Case 16

History: 32-year-old male with palpable abdominal mass.

1. What is the underlying cause for wandering spleen?
   A. Internal hernia
   B. Malrotation
   C. Abnormal suspensory ligaments
   D. Absent vascular pedicle
2. What is the management for wandering spleen?
   A. Conservative
   B. Follow-up imaging
   C. Surgery
   D. Angiography

3. Which underlying conditions may be present in the setting of wandering spleen? (Choose all that apply.)
   A. Mononucleosis
   B. Lymphoma
   C. Sickle cell disease
   D. Pregnancy
4. Which nuclear medicine exam can easily identify the abnormal location of the spleen in wandering spleen?
   A. Sestamibi scan
   B. Sulfur colloid scan
   C. MIBG scan
   D. Gallium scan

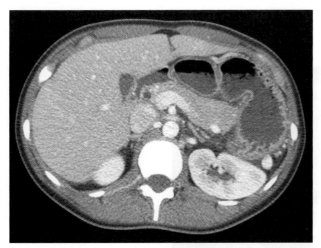

Fig. 16.1

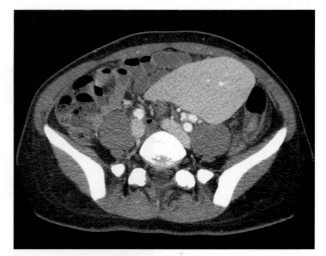

Fig. 16.2

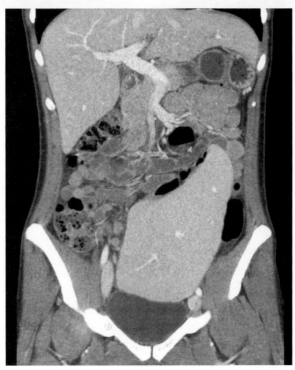

Fig. 16.3

Case 17

History: 33-year-old male with abdominal pain following a motor vehicle collision.

1. What is the most commonly injured abdominal organ following blunt trauma?
   A. Liver
   B. Spleen
   C. Pancreas
   D. Adrenal glands
2. Patients who undergo splenectomy for blunt trauma are at risk for infection with what type of organism?
   A. Encapsulated bacteria
   B. Unencapsulated bacteria
   C. Fungal
   D. Viral

3. Which imaging modality is utilized to triage hemodynamically stable patients with potential traumatic splenic injury?
   A. Plain radiography
   B. Ultrasound
   C. Computed tomography (CT)
   D. Magnetic resonance imaging (MRI)
4. What is the best phase of contrast for evaluating injury to the splenic parenchyma?
   A. Noncontrast
   B. Arterial
   C. Portal venous
   D. 3-minute delay

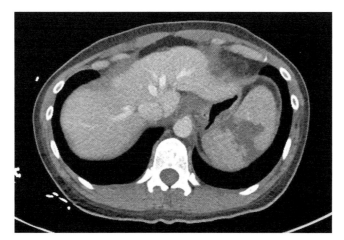

Fig. 17.1

Case 18

History: 76-year-old female has incidentally discovered mass by computed tomography (CT) on staging scan for colon carcinoma.

1. Which of the following would be included in the differential diagnosis for the imaging findings presented? (Choose all that apply.)
   A. Adrenal adenoma
   B. Metastasis from colon carcinoma
   C. Adrenal myelolipoma
   D. Renal angiomyolipoma
2. Which of the following is the most appropriate next diagnostic examination for this lesion?
   A. No further diagnostic workup
   B. Indium (In)–111 pentetreotide imaging (OctreoScan)
   C. Adrenal vein sampling
   D. Percutaneous biopsy
3. Which of the following is the most common presentation of this lesion?
   A. Hypertension
   B. Acute hemorrhage
   C. Hematuria
   D. Incidental finding on imaging studies
4. Presence of intracytoplasmic fat on chemical shift imaging may be a pitfall to diagnosis of adrenal metastasis in which tumor?
   A. Lung cancer
   B. Colon cancer
   C. Renal cell carcinoma
   D. Melanoma

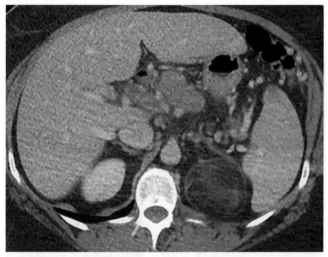

Fig. 18.1

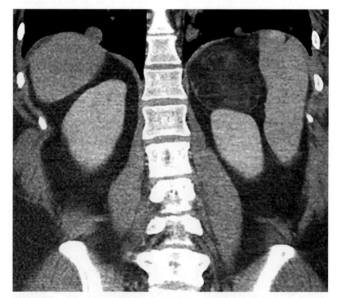

Fig. 18.2

Case 19 is online only and accessible at www.expertconsult.com.

Case 20

History: 30-year-old female with incidental adrenal mass found on imaging study.

1. What should be included in the differential diagnosis of the imaging findings in Fig. 20.1 (noncontrast computed tomography [CT]) and Fig. 20.2 (postcontrast at 60 seconds)? (Choose all that apply.)
   A. Adrenal metastasis
   B. Pheochromocytoma
   C. Adrenal adenoma
   D. Myelolipoma
2. Which attenuation value at unenhanced CT is used to definitively determine an incidental adrenal mass as an adenoma?
   A. <0 Hounsfield units (HU)
   B. <10 HU
   C. <20 HU
   D. <30 HU
3. The left adrenal mass measured 25 HU on unenhanced CT, 85 HU on venous phase postcontrast CT at 60 seconds, and 45 HU on delayed postcontrast CT at 15 minutes. Which of the following is the absolute washout and relative washout for this mass?
   A. Absolute washout 77% (85/110) and relative washout 29% (25/85)
   B. Absolute washout 67% (77/60) and relative washout 47% (40/85)
   C. Absolute washout 113% (60/45) and relative washout 44% (20/45)
   D. Absolute washout 84% (110/130) and relative washout 44% (20/45)
4. All of the following can potentially show absolute or relative washout characteristics that overlap with those of lipid poor adenomas, EXCEPT:
   A. Pheochromocytoma
   B. Adrenal hematoma
   C. Adrenal metastasis from renal cell carcinoma
   D. Adrenal metastasis from hepatocellular carcinoma

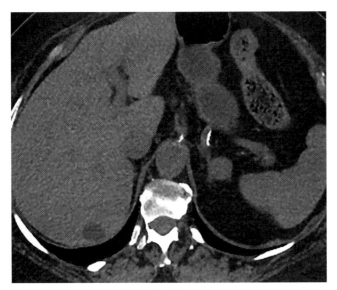

Fig. 20.1

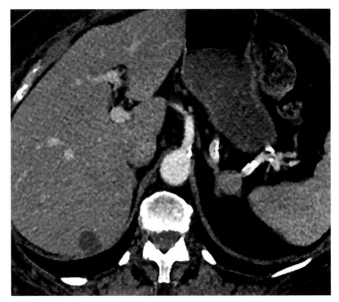

Fig. 20.2

Case 21

History: 42-year-old person with trauma was brought into the emergency department after a fall from a height.

1. Which of the following findings are seen in the figures presented? (Choose all that apply.)
   A. Superficial renal laceration
   B. Deep renal laceration
   C. Active bleeding
   D. Renal artery pseudoaneurysm
2. Which of the following is the best imaging study for this patient with suspected renal injury with bleeding?
   A. Intravenous urography
   B. Noncontrast computed tomography (CT)
   C. Single-phase contrast-enhanced CT
   D. Dual-phase contrast-enhanced CT

3. Which of the following categories of the American Association for the Surgery of Trauma (AAST) grading system is this renal injury classified as, assuming there is no injury to the renal collecting system?
   A. Grade I
   B. Grade II
   C. Grade III
   D. Grade IV/V
4. Which of the following is the absolute indication of operative management of renal injury?
   A. Renal contusion
   B. Expanding or pulsatile hematoma
   C. Subsegmental renal infarct
   D. Free fluid in the abdomen

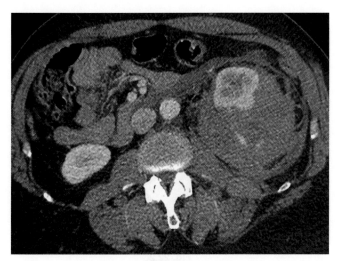

Fig. 21.1

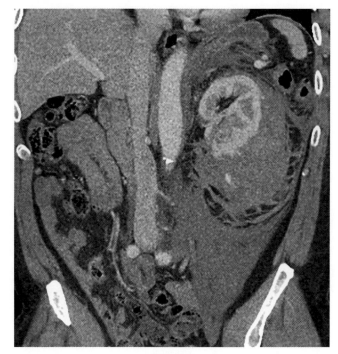

Fig. 21.2

Case 22

History: 56-year-old woman with acute left flank pain with nausea and diaphoresis.

1. Which of the following would be included in the differential diagnosis for the imaging findings presented? (Choose all that apply.)
   A. Retroperitoneal fibrosis
   B. Obstructing calculus at the ureterovesical junction
   C. Calculus that has recently passed into the bladder
   D. Retroperitoneal hematoma
2. Which of the following modalities is most sensitive for detection of urinary calculi?
   A. Plain radiograph
   B. Ultrasound
   C. Computed tomography
   D. Magnetic resonance imaging

3. Which of the following are indirect computed tomography (CT) findings of acute obstructing ureteral calculus? (Choose all that apply.)
   A. Perinephric stranding
   B. Renal atrophy
   C. Enlarged kidney
   D. Hydronephrosis and hydroureter
4. Which of the following types of stones are invisible on CT?
   A. Calcium phosphate
   B. Uric acid stone
   C. Indinavir stone
   D. Cystine stone

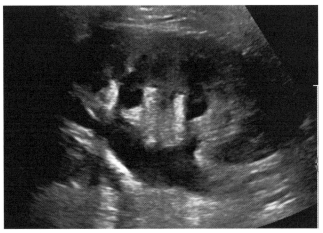

Fig. 22.1

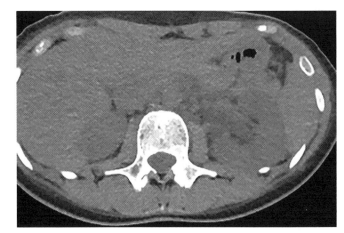

Fig. 22.2

Case 23

History: 28-year-old woman with fever, abdominal pain, nausea, and vomiting.

1. Which of the following would be included in the differential diagnosis for the imaging findings presented? (Choose all that apply.)
   A. Renal infarct
   B. Acute pyelonephritis
   C. Renal contusion
   D. Renal lymphoma
2. Striated nephrogram can be seen in which of the following conditions? (Choose all that apply.)
   A. Acute high-grade ureteral obstruction
   B. Acute renal vein thrombosis
   C. Renal lymphoma
   D. Hypertension
3. The following can commonly cause acute pyelonephritis in an asymptomatic young woman, EXCEPT:
   A. Ascending infection from bladder
   B. Vesicoureteral reflux
   C. Hematogenous spread
   D. Abnormal ureteral insertion
4. In which of the following situations is imaging study least likely indicated?
   A. An elderly patient with a history of diabetes mellitus who has symptoms of severe acute pyelonephritis
   B. A young adult patient with clinical and laboratory findings compatible with uncomplicated acute pyelonephritis
   C. A young boy with first documented urinary tract infection
   D. An adult patient with recent diagnosis of acute pyelonephritis who does not respond to appropriate antibiotic therapy within the first 72 hours

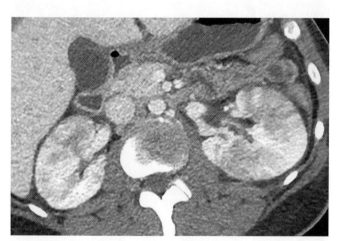

Fig. 23.1

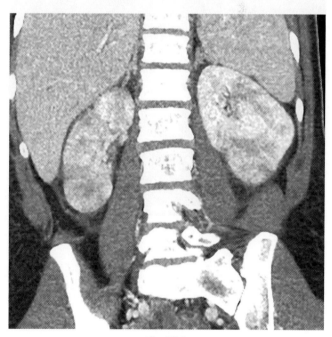

Fig. 23.2

Case 24

History: 28-year-old female with recurrent urinary tract infection.

1. What is the most common anatomic site of fusion in horse-shoe kidney?
   A. Renal pelvis
   B. Upper pole
   C. Interpolar
   D. Lower pole
2. Horseshoe kidney is usually located in the lower abdomen because it is unable to ascend to its normal position in the renal fossa as the isthmus becomes stuck on what anatomic structure during cranial migration?
   A. Renal artery
   B. Celiac axis
   C. Superior mesenteric artery
   D. Inferior mesenteric artery
3. Patients with horseshoe kidney are predisposed to which of the following conditions? (Choose all that apply.)
   A. Stone formation
   B. Renal malignancy
   C. Hydronephrosis
   D. Polyureteritis cystica
4. Which of the following chromosomal abnormalities is most commonly associated with horseshoe kidney?
   A. Down syndrome
   B. Turner syndrome
   C. Klinefelter syndrome
   D. Edwards syndrome

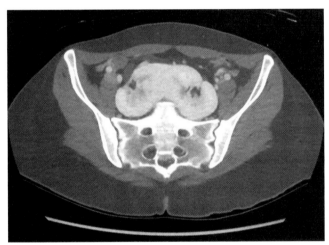

Fig. 24.1

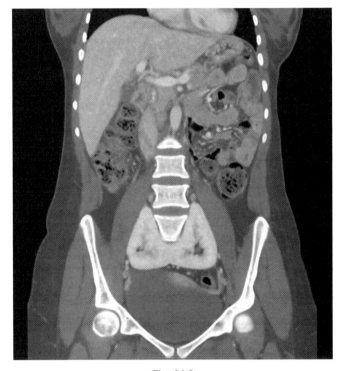

Fig. 24.2

Case 25

History: 39-year-old woman with abdominal pain and hematuria.

1. Which of the following are considered as differential diagnosis for the imaging findings shown? (Choose all that apply.)
   A. Unilateral renal agenesis
   B. Horseshoe kidney
   C. Duplicated renal collecting system
   D. Crossed fused renal ectopia
2. Which of the following is true regarding the renal anomalies in the figures shown?
   A. It is the most common type of renal fusion anomaly
   B. The ureteral insertion of the kidney across the midline is at its normal location in the bladder
   C. Blood supply to the kidney across a midline is in its normal location from the renal artery from the aorta
   D. The kidney across a midline usually lies above anomaly situated kidney
3. The renal anomaly shown in the figures is more susceptible to all of the following conditions, EXCEPT:
   A. Urinary tract infection
   B. Urolithiasis
   C. Hydronephrosis
   D. Renal cysts
4. According to embryogenesis, the renal anomaly shown occurs in which time period during fetal development?
   A. 4 to 8 weeks
   B. 8 to 12 weeks
   C. 12 to 16 weeks
   D. 16 to 20 weeks

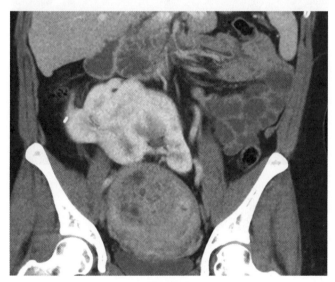

Fig. 25.1

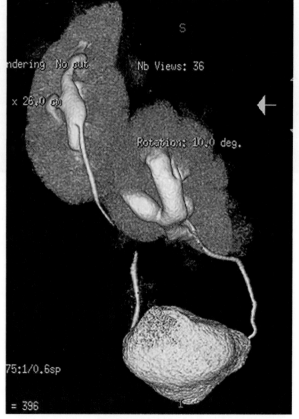

Fig. 25.2

Case 26 is online only and accessible at www.expertconsult.com.

Case 27

History: 45-year-old male with right flank pain.

1. The best diagnosis regarding this abdominal radiograph is:
   A. Normal abdominal radiograph
   B. Bowel obstruction
   C. Pneumoperitoneum
   D. Renal stone
2. Of the following renal stone compositions, the most likely to be radiolucent is:
   A. Calcium oxalate
   B. Calcium phosphate
   C. Uric acid
   D. Struvite
3. What is the most common composition of renal stones?
   A. Calcium oxalate
   B. Pure calcium phosphate
   C. Struvite
   D. Uric acid
4. Ureteral stones above what size may necessitate urologic intervention?
   A. 3 mm
   B. 5 mm
   C. 7 mm
   D. 10 mm

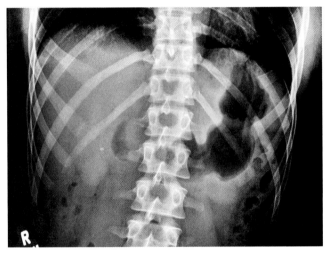

Fig. 27.1

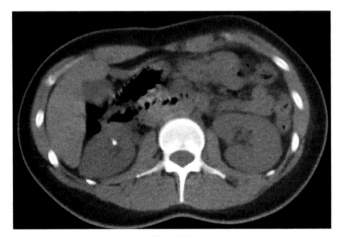

Fig. 27.2

Case 28 is online only and accessible at www.expertconsult.com.

Case 29

History: 58-year-old male with history of painless gross hematuria. The patient has remote history of prostate cancer.

1. Which of the following would be included in the differential diagnosis for the imaging findings presented? (Choose all that apply.)
   A. Radiation cystitis
   B. Primary bladder cancer
   C. Infectious cystitis
   D. Metastatic bladder cancer
2. Which of the following is the most common histologic type of primary bladder neoplasm?
   A. Squamous cell carcinoma
   B. Adenocarcinoma
   C. Transitional cell carcinoma (TCC)
   D. Small cell carcinoma
3. Which of the following imaging modality is most helpful for evaluation of depth of invasion of the bladder tumor?
   A. Excretory urography
   B. Ultrasonography
   C. Computed tomography (CT)
   D. Magnetic resonance imaging (MRI)
4. Which of the following areas in the bladder show early enhancement on dynamic postcontrast magnetic resonance imaging (MRI)?
   A. Adventitial layer, mucosa, and detrusor muscle
   B. Detrusor muscle, adventitial layer, and submucosa
   C. Bladder tumor, mucosa, and submucosa
   D. Mucosa, submucosa, and adventitial layer

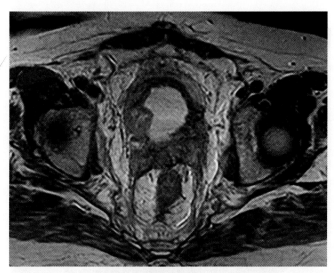

Fig. 29.1

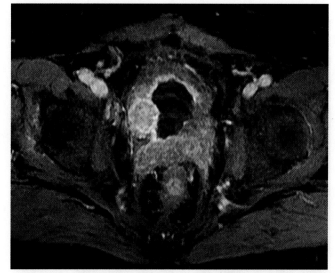

Fig. 29.2

Case 30

History: 49-year-old woman complains of dyspareunia and dribbling incontinence.

1. Which of the following would be included in the differential diagnosis for the imaging findings presented? (Choose all that apply.)
   A. Vaginal cyst
   B. Urethral diverticulum
   C. Bladder diverticulum
   D. Bladder carcinoma
2. Which one of the following is a typical location in the urethra for the disease shown in the figures?
   A. Close to bladder base
   B. Midurethra
   C. At introitus
   D. Throughout the whole urethra
3. Which one of the following imaging features is considered pathognomonic for the diagnosis of urethral adenocarcinoma?
   A. Location of the mass close to the bladder
   B. Calcifications in the mass
   C. Enhancement and soft tissue components in the mass
   D. Nonenhancing septations in the mass
4. Which of the following complications are typically seen in this disease?
   A. Infection
   B. Rupture
   C. Calculus formation
   D. Malignancy

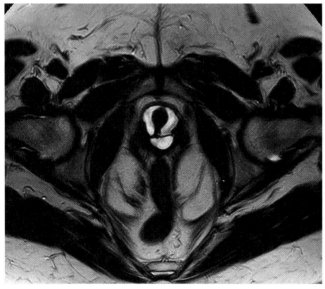

Fig. 30.1

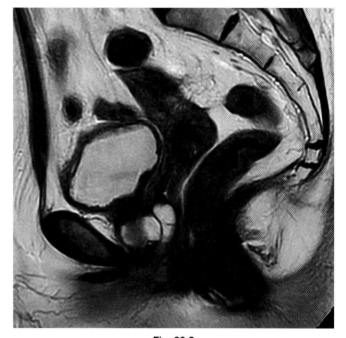

Fig. 30.2

Case 31

History: 60-year-old woman with history of diabetes presents with dysuria and pelvic pain.

1. Which of the following would be included in the differential diagnosis for the imaging findings presented in the figures? (Choose all that apply.)
   A. Subcutaneous emphysema
   B. Pelvic abscess
   C. Post–cesarean section air in the uterus
   D. Emphysematous cystitis
2. Which of the following is considered a risk factor for development of emphysematous cystitis?
   A. Bladder calculus
   B. Diabetes mellitus
   C. Malignant involvement
   D. Fistulization with adjacent bowel

3. Which of the following are considered features of emphysematous cystitis seen on computed tomography (CT)? (Choose all that apply.)
   A. Bladder calculi
   B. Bladder wall thickening
   C. Air in bladder wall
   D. Air in bladder lumen
4. Which of the following is not a complication of untreated emphysematous cystitis? (Choose all that apply.)
   A. Ureteritis
   B. Renal pyelitis
   C. Rupture
   D. Fistula formation

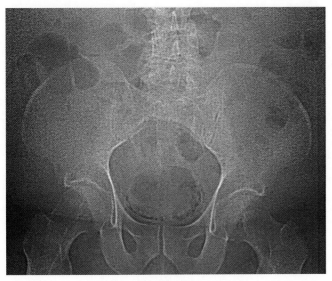

Fig. 31.1

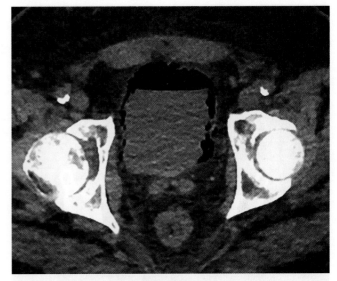

Fig. 31.2

Case 32

History: 51-year-old man presents with hematuria after abdominal trauma. A computed tomography (CT) cystogram is performed.

1. The provided figures demonstrate:
   A. Pelvic organ injury
   B. Pelvic vascular injury
   C. Pelvic fracture
   D. Pelvic mass
2. In the provided figures, abnormal contrast opacification is shown in:
   A. Morison pouch
   B. Pouch of Douglas
   C. Space of Retzius
   D. Rectovesical space

3. From the provided figures, the visceral organ injury can be classified as:
   A. Contusion
   B. Intraperitoneal rupture
   C. Extraperitoneal rupture
   D. Combined injury
4. From the provided figures, a potential mechanism of injury is:
   A. Blunt abdominal trauma
   B. Penetrating abdominal trauma
   C. Motor vehicle crash
   D. Both A and C

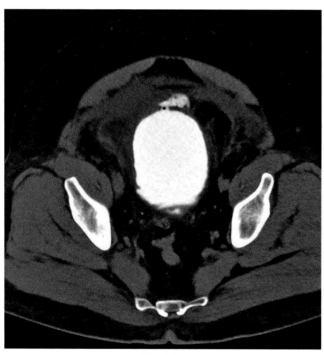

Fig. 32.1

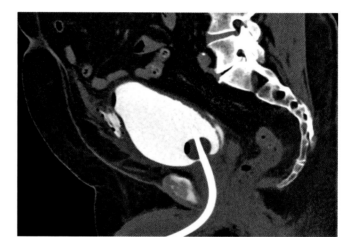

Fig. 32.2

Case 33 is online only and accessible at www.expertconsult.com.

Case 34

History: 28-year-old woman with right lower quadrant pain.

1. Which of the following would be included in the differential diagnosis for the imaging findings presented? (Choose all that apply.)
   A. Hemorrhagic cyst
   B. Fibroid
   C. Mature cystic teratoma
   D. Cystadenoma
2. What is the most specific sign for diagnosis of an ovarian mature cystic teratoma?
   A. High signal intensity on T1 weighted images
   B. High signal intensity on T2 weighted images
   C. Low signal on T2 weighted images
   D. Low signal on fat suppressed T1 weighted images
3. Difference between immature and mature cystic teratoma includes which of the following?
   A. Immature teratomas are more common than mature cystic teratomas
   B. Immature teratomas occur in older age group females
   C. Have immature or embryonic tissues in them
   D. Demonstrate clinically benign behavior
4. What is the most common complication in mature cystic teratoma?
   A. Torsion
   B. Malignant degeneration
   C. Rupture
   D. Hemorrhage

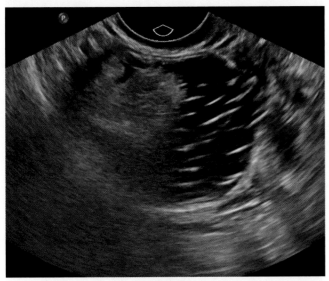

Fig. 34.1

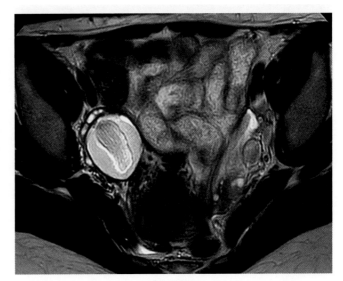

Fig. 34.2

Case 35

History: 24-year-old woman presented with infertility.

1. Which uterine anomalies are the result of müllerian duct defects? (Choose all that apply.)
   A. Uterus unicornis
   B. Uterus didelphys
   C. Uterus bicornis
   D. Uterus septate
2. Which imaging modalities are most effective in diagnosing uterus bicornis?
   A. Computed tomography (CT)
   B. Hysterosalpingography
   C. Magnetic resonance imaging (MRI)
   D. Two-dimensional transvaginal ultrasonography
3. Which particular sign has been suggested to be most sensitive and specific for diagnosis of uterine didelphys on MRI?
   A. Fundal cleft <1 cm
   B. Fundal cleft >1 cm
   C. Absence of fundal cleft
   D. Presence of two uterine horns
4. Which particular symptoms are most commonly seen in patients with uterine didelphys? (Choose all that apply.)
   A. Asymptomatic
   B. Dysparenuia
   C. Infertility
   D. Preterm birth

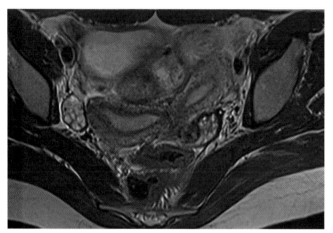

Fig. 35.1

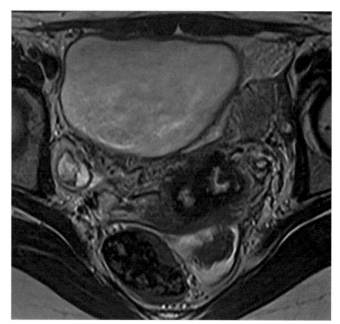

Fig. 35.2

Case 36

History: 35-year-old woman with difficulty urinating and a mass felt on vaginal palpation.

1. Which of the following would be included in the differential diagnosis for the imaging findings presented? (Choose all that apply.)
   A. Urethral diverticulum
   B. Gartner duct cyst
   C. Cystocele
   D. Bartholin cyst
2. Which one of the following is the best modality for imaging of vaginal wall cysts?
   A. Hysterosonogram
   B. Ultrasound (US)
   C. Computed tomography (CT)
   D. Magnetic resonance imaging (MRI)
3. Which one of the following imaging features is considered pathognomonic for the presence of infection in the cyst shown?
   A. Location of the cyst
   B. T2 hyperintense signal
   C. Wall enhancement
   D. Fluid level
4. Which particular imaging plane is most helpful for evaluation of vaginal wall cysts?
   A. Sagittal
   B. Coronal
   C. Axial
   D. Oblique

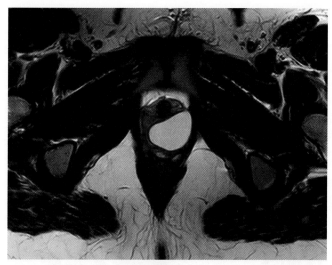

Fig. 36.1

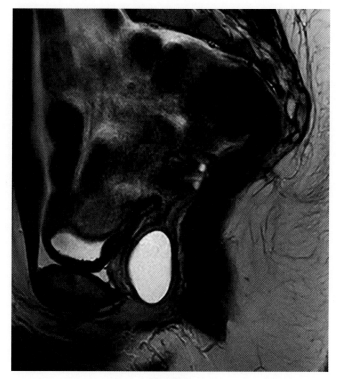

Fig. 36.2

Case 37 is online only and accessible at www.expertconsult.com.

Case 38

History: 54-year-old woman presented with postmenopausal vaginal bleeding.

1. Which of the following would be included in the differential diagnosis for the imaging findings presented in the figure? (Choose all that apply.)
   A. Endometrial polyp
   B. Endometrial hyperplasia
   C. Endometrial carcinoma
   D. Cervical carcinoma
2. On ultrasound, what is the threshold for endometrial thickness in postmenopausal women with vaginal bleeding that warrants biopsy?
   A. 3 mm
   B. 5 mm
   C. 8 mm
   D. 11 mm
3. Which uterine structure visualized on magnetic resonance imaging (MRI) is most helpful in the evaluation of myometrial invasion by the endometrial carcinoma?
   A. Cervical stroma
   B. Junctional zone
   C. Serosa
   D. Lymphovascular plexus
4. Which of the following are risk factors for development of endometrial carcinoma? (Choose all that apply.)
   A. Hormonal replacement therapy
   B. Obesity
   C. Nulliparity
   D. Tamoxifen therapy

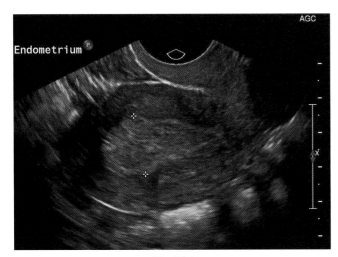

Fig. 38.1

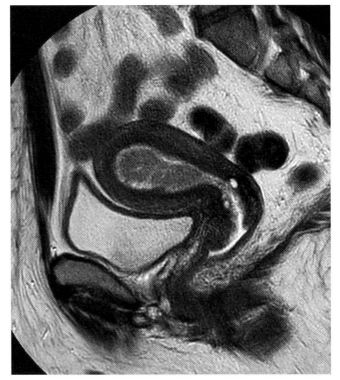

Fig. 38.2

Case 39

History: 36-year-old nulligravid woman with recurrent pelvic pain.

1. Which of the following would be included in the differential diagnosis for the imaging findings presented? (Choose all that apply.)
   A. Hemorrhagic cysts
   B. Simple cysts
   C. Dermoid
   D. Endometriosis
2. What is the association between endometriosis and adenomyosis?
   A. Increased incidence of adenomyosis among infertile women with endometriosis
   B. Less than 1% of women with endometriosis have concomitant adenomyosis
   C. Endometriosis and adenomyosis are not related
   D. All women with endometriosis also have concomitant adenomyosis
3. What is the incidence of malignant transformation in endometriomas?
   A. 1%
   B. 5%
   C. 10%
   D. 15%
4. In which of the following situations would endometriomas undergo decidualization? (Choose all that apply.)
   A. Malignant degeneration
   B. Pregnancy
   C. Postmenopausal status
   D. Coexistent adenomyosis

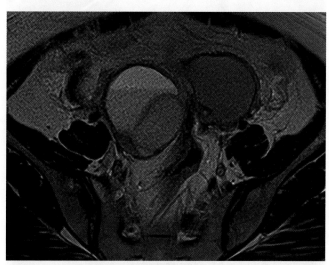

Fig. 39.1

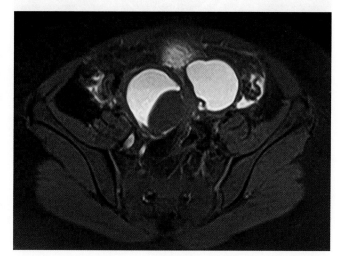

Fig. 39.2

Case 40

History: 36-year-old woman with intermenstrual bleeding.

1. Which of the following would be included in the differential diagnosis for the findings presented on the first figure? (Choose all that apply.)
   A. Uterine rupture
   B. Cesarean section scar
   C. Fibroid
   D. Adhesion
2. Which orientation of the figures is best for imaging this abnormality on ultrasound (US)?
   A. Axial
   B. Coronal
   C. Sagittal
   D. Oblique

3. What is a common presentation of patients with this abnormality?
   A. Pelvic pain
   B. Postmenstrual spotting
   C. Infertility
   D. Amenorrhea
4. Cesarean scar niche is best evaluated on which imaging modality?
   A. Ultrasound
   B. Computed tomography
   C. Magnetic resonance imaging
   D. Sonohysterography

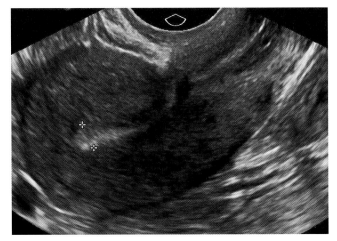

Fig. 40.1

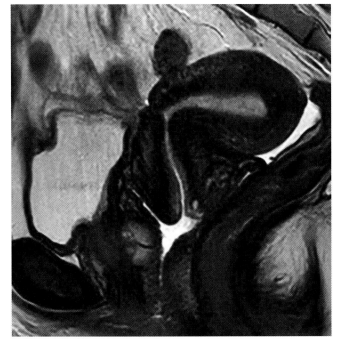

Fig. 40.2

Case 41

History: 45-year-old woman with pelvic pain and heaviness.

1. Which of the following would be included in the differential diagnosis for the imaging findings presented? (Choose all that apply.)
   A. Fibroids
   B. Adenomyosis
   C. Normal uterus
   D. Endometrial carcinoma
2. Which of the following statements given about fibroids is correct?
   A. Not influenced by estrogen
   B. Increase in size during pregnancy
   C. Increase in size after menopause
   D. Not influenced by progesterone
3. Which of the following types of fibroids are typically most symptomatic?
   A. Subserosal
   B. Intramural
   C. Submucosal
   D. Pedunculated subserosal
4. Which of the following types of degenerated fibroids have high signal intensity of T2 weighted images on magnetic resonance imaging (MRI)? (Choose all that apply.)
   A. Hyaline
   B. Cystic
   C. Myxoid
   D. Lipomatous

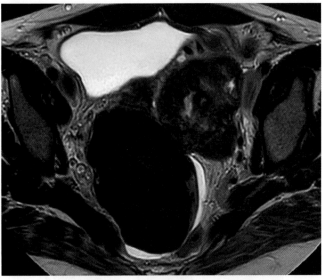

Fig. 41.1

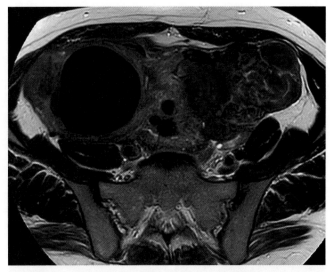

Fig. 41.2

Case 42

History: 34-year-old woman recently underwent a cesarean delivery and presented with new left-sided pelvic pain.

1. Which of the following would be included in the differential diagnosis for the imaging findings presented? (Choose all that apply.)
   A. Retroperitoneal hematoma
   B. Dilated ureter
   C. Mixing flow artifact in the ovarian vein
   D. Ovarian vein thrombosis
2. All of the following are predisposing factors to this condition, EXCEPT:
   A. Obstructing ureteral stone
   B. Stasis of blood flow
   C. Hypercoagulability
   D. Recent cesarean section
3. All of the following are common presenting signs and symptoms of the condition, EXCEPT:
   A. Fever
   B. Abdominal pain
   C. Palpable mass
   D. Hematuria
4. Which of the following is correct regarding the lesion seen in the figures?
   A. It is best detected by grayscale and color Doppler ultrasound
   B. It occurs more commonly in females than in males
   C. It occurs more frequently on the left side
   D. It occurs most commonly during early pregnancy

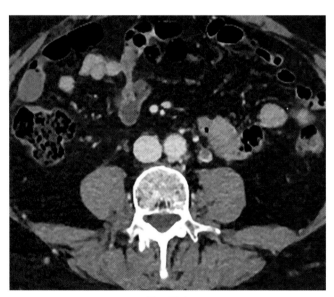

Fig. 42.1

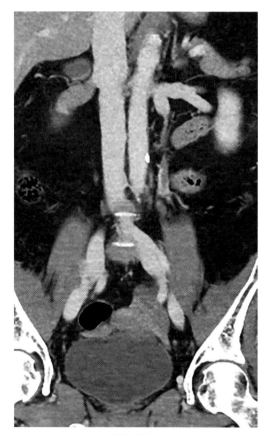

Fig. 42.2

Case 43

History: 35-year-old woman with left pelvic pain.

1. Which of the following are true regarding cyclic changes in the ovary? (Choose all that apply.)
   A. All follicles are large in the follicular phase
   B. Hemorrhagic cyst is more likely seen in the secretary phase
   C. Ovarian stroma becomes intimate in the proliferative phase
   D. Corpus luteum is visualized in the luteal phase
2. Which magnetic resonance image sequence shows the ovarian anatomy best?
   A. T2 weighted
   B. T1 weighted
   C. Gradient echo in phase
   D. Diffusion weighted
3. What is a luteal cyst?
   A. Functional system develops when the corpus luteum fails to regress
   B. Functional cyst resulting from persistence of an unruptured graafian follicle.
   C. Fluid accumulation in the corpus albicans
   D. Functional cyst developing under influence of gonadotropin
4. What is the ring of fire sign?
   A. Peripheral hyperdensity on computed tomography (CT)
   B. Ringlike enhancement on magnetic resonance imaging
   C. ^{18}F-fluorodeoxyglucose (FDG) avid rim on positron emission tomography (PET)
   D. Vascular ring on color Doppler imaging

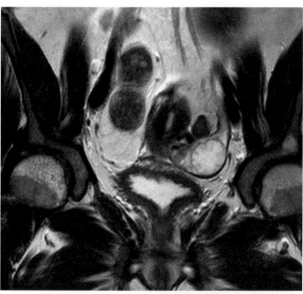

Fig. 43.1

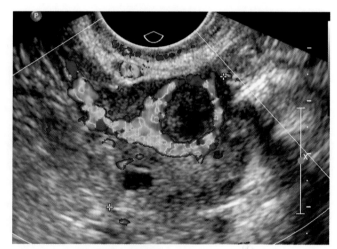

Fig. 43.2

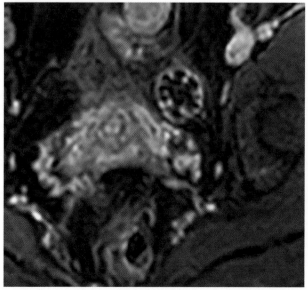

Fig. 43.3

Case 44

History: 33-year-old female presents for evaluation of infertility.

1. A hysterosalpingogram is performed. The final figure is shown. Based on these imaging findings, the conclusion regarding tubal patency is:
   A. Right patent, left patent
   B. Right occluded, left patent
   C. Right patent, left occluded
   D. Right occluded, left occluded
2. The finding shown at the left adnexa likely represents:
   A. Intraperitoneal free spill of contrast
   B. Hydrosalpinx
   C. Ovarian cyst
   D. Pelvic sidewall lymph node

3. The sequential order of passage of an ovum is:
   A. Ovary – infundibulum – ampulla – isthmus
   B. Ovary – ampulla – isthmus – infundibulum
   C. Ovary – isthmus – ampulla – infundibulum
   D. Ovary – isthmus – infundibulum – ampulla
4. Hysterosalpingography is typically performed at what phase of the menstrual cycle?
   A. Days 1 to 6
   B. Days 7 to 10
   C. Days 11 to 14
   D. Days 14 to 28

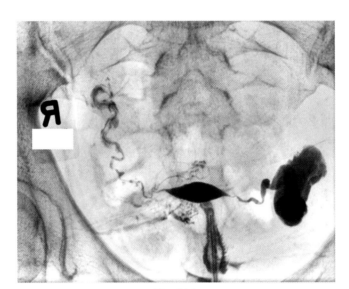

Fig. 44.1

Case 45

History: 38-year-old woman with menorrhagia and dysmenorrhea.

1. Which of the following would be included in the differential diagnosis for the imaging findings presented?
   A. Adenomyosis
   B. Fibroids
   C. Endometrial carcinoma
   D. Myometrial contraction
2. What is the most specific feature of adenomyosis on magnetic resonance imaging (MRI)?
   A. T2 bright foci in the myometrium
   B. T1 low signal intensity foci in the myometrium
   C. T1 low signal intensity area in the endometrium
   D. T2 low signal intensity foci in the endometrium

3. What is the junctional zone on MRI?
   A. An interface on T1 weighted images between the inner and outer myometrium
   B. A high signal layer on T2 weighted images between endometrium and myometrium
   C. An interface on T2 weighted images between the outer myometrium and serosa
   D. A low signal layer on T2 weighted images between endometrium and myometrium
4. The threshold for thickening of the junctional zone as a strong indicator of adenomyosis is at:
   A. 1 mm
   B. 5 mm
   C. 8 mm
   D. 12 mm

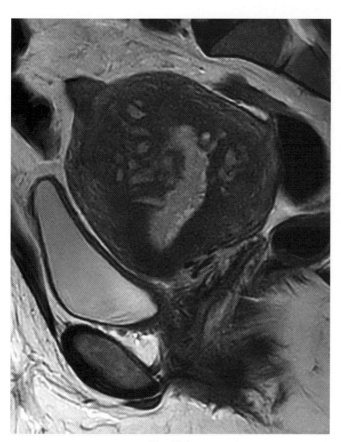

Fig. 45.1

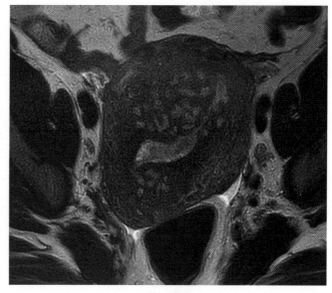

Fig. 45.2

Case 46

History: 27-year-old man has acute right scrotal pain approximately 8 hours in duration.

1. Which of the following would be in the differential diagnosis for the color Doppler ultrasound findings of the right testes presented? (Choose all that apply.)
   A. Epididymoorchitis
   B. Testicular torsion
   C. Testicular neoplasm
   D. Torsion of the testicular appendage
2. Which of the following is a congenital anomaly of the testis/scrotum predisposed to the illustrated disease?
   A. Klippel-Feil deformity
   B. Mondini deformity
   C. Madelung deformity
   D. Bell clapper deformity

3. Which of the following is the maximum duration from the onset of symptoms to appropriate treatment to achieve nearly 100% testicular salvage rate for the illustrated disease?
   A. 2 hours
   B. 6 hours
   C. 12 hours
   D. 24 hours
4. Which of the following is true regarding the illustrated disease?
   A. Venous flow within the testes is first compromised before arterial flow
   B. Testicular artery arises from the ipsilateral internal iliac artery
   C. Grayscale ultrasound is more sensitive than color Doppler ultrasound and the diagnosis of this condition
   D. Grayscale ultrasound often shows diffusely hypoechoic testes immediately after onset of symptoms

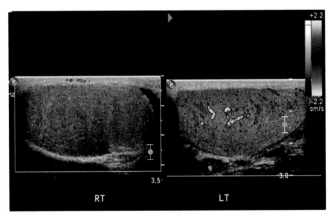

Fig. 46.1

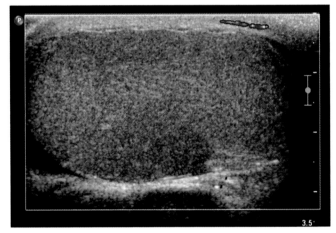

Fig. 46.2

Case 47

History: 65-year-old man with history of metastatic renal cell carcinoma has altered mental status.

1. Which of the following are differential diagnostic considerations for the condition visualized on the figures shown? (Choose all that apply.)
   A. Recent surgical procedure
   B. Penetrating trauma
   C. Decubitus ulcer
   D. Fournier gangrene

2. Which of the following is the most common predisposing factor associated with the condition shown?
   A. Neurogenic bladder
   B. Diabetes mellitus
   C. Malignant neoplasms
   D. Renal insufficiency

3. Which of the following urologic examinations is the most useful for the diagnosis of the condition shown?
   A. Plain radiography
   B. Ultrasonography
   C. Computed tomography (CT)
   D. Magnetic resonance imaging (MRI)

4. Which of the following statements is true regarding the condition shown?
   A. Broad-spectrum intravenous antibiotics obviates the need for surgery
   B. It is usually caused by multiple microorganisms
   C. Infection in this condition is limited to the genitalia and does not extend into the abdominal wall, retroperitoneum, or thigh
   D. Men and women are equally affected

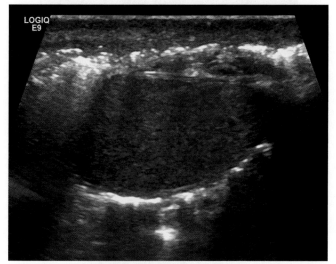

Fig. 47.1

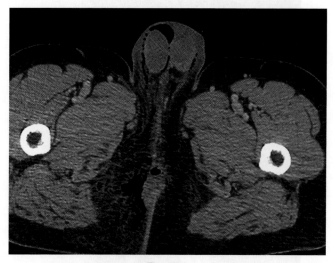

Fig. 47.2

Case 48

History: 55-year-old man with a history of smoking and alcohol use presents for evaluation of dysphagia; additional history withheld.

1. The most likely underlying cause of this finding is:
   A. Vascular
   B. Muscular
   C. Malignant
   D. Inflammatory
2. This most likely represents:
   A. Adenocarcinoma
   B. Squamous cell carcinoma
   C. Achalasia
   D. Herpes esophagitis
3. Unlike squamous cell carcinoma, a risk factor for esophageal adenocarcinoma is:
   A. Smoking
   B. Alcohol use
   C. Barrett esophagus
   D. Caustic esophagitis
4. This patient would benefit from:
   A. Chest computed tomography (CT) with intravenous contrast
   B. Surgical consultation
   C. Endoscopic intervention
   D. Vascular interventional radiology consultation

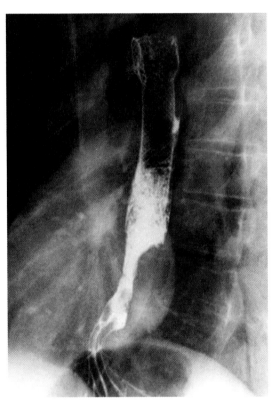

Fig. 48.1

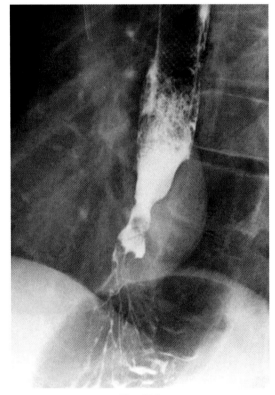

Fig. 48.2

Case 49

History: 69-year-old woman presents with dysphagia.

1. The underlying cause of this finding is:
   A. Vascular
   B. Muscular
   C. Malignant
   D. Inflammatory
2. This finding typically is seen at the level of:
   A. C1–C3
   B. C4–C6
   C. T4–T6
   D. L4–L5

3. Descriptors of this finding are:
   A. Smooth; mobile
   B. Smooth; fixed
   C. Irregular; mobile
   D. Irregular; fixed
4. The finding represented in the figure is a:
   a. Cricopharyngeal bar
   b. Squamous cell carcinoma
   c. Barrett esophagus
   d. Benign ulcer

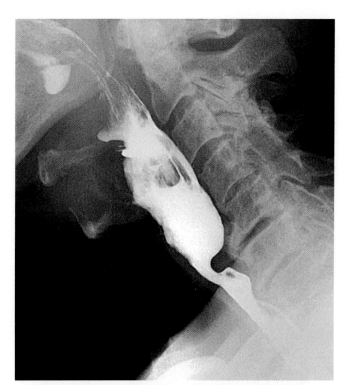

Fig. 49.1

Case 50

History: 47-year-old patient presents with dysphagia.

1. In the fluoroscopic image provided, the abnormal finding is best described as a/an:
   A. Filling defect
   B. Outpouching
   C. Contrast extravasation
   D. Air-fluid level
2. Additional descriptors of the abnormality depicted in the figure are:
   A. Smooth
   B. Smooth; circumferential
   C. Irregular
   D. Irregular; circumferential

3. The finding most likely represents:
   A. Schzatki ring
   B. Barrett esophagus
   C. Nissen fundoplication
   D. Toupet fundoplication
4. The etiology of this finding is:
   A. Vascular
   B. Malignant
   C. Infectious
   D. Idiopathic

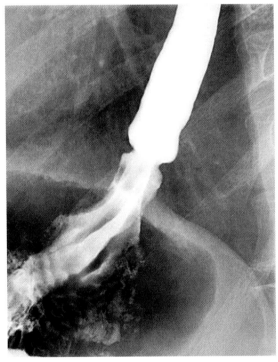

Fig. 50.1

Case 51 is online only and accessible at www.expertconsult.com.

Case 52

History: 83-year-old man presents with abdominal distension. An abdominopelvic computed tomography (CT) was reported with abnormal findings (not shown), and a contrast enema was subsequently performed. A scout image was obtained (Fig. 52.1). Rectal contrast was administered, without opacification of proximal colon; the final fluoroscopic spot image is shown (Fig. 52.2).

1. On radiographs, small bowel can typically be distinguished from large bowel by these characteristics, EXCEPT:
   A. Caliber
   B. Position
   C. Fold appearance
   D. Angulation
2. Small bowel folds are termed _____; large bowel folds are termed _____.
   A. Haustra; valvulae conniventes
   B. Valvulae conniventes; haustra
   C. Rugae; haustra
   D. Rugae; valvulae conniventes
3. In the figures provided, the most likely diagnosis is:
   A. Diffuse ileus
   B. Large bowel obstruction
   C. Diverticulosis
   D. Sigmoid volvulus
4. Underlying etiologies of large bowel obstruction include:
   A. Chronic inflammation
   B. Colorectal malignancy
   C. Peritoneal metastasis
   D. All of these

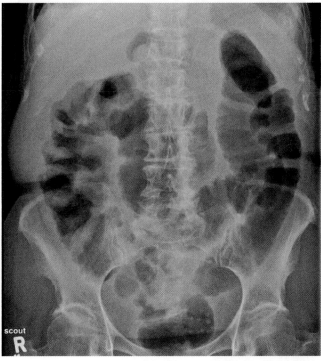

Fig. 52.1

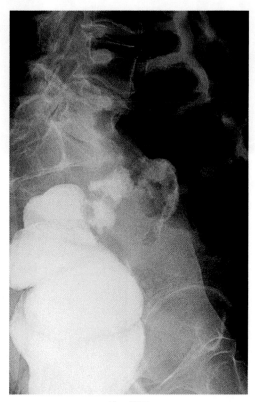

Fig. 52.2

Case 53

History: 62-year-old female with left lower quadrant pain.

1. The findings on contrast enema in Fig. 53.3 corroborate what computed tomography (CT) abnormalities, which may be suspected in Figs. 53.1 and 53.2?
   A. Pelvic abscess
   B. Sigmoid colon stricture
   C. Colovesical fistula
   D. Colon cancer
2. Which segment of colon demonstrates the highest incidence of diverticular disease?
   A. Cecum
   B. Transverse colon
   C. Descending colon
   D. Sigmoid colon
3. Which of the following are potential complications of diverticulitis? (Choose all that apply.)
   A. Abscess
   B. Peritonitis
   C. Stricture
   D. Bowel obstruction
4. What is the imaging modality of choice for suspected diverticulitis?
   A. Plain film
   B. Computed tomography
   C. Magnetic resonance imaging
   D. Fluoroscopy

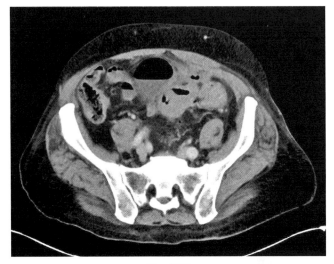

Fig. 53.1

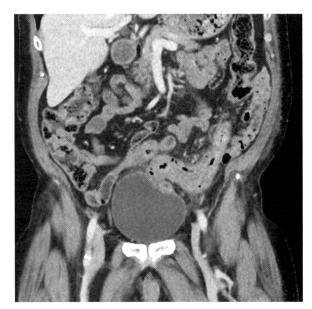

Fig. 53.2

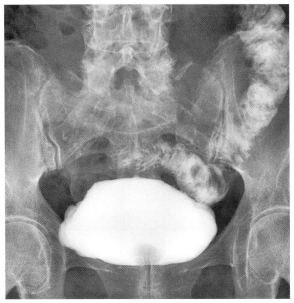

Fig. 53.3

Case 54

History: 74-year-old patient presents with a month-long history of weight loss and bloody stool.

1. The most prevalent segment of colon cancer is:
   A. Cecum/ascending colon
   B. Transverse colon
   C. Descending colon
   D. Rectosigmoid
2. The most common site of colon cancer metastases is:
   A. Lung
   B. Brain
   C. Bone
   D. Liver

3. What serum biochemical marker can be used in the follow-up evaluation of treated colon cancer?
   A. CA 19-9
   B. CA 125
   C. CEA
   D. 5-HIAA
4. According to the CT Colonography Reporting and Data System, a small polyp is defined by what size?
   A. 3 to 6 mm
   B. 6 to 9 mm
   C. 10 to 30 mm
   D. <30 mm

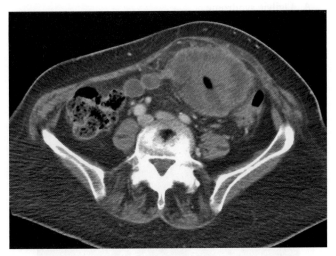

Fig. 54.1

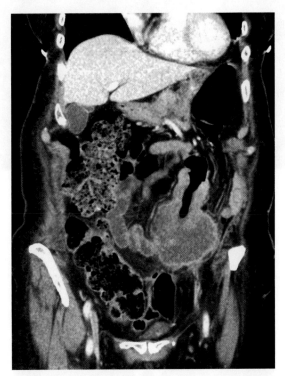

Fig. 54.2

Case 55

History: 51-year-old male with abdominal pain and diarrhea.

1. The thickened haustra of the transverse colon depicted in Fig. 55.1 account for which radiologic sign?
   A. Comb sign
   B. Thumbprinting
   C. Double bubble
   D. Steinstrasse

2. Pancolitis in an acutely ill patient with cross-sectional findings as seen in the figures most likely represents which condition?
   A. Crohn's disease
   B. Ischemic colitis
   C. Pseudomembranous colitis
   D. Typhlitis

3. Which of the following are treatment options for pseudomembranous colitis? (Choose all that apply.)
   A. Antibiotics
   B. Colonic resection
   C. Fecal transplant
   D. Chemotherapy

4. Dilation of the transverse colon exceeding 6 cm in caliber is concerning for potential impending perforation due to what condition?
   A. Ogilvie syndrome
   B. Toxic megacolon
   C. Pneumatosis
   D. Accordion sign

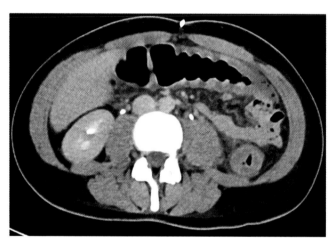

Fig. 55.1

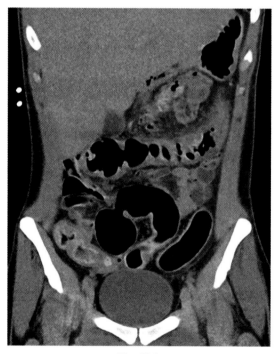

Fig. 55.2

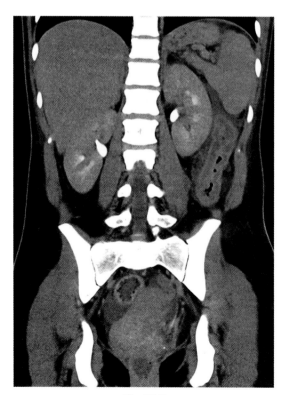

Fig. 55.3

Case 56

History: 35-year-old man with history of acute right to a quadrant abdominal pain with nausea, vomiting, and fever.

1. What is the best diagnosis based on the imaging findings presented? (Choose all that apply.)
   A. Ileitis
   B. Appendicitis
   C. Ureteric colic
   D. Right-sided colitis
2. High-density area seen within this structure in the right lower quadrant (*arrows*) is best characterized as:
   A. Ureteric calculus
   B. Phleboliths
   C. Diverticolith
   D. Appendicolith

3. Which of the following is not a specific sign of appendicitis on computed tomography (CT)?
   A. Appendiceal dilatation >6 mm in diameter
   B. Wall thickening >3 mm and enhancement
   C. Appendicolith
   D. Periappendiceal inflammation seen as fat stranding
4. Which of the following statements about imaging of acute appendicitis is true?
   A. Plain abdominal radiograph usually reveals nonspecific localized right lower quadrant paralytic ileus
   B. An appendicolith is visible on plain radiography in 20% to 25% of cases
   C. Ultrasound is a modality of choice for children and young women
   D. Radionuclide scanning with ^{99m}Technetium pertechnetate is highly sensitive and specific for the diagnosis of appendicitis

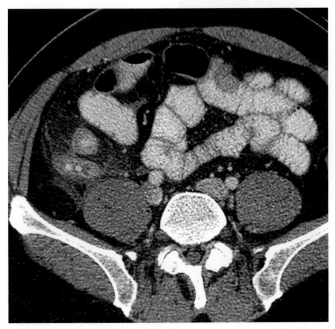

Fig. 56.1

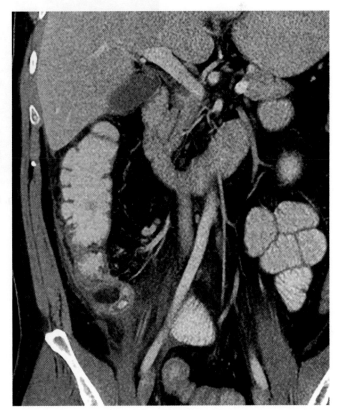

Fig. 56.2

Cases 57–59 are online only and accessible at www.expertconsult.com.

Case 60

1. The best diagnosis regarding this abdominal radiograph is:
   A. Normal abdominal radiograph
   B. Bowel obstruction
   C. Pneumoperitoneum
   D. Iatrogenic complication
   E. Renal stone
2. The radiograph was likely obtained with the patient in what position?
   A. Supine
   B. Erect
   C. Decubitus

3. The radiographic signs that are shown on this radiograph include:
   A. Rigler sign
   B. Continuous diaphragm sign
   C. Falciform ligament sign
   D. Both A and B
   E. A, B, and C
4. The most sensitive radiographic technique for the detection of intraperitoneal free air is:
   A. Upright chest radiograph
   B. Supine abdominal radiograph
   C. Prone abdominal radiograph
   D. Right lateral decubitus abdominal radiograph

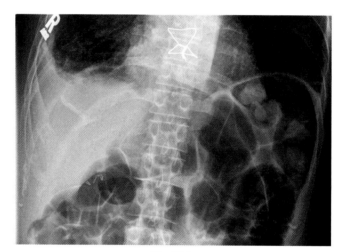

Fig. 60.1

Case 61

History: 68-year-old male with chronic hepatitis C, presenting with abdominal pain and weight loss.

1. The imaging characteristics seen on this computed tomography (CT) and magnetic resonance image (MRI) favor what disease process?
   A. Hepatocellular carcinoma
   B. Neuroendocrine tumor metastases
   C. Hepatic adenoma
   D. Cholangiocarcinoma
2. What is the leading cause of hepatocellular carcinoma worldwide?
   A. Alcohol
   B. Hepatitis B
   C. Hepatitis C
   D. Fatty liver

3. Which of the following are classified as major diagnostic features of hepatocellular carcinoma (HCC) on cross-sectional imaging? (Choose all that apply.)
   A. Arterial enhancement
   B. Washout
   C. Capsule
   D. Threshold growth
4. Which tumor marker is elevated in the majority of patients with hepatocellular carcinoma?
   A. CEA
   B. CA 19-9
   C. CA-125
   D. AFP

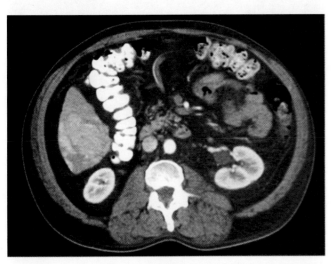

Fig. 61.1

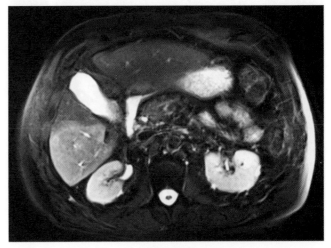

Fig. 61.2

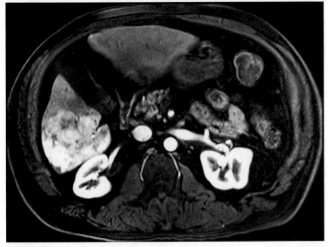

Fig. 61.3

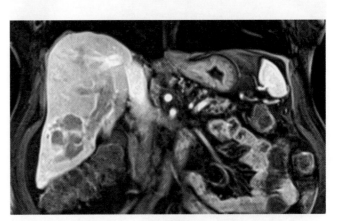

Fig. 61.4

Case 62

History: 55-year-old man with melanoma presents for staging assessment.

1. In the provided figures, the finding shown in the liver, adjacent to the falciform ligament *(arrow on Fig. 62.1)*, most likely represents:
   A. Normal liver
   B. Focal fat deposition
   C. Hemangioma
   D. Metastasis

2. In the provided figures, there is evidence of what diffuse liver condition?
   A. None; normal liver
   B. Fatty liver
   C. Hepatitis
   D. Cirrhosis

3. For hepatic or portal venous phase postcontrast computed tomography (CT) imaging of the abdomen, typical postcontrast injection timing is:
   A. 15–20 seconds
   B. 35–40 seconds
   C. 70–80 seconds
   D. 100–120 seconds

4. The following malignancies are associated with hypervascular liver metastases, EXCEPT:
   A. Melanoma
   B. Lung adenocarcinoma
   C. Renal cell carcinoma
   D. Neuroendocrine tumors

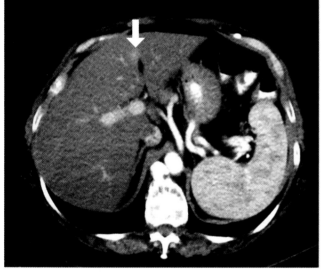

Fig. 62.1

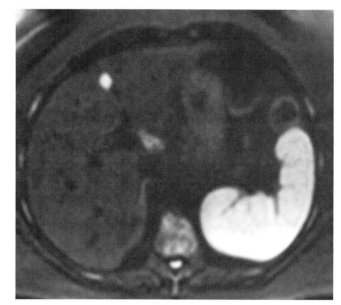

Fig. 62.2

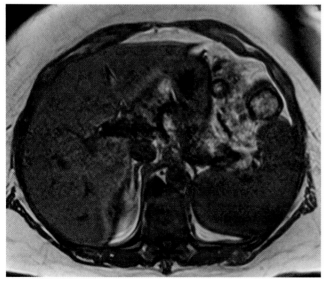

Fig. 62.3

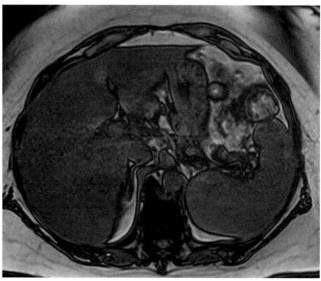

Fig. 62.4

Case 63

History: 68-year-old male with a history of chronic liver disease.

1. The magnetic resonance imaging (MRI) appearance of this liver lesion is most compatible with which entity?
   A. Hemangioma
   B. Hepatocellular carcinoma
   C. Cholangiocarcinoma
   D. Metastasis
2. Patients from which region of the world demonstrate a higher incidence of cholangiocarcinoma?
   A. North America
   B. South America
   C. Sub-Saharan Africa
   D. Southeast Asia

3. Which of the following are known risk factors for developing cholangiocarcinoma? (Choose all that apply.)
   A. Choledochal cysts
   B. Thorotrast exposure
   C. Primary sclerosing cholangitis
   D. *Clonorchis sinensis*
4. Which of the following features are classically seen with intrahepatic cholangiocarcinoma on cross-sectional imaging? (Choose all that apply.)
   A. Capsular retraction
   B. Intrahepatic biliary dilation
   C. T2 hyperintensity
   D. Rim enhancement with central fill-in

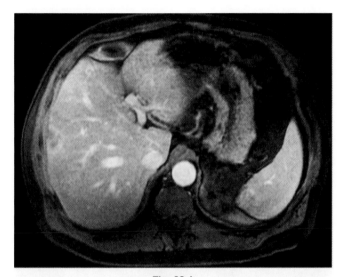

Fig. 63.1

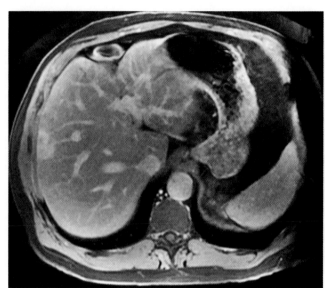

Fig. 63.2

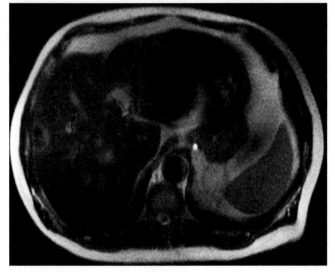

Fig. 63.3

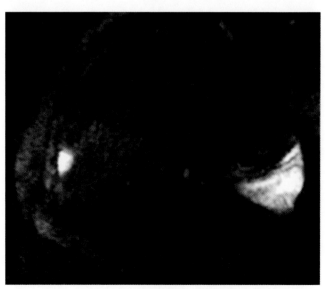

Fig. 63.4

Case 64 is online only and accessible at www.expertconsult.com.

Case 65

History: 64-year-old woman with recurrent abdominal pain, dyspepsia, and nausea.

1. Which of the following would be included in the differential diagnosis for the imaging findings presented?
   A. Polyps
   B. Adherent calculi
   C. Adenomyosis
   D. Gallbladder carcinoma
2. What is the most common type of gallbladder cancer histology?
   A. Adenocarcinoma
   B. Squamous cell carcinoma
   C. Undifferentiated carcinoma
   D. Adenosquamous carcinoma
3. Which of the following are considered risk factors for development of gallbladder carcinoma? (Choose all that apply.)
   A. Porcelain gallbladder
   B. Polyps >10 mm
   C. Primary sclerosing cholangitis (PSC)
   D. Indian ethnicity
4. What are the reasons for poor prognosis in patients with gallbladder carcinoma? (Choose all that apply.)
   A. Lymphatic involvement
   B. Hepatic involvement
   C. Early transperitoneal spread
   D. Lack of symptoms

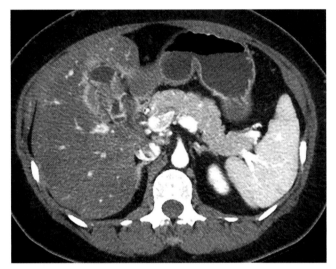

Fig. 65.1

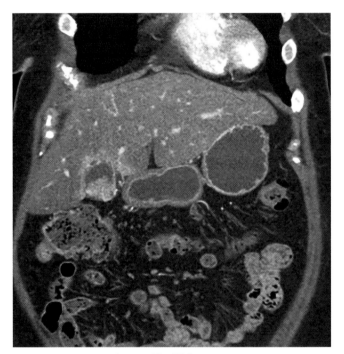

Fig. 65.2

Case 66

History: 75-year-old woman presents with abdominal pain and fever.

1. Which of the following would be included in the differential diagnosis for the imaging findings presented in Fig. 66.1?
   A. Hepatic abscess
   B. Pneumatosis coli
   C. Pneumatosis intestinalis
   D. Emphysematous cholecystitis
   E. Emphysematous pyelonephritis
2. Which organisms typically produce the process shown in these images of the right upper quadrant?
   A. *Escherichia coli*
   B. Cytomegalovirus
   C. *Coliform* species
   D. *Clostridium* species

3. What underlying condition does this patient probably have?
   A. Acquired immunodeficiency syndrome (AIDS)
   B. Emphysema
   C. Atherosclerosis
   D. Diabetes mellitus
4. What is the major complication leading to high mortality rate seen in this condition?
   A. Perforation
   B. Pancreatitis
   C. Cystic duct obstruction
   D. Common bile duct obstruction

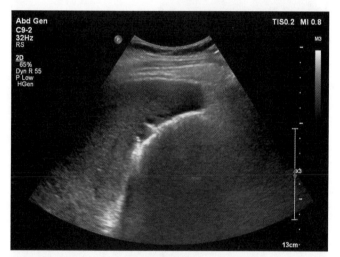

Fig. 66.1

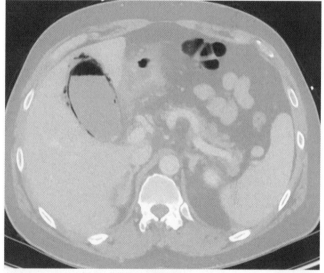

Fig. 66.2

Case 67

History: 54-year-old female with acute right upper quadrant pain and nausea.

1. What should be included in the differential diagnosis of the imaging finding shown in Fig. 67.1? (Choose all that apply.)
   A. Mirizzi syndrome
   B. Lymphadenopathy
   C. Bouveret syndrome
   D. Cholangiocarcinoma carcinoma
   E. Gallbladder carcinoma
2. What is the mechanism of Mirizzi syndrome?
   A. Gallstone eroded into the common hepatic duct
   B. Gallstone passed into the common bile duct
   C. Gallstone impacted in the cystic duct
   D. Gallstone eroded into the duodenum

3. What major iatrogenic complication is associated with this condition?
   A. Surgical ligation of the common hepatic duct
   B. Cholecystoduodenal fistula formation
   C. Perforation of the gallbladder
   D. Portal vein thrombosis
4. What is the most common cause of obstructive jaundice?
   A. Viral hepatitis
   B. Choledocholithiasis
   C. Cholangiocarcinoma
   D. Pancreatic carcinoma

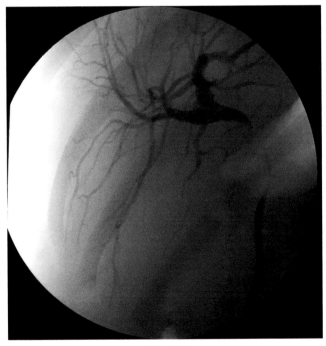

Fig. 67.1

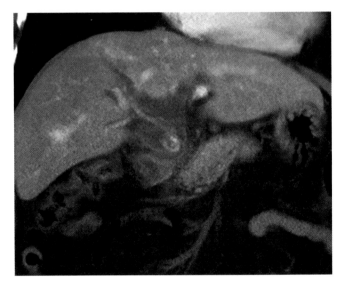

Fig. 67.2

Case 68

History: 36-year-old man with known Crohn's disease with new elevated bilirubin levels.

1. Which of the following would be included in the differential diagnosis for the imaging findings presented? (Choose all that apply.)
   A. Acquired immunodeficiency syndrome (AIDS)–related cholangitis
   B. Ascending cholangitis
   C. Oriental cholangiohepatitis
   D. Primary sclerosing cholangitis
2. Which of the following statements describes the "beaded appearance" seen in primary sclerosing cholangitis (PSC)?
   A. Long segment of stricture
   B. Multifocal annular short segmental strictures alternating with normal ducts
   C. Multiple cysts in the liver
   D. Short segment of stricture in the common bile duct

3. Which of the following are complications seen in PSC? (Choose all that apply.)
   A. Biliary stones
   B. Bacterial cholangitis
   C. Gallbladder carcinoma
   D. Cholangiocarcinoma
4. Which of the following is the definitive treatment for liver complications seen in PSC?
   A. Oral ursodeoxycholic acid
   B. Lithotripsy of biliary stones
   C. Liver transplantation
   D. Percutaneous transhepatic biliary drainage (PTBD)

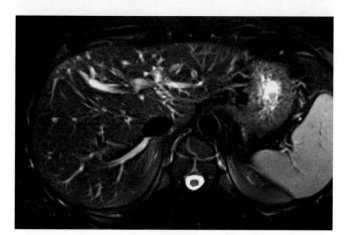

Fig. 68.1

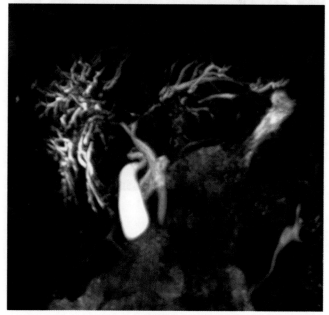

Fig. 68.2

Case 69

History: 52-year-old male with recurrent pancreatitis.

1. The images demonstrate what form of variant anatomy, thought to be a cause of idiopathic pancreatitis?
   A. Annular pancreas
   B. Pancreas divisum
   C. Ansa pancreatica
   D. Autoimmune pancreatitis
2. What is the most common form of pancreas divisum?
   A. Type 1
   B. Type 2
   C. Type 3
   D. Reverse

3. What is the gold standard for diagnosis of pancreas divisum?
   A. Ultrasound (US)
   B. Computed tomography (CT)
   C. Magnetic resonance cholangiopancreatography (MRCP)
   D. Endoscopic retrograde cholangiopancreatography (ERCP)
4. What is the management of pancreas divisum in the majority of cases?
   A. Nonoperative
   B. Pancreatic enzymes
   C. Minor papillectomy
   D. Minor papilla stenting

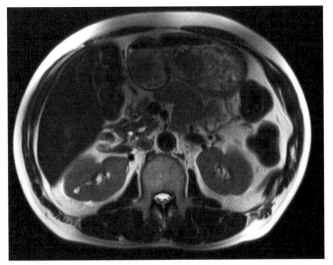

Fig. 69.1

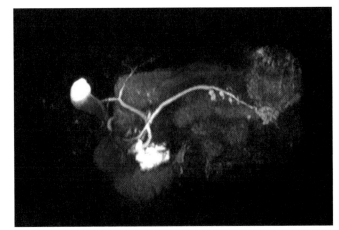

Fig. 69.2

Case 70

History: 64-year-old male with abdominal discomfort and early satiety.

1. Which of the following syndromes may be associated with the development of pancreatic neuroendocrine tumors? (Choose all that apply.)
   A. Multiple endocrine neoplasia type 1
   B. von Hippel-Lindau disease
   C. Tuberous sclerosis
   D. Neurofibromatosis type 1
2. Which of the following is the most common form of functional pancreatic neuroendocrine tumor?
   A. Insulinoma
   B. Gastrinoma
   C. Glucagonoma
   D. VIPoma
3. Which type of functional pancreatic neuroendocrine tumor is associated with the "4 Ds"?
   A. Insulinoma
   B. Gastrinoma
   C. Glucagonoma
   D. VIPoma
4. Which imaging modality demonstrates the highest overall sensitivity for detection of pancreatic neuroendocrine tumors?
   A. Magnetic resonance imaging (MRI)
   B. In-111 octreotide scan
   C. F-18 positron emission tomography (PET) computed tomography (CT)
   D. Ga-68 dotatate scan

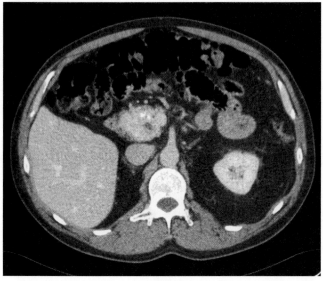

Fig. 70.1

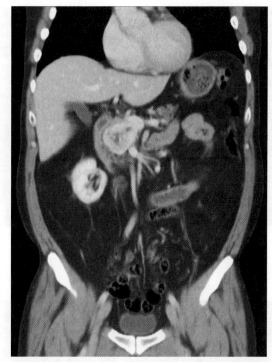

Fig. 70.2

Case 71 is online only and accessible at www.expertconsult.com.

Case 72

History: 62-year-old male with abdominal pain and nausea.

1. Which of the following is the most common primary nonhematolymphatic malignancy of the spleen?
   A. Melanoma
   B. Squamous cell carcinoma
   C. Angiosarcoma
   D. Carcinosarcoma

2. What is the most common site of metastatic spread from splenic angiosarcoma?
   A. Omentum
   B. Liver
   C. Lungs
   D. Bones

3. Which of the following interventions may decrease risk of spontaneous hemorrhage from splenic angiosarcoma?
   A. Splenectomy
   B. Bland embolization
   C. Radioembolization
   D. Cryoablation

4. Which of the following exposures is associated with increased risk of splenic angiosarcoma?
   A. Thorotrast
   B. Vinyl chloride
   C. Arsenic
   D. None of these

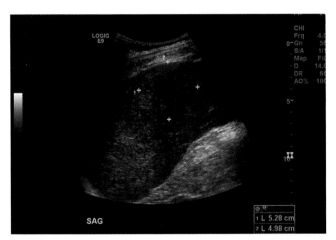

Fig. 72.1

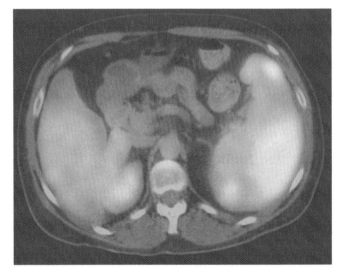

Fig. 72.2

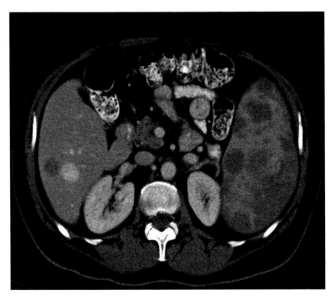

Fig. 72.3

Case 73

History: 48-year-old male with chronic abdominal pain.

1. Multiple splenic hamartomas can be seen in association with which syndrome? (Choose all that apply.)
   A. von Hippel-Lindau
   B. Tuberous sclerosis
   C. Wiskott-Aldrich syndrome
   D. Birt-Hogg-Dube syndrome
2. Which splenic lesion may represent a fibrosing variation of splenic hamartoma?
   A. Littoral cell angioma
   B. Hemangioma
   C. Lymphoma
   D. Sclerosing adenomatoid nodular transformation

3. Which phase is most helpful in distinguishing a hamartoma from background splenic parenchyma?
   A. Arterial phase
   B. Portal venous phase
   C. Enteric phase
   D. 3-minute delay
4. Beyond the pattern of contrast enhancement, which magnetic resonance imaging (MRI) signal characteristic can be helpful in differentiating a splenic hamartoma from background splenic parenchyma?
   A. T1 hypointensity
   B. T2 hyperintensity
   C. Restricted diffusion
   D. Signal drop on out-of-phase imaging

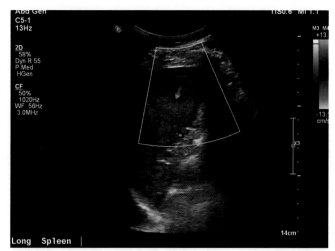

Fig. 73.1

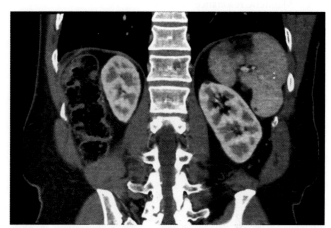

Fig. 73.2

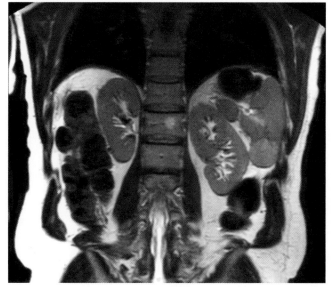

Fig. 73.3

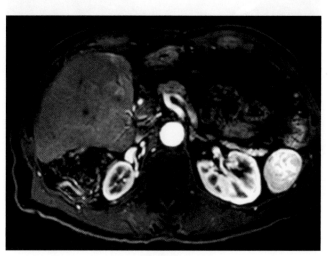

Fig. 73.4

Case 74

History: 28-year-old patient with history of multiple gunshot wounds, postlaparotomy with history of bilateral multiple pulmonary embolisms, placed on heparin therapy. One week after Fig. 74.1, the patient developed acute abdominal pain and hypotension; repeat computed tomography (CT) image shown in Fig. 74.2.

1. Which of the following would be included in the differential diagnosis for the imaging findings presented in Fig. 74.2? (Choose all that apply.)
   A. Adrenal lymphoma
   B. Adrenal metastasis
   C. Adrenal adenomas
   D. Adrenal hemorrhage
2. Which imaging modality is most useful for specific diagnosis of this condition shown in Fig. 74.2?
   A. Ultrasound
   B. Computed tomography
   C. Magnetic resonance imaging
   D. Angiography

3. Which of the following conditions more likely causes unilateral adrenal involvement than bilateral involvement in the condition shown in Fig. 74.2?
   A. Trauma
   B. Anticoagulation
   C. Heparin-induced thrombocytopenia
   D. Severe stress
4. Which of the following is a rare but serious complication of the condition shown in Fig. 74.2 if both adrenal glands are involved?
   A. Acute adrenal insufficiency
   B. Hypertensive crisis
   C. Hypernatremia
   D. Hyperglycemia

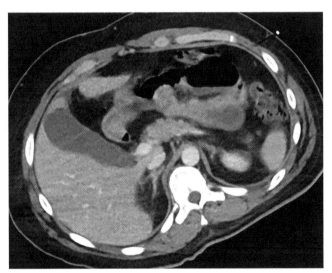

Fig. 74.1

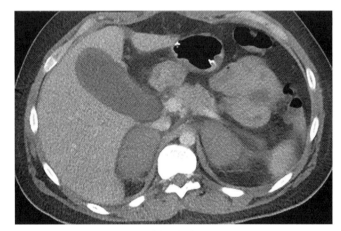

Fig. 74.2

Case 75

History: 61-year-old woman with history of hypertension, tremors, and palpitations.

1. Which of the following would be included in the differential diagnosis for the imaging findings presented? (Choose all that apply.)
   A. Fat-poor adrenal adenoma
   B. Pheochromocytoma
   C. Adrenal metastasis
   D. Adrenocortical carcinoma
2. This patient had elevated catecholamine levels. Which of the following is the most specific imaging modality for the diagnosis of catecholamine producing adrenal mass seen in the figures?
   A. Computed tomography (CT)
   B. Magnetic resonance imaging (MRI)
   C. Ultrasonography
   D. Iodine-131 metaiodobenzylguanidine (^{131}I-MIBG)

3. How often are the tumors shown in the figures malignant?
   A. <5%
   B. 10%
   C. 50%
   D. 80%
4. Which of the following is not recommended as the next diagnostic step for the patient shown in the figures?
   A. Plasma catecholamine levels
   B. Percutaneous biopsy
   C. 24-hour urine catecholamines, normetanephrines, and metanephrines
   D. Correlation with clinical signs and symptoms of hypertension, palpitation, and sweating

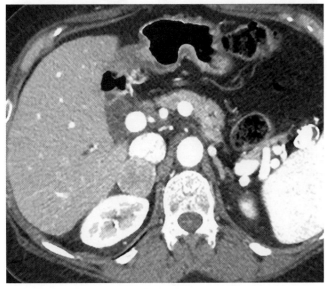

Fig. 75.1

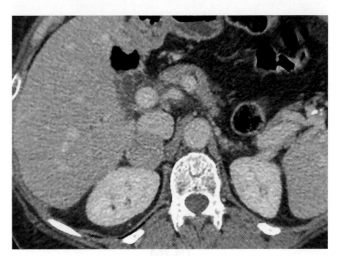

Fig. 75.2

Case 76

History: 58-year-old female with right flank pain.

1. Which of the following would be included in the differential diagnosis for the imaging findings presented? (Choose all that apply.)
   A. Hemorrhagic renal cyst
   B. Calculi
   C. Arteriovenous malformation
   D. Renal cell carcinoma
2. Which of the following is recommended as the favored treatment for this entity?
   A. Surgical resection
   B. Percutaneous embolization
   C. Nephrectomy
   D. Medical management
3. Hypertension seen in this entity is usually due to which mechanism?
   A. Iatrogenic
   B. Associated renal artery stenosis
   C. Ischemia in the renal parenchyma with renin release
   D. Secretion of renin by the lesion
4. Early enhancement of which structure is seen in this entity?
   A. Renal artery
   B. Renal parenchyma
   C. Renal collecting system
   D. Renal vein

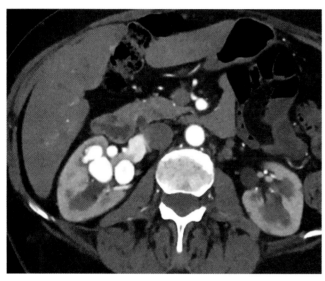

Fig. 76.1

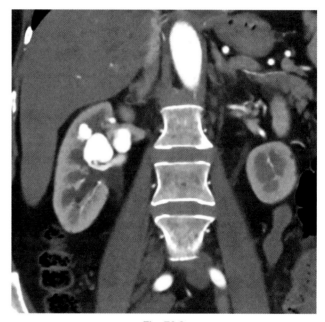

Fig. 76.2

Case 77

History: 38-year-old woman has history of hypertension that is refractory to medical therapy.

1. Which of the following would be included in the differential diagnosis for the imaging findings presented? (Choose all that apply.)
   A. Atherosclerosis
   B. Vasculitis
   C. Fibromuscular dysplasia (FMD)
   D. Segmental arterial mediolysis (SAM)
2. Which of the following is the commonest site of involvement in the arterial system by the entity illustrated in the figures?
   A. Renal
   B. Carotid
   C. Mesenteric vessels
   D. Iliac arteries

3. Which of the following is the most appropriate next diagnostic examination for this lesion?
   A. No further diagnostic workup is necessary
   B. Angiography
   C. Adrenal vein sampling
   D. Ultrasound
4. Which of the following is correct regarding the lesion seen in the figures? (Choose all that apply.)
   A. Most commonly seen in young males
   B. Most commonly affected layer of the artery is the medial layer
   C. The lesion is typically seen in the middle to the distal portion of the renal artery
   D. Has a relapsing and remitting course

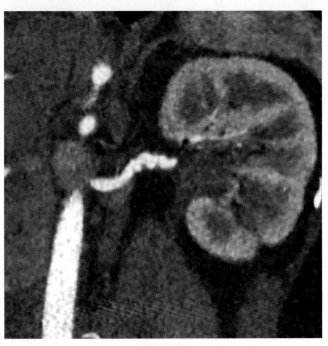

Fig. 77.1

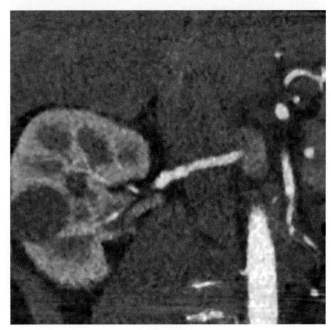

Fig. 77.2

Case 78 is online only and accessible at www.expertconsult.com.

Case 79

History: 60-year-old man with abdominal pain and leg swelling.

1. Which of the following would be included in the differential diagnosis for the imaging findings presented?
   A. Leiomyosarcoma
   B. Renal cell carcinoma
   C. Hepatocellular carcinoma
   D. Angiomyolipoma
2. Based on the imaging features shown, the tumor stage for this lesion is which of the following?
   A. T0
   B. T1
   C. T2
   D. T3

3. Invasion of the Gerota fascia suggests which tumor stage?
   A. T1
   B. T2
   C. T3
   D. T4
4. Which of the following suggests perinephric spread on computed tomography (CT)? (Choose all that apply.)
   A. An indistinct tumor margin
   B. Blurring of the renal outline
   C. Focal thickening of Gerota fascia contiguous with the tumor
   D. Invasion of the inferior vena cava (IVC)

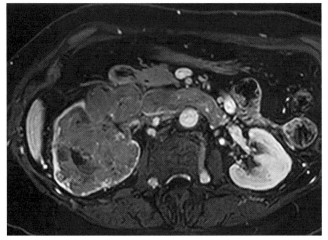

Fig. 79.1

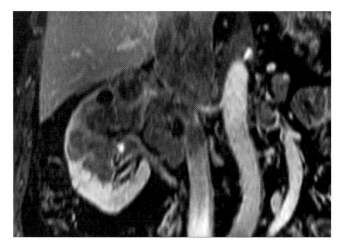

Fig. 79.2

Case 80

History: 35-year-old person with trauma was brought into the emergency department after vehicular trauma.

1. Which of the following findings are seen in the imaging presented? (Choose all that apply.)
   A. Superficial renal laceration
   B. Deep renal laceration
   C. Renal artery pseudoaneurysm
   D. Devascularization
2. Which of the following is the best imaging study for this patient with suspected renal injury with bleeding?
   A. Intravenous urography
   B. Noncontrast computed tomography (CT)
   C. Single phase contrast enhanced CT
   D. Contrast enhanced CT with a delayed phase scan

3. In which of the following categories of the American Association for the Surgery of Trauma (AAST) grading system is this renal injury classified?
   A. Grade II
   B. Grade III
   C. Grade IV
   D. Grade V
4. Which of the following is the appropriate treatment for this patient with the imaging findings presented?
   A. Conservative management
   B. Conservative management with observation
   C. Surgical management
   D. Angiographic embolization

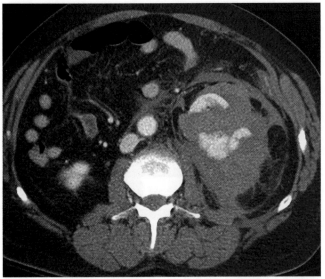

Fig. 80.1

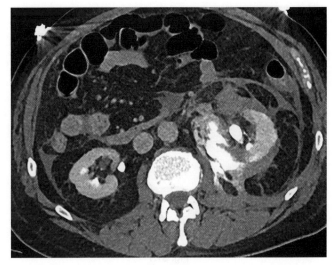

Fig. 80.2

Case 81

History: 38-year-old man with abdominal pain.

1. Which of the following would be included in the differential diagnosis for the imaging findings presented?
   A. Transitional cell carcinoma
   B. Renal cell carcinoma
   C. Lymphoma
   D. Metastases
2. What is the most common presentation of renal lymphoma?
   A. Unilateral single mass
   B. Multifocal renal masses
   C. Perirenal involvement
   D. Diffuse infiltration

3. Which of the following are considered features of renal lymphoma seen on computed tomography (CT)? (Choose all that apply.)
   A. Unilateral single mass
   B. Multifocal renal masses
   C. Perirenal involvement
   D. Diffuse infiltration
4. What is the role of positron emission tomography (PET)/computed tomography (CT) in renal lymphoma? (Choose all that apply.)
   A. Diagnosis
   B. Evaluation of extranodal disease
   C. Follow-up staging
   D. Biopsy

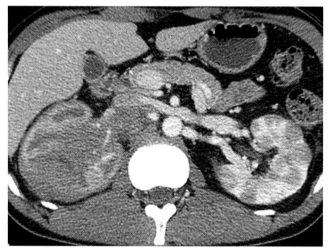

Fig. 81.1

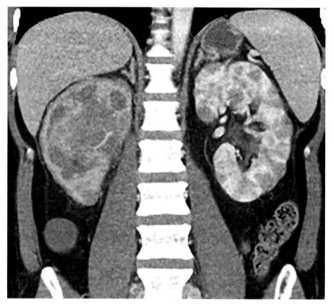

Fig. 81.2

Case 82

History: 46-year-old woman with acute right upper quadrant pain.

1. Which of the following would be included in the differential diagnosis for the imaging findings presented?
   A. Renal cell carcinoma (RCC)
   B. Angiomyolipoma (AML)
   C. Renal cyst
   D. Renal abscess
2. Which of the following is considered the most specific feature of AML on a noncontrast computed tomography (CT)?
   A. Presence of regions of interest (ROIs) containing attenuations of <−10 HU
   B. Presence of ROIs containing attenuations of >10 HU
   C. Presence of ROIs containing attenuations of >60 HU
   D. Presence of ROIs containing attenuations between 10 and 60 HU

3. Which of the following are considered syndromic causes of AML? (Choose all that apply.)
   A. Tuberous sclerosis
   B. Neurofibromatosis
   C. Lymphangioleiomyomatosis
   D. Autosomal dominant polycystic kidney disease
4. Which of the following is considered the most specific feature of AML on magnetic resonance imaging (MRI)? (Choose all that apply.)
   A. T2 hyperintensity
   B. T1 hyperintensity
   C. T1 hypointense with and T1 hyperintense without fat suppression
   D. India ink artifact at the interface between fat and nonfat components on out of phase images

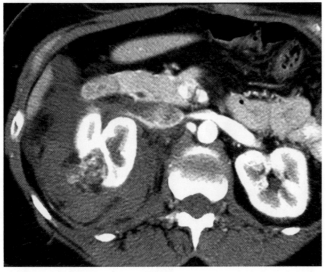

Fig. 82.1

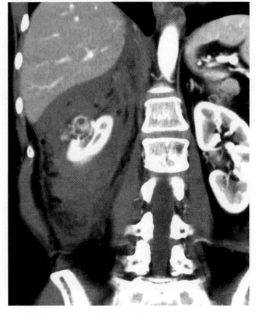

Fig. 82.2

Case 83 is online only and accessible at www.expertconsult.com.

Case 84

History: 45-year-old man with acute right flank pain, nausea, and diaphoresis.

1. Which of the following would be included in the differential diagnosis for the imaging findings presented? (Choose all that apply.)
   A. Delayed nephrogram
   B. Forniceal rupture
   C. Perinephric edema
   D. Renal infarction
2. What is the most susceptible part of the renal collecting system to rupture from increased pressure?
   A. Renal calyx
   B. Renal fornix
   C. Pyramid
   D. Midureter

3. In which condition(s) can a delayed nephrogram be seen? (Choose all that apply.)
   A. Obstructive uropathy
   B. Renal vein thrombosis
   C. Renal artery stenosis
   D. Extrinsic compression
4. Imaging findings of forniceal rupture include all of the following, EXCEPT:
   A. Perinephric edema
   B. Obstructing calculus
   C. Urinoma
   D. Wedge-shaped area of decreased renal cortical enhancement

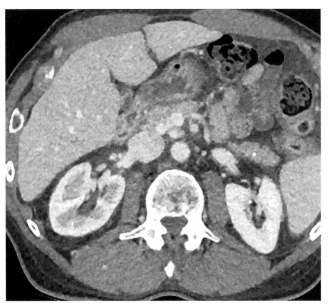

Fig. 84.1

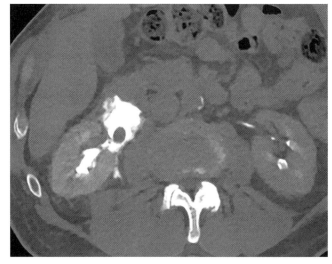

Fig. 84.2

Case 85

History: 32-year-old person with trauma was brought into the emergency department after sustaining abdominal injury due to a fall from a height.

1. Which of the following findings are seen in the imaging presented? (Choose all that apply.)
   A. Superficial renal laceration
   B. Deep renal laceration
   C. Renal artery pseudoaneurysm
   D. Devascularization

2. Which of the following is the best imaging study for this patient with suspected renal injury with bleeding?
   A. Intravenous urography
   B. Noncontrast computed tomography (CT)
   C. Single phase contrast enhanced CT
   D. Dual phase contrast enhanced CT

3. In which of the following categories of the American Association for the Surgery of Trauma (AAST) grading system is this renal injury classified?
   A. Grade II
   B. Grade III
   C. Grade IV
   D. Grade V

4. Which of the following is the appropriate treatment for this patient with the imaging findings presented?
   A. Conservative management
   B. Conservative management with observation
   C. Surgical management
   D. Angiographic embolization

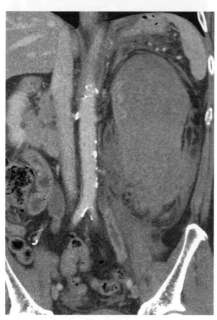

Fig. 85.1

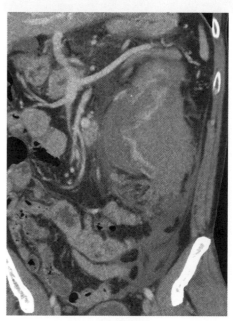

Fig. 85.2

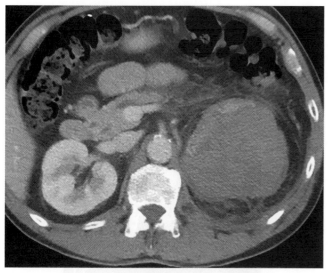

Fig. 85.3

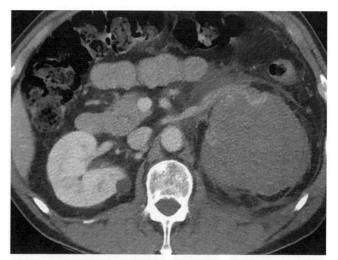

Fig. 85.4

Case 86

History: 56-year-old man with abdominal pain.

1. Which of the following would be included in the differential diagnosis for the imaging findings presented? (Choose all that apply.)
   A. Hematoma
   B. Urachal remnant
   C. Bladder diverticulum
   D. Bladder carcinoma
2. Which one of the following is a reason for poor prognosis in the disease shown in the figures?
   A. Early diagnosis due to easily visible symptoms
   B. Presence of local invasion or metastatic disease at presentation
   C. Difficulty during surgical resection due to the close relationship to the bladder
   D. Presence of calcifications in this mass

3. Which one of the following imaging features is considered pathognomonic for the diagnosis of urachal adenocarcinoma?
   A. Location of the mass superior to the bladder
   B. Calcifications in a midline supravesicular mass
   C. Enhancement and soft tissue components in the mass
   D. Mixed cystic and solid appearance of the mass
4. Which particular imaging plane is most helpful for evaluation of urachal abnormalities?
   A. Sagittal
   B. Coronal
   C. Axial
   D. Oblique

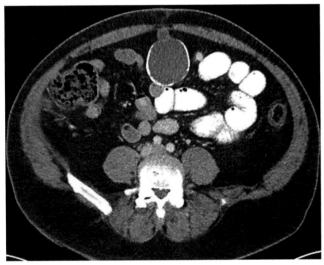

Fig. 86.1

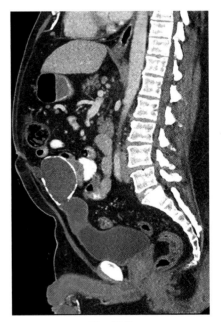

Fig. 86.2

Case 87

History: 64-year-old woman with postvoid dribbling, hematuria, and dysuria.

1. Which of the following would be included in the differential diagnosis for the imaging findings presented? (Choose all that apply.)
   A. Urethral carcinoma
   B. Urethral diverticulum
   C. Bladder diverticulum
   D. Bladder carcinoma
2. Which one of the following malignant lesions can be seen in the female urethral diverticulum?
   A. Adenocarcinoma
   B. Squamous cell carcinoma
   C. Transitional cell carcinoma
   D. Sarcoma

3. Which one of the following imaging features is considered pathognomonic for the diagnosis of urethral adenocarcinoma?
   A. Location of the mass close to the bladder
   B. Calcifications in the mass
   C. Enhancement and soft tissue components in the mass
   D. Nonenhancing septations in the mass
4. Which of the following are the reasons for poor prognosis and urethral diverticulum adenocarcinoma? (Choose all that apply.)
   A. Close proximity to the bladder and vagina
   B. Delayed diagnosis due to lack of pathognomonic signs and symptoms
   C. Early metastasis seen
   D. High grade of the tumor at presentation due to absence or poor muscle layer around the urethral diverticulum

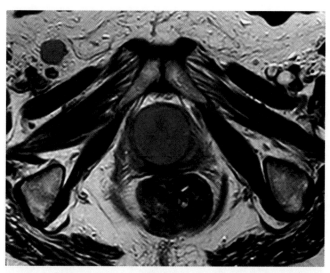

Fig. 87.1

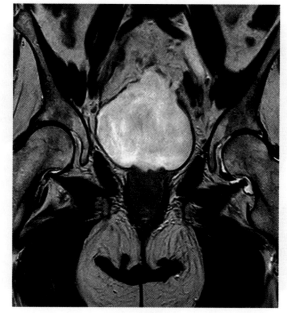

Fig. 87.2

Case 88

History: 35-year-old man with history of motor vehicle accident and hematuria.

1. Which of the following is the most likely type of bladder injury seen in the figures presented?
   A. Bladder contusion
   B. Partial thickness bladder laceration
   C. Extraperitoneal bladder rupture
   D. Intraperitoneal bladder rupture
2. Which of the following locations of contrast accumulation on computed tomography (CT) cystography suggest extraperitoneal bladder rupture?
   A. Space of Retzius
   B. Paracolic gutter
   C. Retrovesical recess
   D. Pouch of Douglas

3. Which of the following is the most appropriate technique for CT cystography to detect bladder rupture?
   A. Clamp Foley catheter and perform at the late phase CT after intravenous administration of contrast material
   B. Hand-inject sterile contrast material into the bladder through Foley catheter with a syringe
   C. Low-gravity drip infusion of diluted contrast material into the bladder through Foley catheter
   D. Instill approximately 100 mL of diluted contrast material into the bladder through Foley catheter with a machine injector
4. When extraperitoneal bladder rupture is present, how often is pelvic fracture seen?
   A. <10%
   B. ~25%
   C. ~50%
   D. >90%

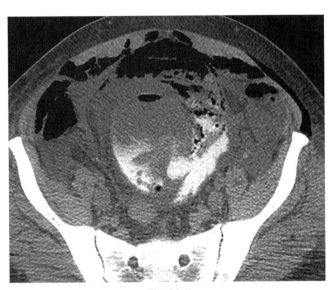

Fig. 88.1

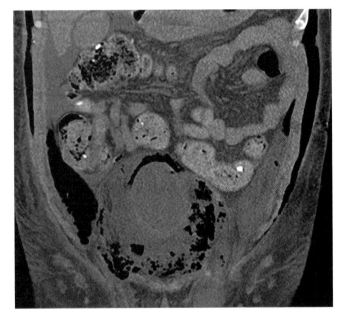

Fig. 88.2

Case 89

History: 40-year-old woman with recent onset of anemia and menorrhagia.

1. What should be included in the differential diagnosis of the imaging finding shown? (Choose all that apply.)
   A. Leiomyoma
   B. Endometrial carcinoma
   C. Leiomyosarcoma
   D. Adenomyosis

2. What types of changes can be seen in the leiomyomas?
   A. Hyaline degeneration
   B. Torsion
   C. Cystic degeneration
   D. Myxoid degeneration

3. Which imaging approach is the first-line modality in the detection of leiomyomas?
   A. Computed tomography (CT)
   B. Laparoscopy
   C. Magnetic resonance imaging (MRI)
   D. Ultrasonography

4. What is the most definitive method for diagnosis of the lesion shown?
   A. Ultrasound
   B. Computed tomography (CT)
   C. Magnetic resonance imaging (MRI)
   D. Histopathology

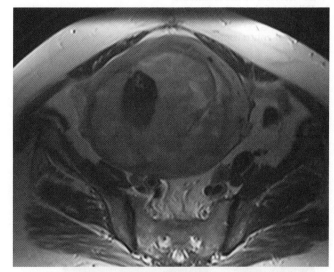

Fig. 89.2

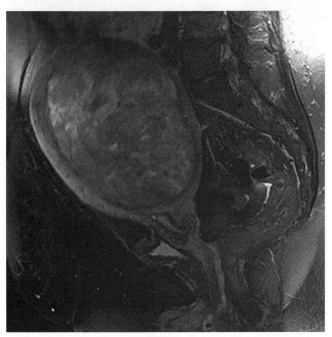

Fig. 89.1

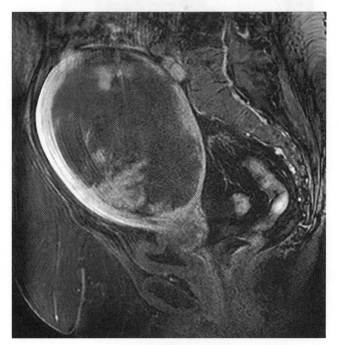

Fig. 89.3

73

Case 90

History: 36-year-old gravida 0 woman with postcoital bleeding.

1. Which of the following would be included in the differential diagnosis for the imaging findings presented? (Choose all that apply.)
   A. Cervical squamous cell carcinoma
   B. Cervical leiomyoma
   C. Nabothian cyst
   D. Cervical adenocarcinoma
2. Which of the following factors appears to lower the risk of developing cervical carcinoma?
   A. Oral contraceptives
   B. Smoking
   C. Human immunodeficiency virus (HIV)
   D. Intrauterine device (IUD)

3. What percentage of cervical carcinomas have concomitant human papillomavirus (HPV) infection?
   A. 95% to 100%
   B. 80% to 90%
   C. 50% to 75%
   D. 25% to 50%
4. Which modality has the highest agreement with disease for delineating cervical carcinoma tumor margins and measuring tumor size?
   A. Computed tomography (CT)
   B. Magnetic resonance imaging (MRI)
   C. Ultrasonography
   D. Positron emission tomography (PET)/computed tomography (CT)

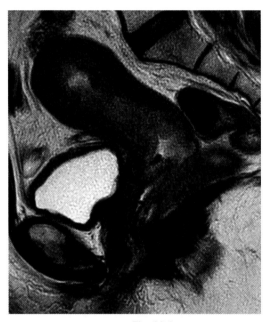

Fig. 90.1

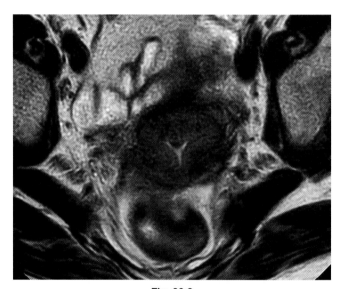

Fig. 90.2

Case 91

History: 36-year-old nulligravid woman with recurrent pelvic pain.

1. Which of the following would be included in the differential diagnosis for the imaging findings presented? (Choose all that apply.)
   A. Adnexal abscess
   B. Endometriosis
   C. Adenomyosis
   D. Ovarian carcinoma

2. What is the association between endometriosis and adenomyosis?
   A. Increased incidence of adenomyosis among infertile women with endometriosis
   B. Less than 1% of women with endometriosis have concomitant adenomyosis
   C. Endometriosis and adenomyosis are not related
   D. All women with endometriosis also have concomitant adenomyosis

3. What is the junctional zone on magnetic resonance imaging (MRI)?
   A. An interface on T1 weighted images between the inner and outer myometrium
   B. A high signal layer on T2 weighted images between the endometrium and myometrium
   C. An interface on T2 weighted images between the outer myometrium and serosa
   D. A low signal layer on T2 weighted images between the endometrium and myometrium

4. The threshold for thickening of the junctional zone as a strong indicator of adenomyosis is at:
   A. 5 mm
   B. 8 mm
   C. 12 mm
   D. 25 mm

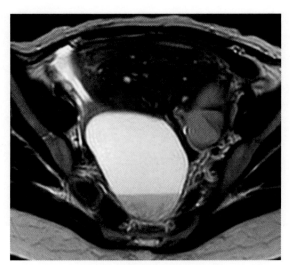

Fig. 91.1

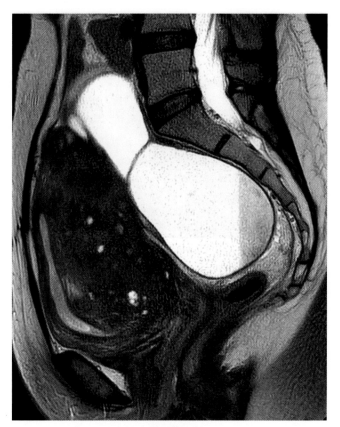

Fig. 91.2

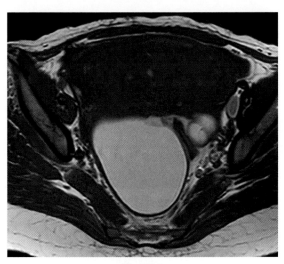

Fig. 91.3

Case 92 is online only and accessible at www.expertconsult.com.

Case 93

History: 39-year-old woman with prior history of cesarean section with slow-growing right lower abdominal wall mass.

1. Which of the following would be included in the differential diagnosis for the imaging findings presented? (Choose all that apply.)
   A. Endometrioma
   B. Desmoid
   C. Abscess
   D. Lipoma
2. What is the incidence of pelvic endometriosis in patients with abdominal wall scar endometriosis?
   A. 5%
   B. 10%
   C. 25%
   D. 50%

3. What is the typical imaging appearance of abdominal wall scar endometriosis on magnetic resonance imaging (MRI)?
   A. Hyperintense nodule on T1 weighted image
   B. Hypointense nodule on T1 weighted image
   C. Hypointense on T2 weighted image
   D. Hypointense on postcontrast T1 weighted image
4. What are the treatment options for patients with abdominal wall endometriosis? (Choose all that apply.)
   A. Surgery
   B. Progesterone
   C. Gonadotropin-releasing hormone (GnRH)
   D. Estrogen

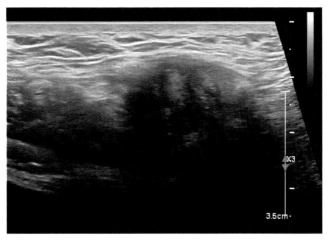

Fig. 93.1

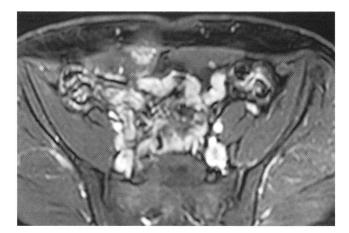

Fig. 93.2

Case 94

History: 23-year-old patient presenting with acute pelvic pain.

1. Which of the following would be included in the differential diagnosis for the imaging findings presented? (Choose all that apply.)
   A. Normal ovary
   B. Fibroma
   C. Ovarian torsion
   D. Cystadenoma
2. Which vessels provide arterial blood supply to the ovaries? (Choose all that apply.)
   A. Ovarian artery
   B. External iliac artery
   C. Uterine artery
   D. Inferior mesenteric artery

3. Which of the following are imaging signs seen on ultrasound in a patient with acute ovarian torsion? (Choose all that apply.)
   A. Twisting pedicle sign
   B. Follicular ring sign
   C. Whirlpool sign
   D. String of pearls sign
4. In acute ovarian torsion, the anatomy of the ovary is altered in which way?
   A. Shrinkage of the ovary due to ischemia and infarction
   B. Shrinkage of the ovary stroma with enlargement of the peripheral follicles
   C. Enlargement of the ovary with follicles separated by edematous stroma
   D. Enlargement of the ovary due to enlargement of follicles

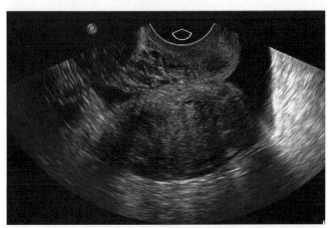

Fig. 94.1

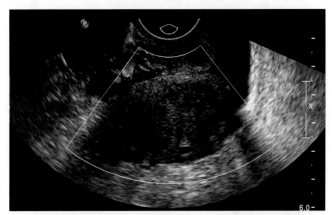

Fig. 94.2

Case 95

History: 22-year-old with amenorrhea since puberty.

1. Which conditions are associated with the imaging findings presented? (Choose all that apply.)
   A. 46,XX karyotype
   B. Abnormal secondary sexual characteristics
   C. Unilateral renal agenesis
   D. Uterovaginal agenesis

2. According to the American Society of Reproductive Medicine classification of müllerian anomalies, which class anomaly is illustrated in the figures?
   A. I
   B. II
   C. III
   D. IV

3. Which organ is not typically affected in the illustrated anomaly?
   A. Kidney
   B. Ovary
   C. Uterus
   D. Vagina

4. Which imaging approach is most effective in the detection of ovaries?
   A. Computed tomography (CT)
   B. Laparoscopy
   C. Magnetic resonance imaging (MRI)
   D. Ultrasonography

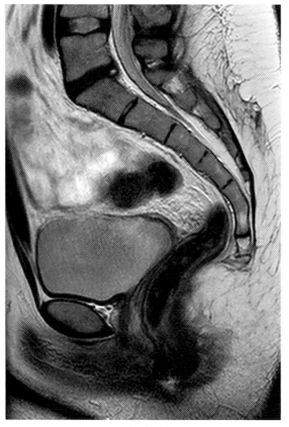

Fig. 95.1

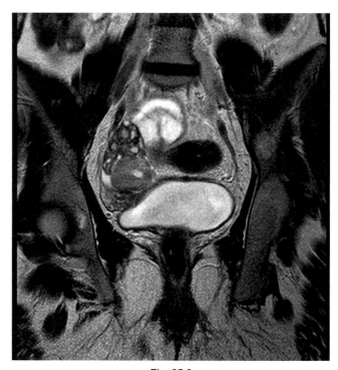

Fig. 95.2

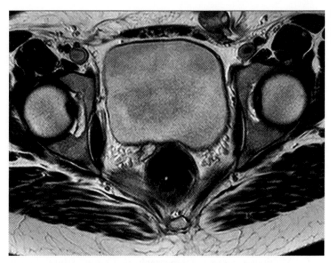

Fig. 95.4

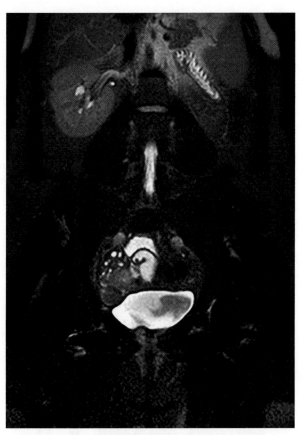

Fig. 95.3

Case 96

History: 31-year-old man has a history of abdominal pain.

1. Which of the following would be included in the differential diagnosis for the computed tomography (CT) imaging findings presented? (Choose all that apply.)
   A. Primary retroperitoneal neoplasm
   B. Metastatic adenopathy
   C. Lymphoma
   D. Mycobacterial infection
2. The patient has a palpable mass in the scrotum. Which of the following is the most useful next step?
   A. Magnetic resonance imaging (MRI)
   B. Testicular ultrasonography
   C. Multiphase computed tomography (CT) scan of the abdomen
   D. Bone scan

3. Which of the following is the initial site of metastasis from testicular germ cell tumor?
   A. Lung
   B. Liver
   C. Inguinal lymph nodes
   D. Retroperitoneal lymph nodes at the level of the renal hilum
4. All the following tumor markers are used for the diagnosis, staging, and follow-up for testicular germ cell tumors, EXCEPT:
   A. Carcinoembryonic antigen (CEA)
   B. Alpha-fetoprotein
   C. Human chorionic gonadotropin (HCG)
   D. Lactate dehydrogenase (LDH)

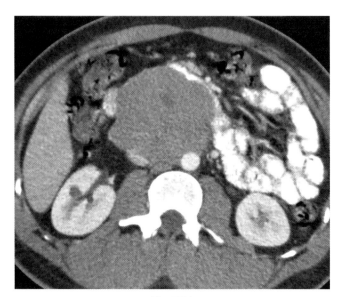

Fig. 96.1

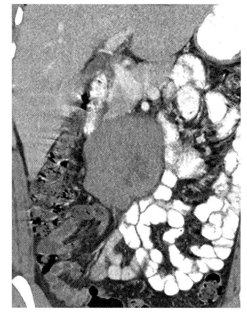

Fig. 96.2

Case 97 is online only and accessible at www.expertconsult.com.

Case 98

History: 72-year-old male with fever and dysuria.

1. What is the condition depicted on these computed tomography (CT) and magnetic resonance (MR) images?
   A. Benign prostatic hyperplasia
   B. Utricle cyst
   C. Seminal vesicle cyst
   D. Prostate abscess
2. Prostate abscess is most commonly a complication of which underlying process?
   A. Acute bacterial prostatitis
   B. Benign prostatic hyperplasia
   C. Clinically insignificant prostate cancer
   D. Clinically significant prostate cancer

3. Prostate abscess most commonly occurs in patients with which underlying condition? (Choose all that apply.)
   A. Diabetes
   B. Immunosuppression
   C. Prostate cancer
   D. Bladder cancer
4. What is the treatment of choice for patients with prostate abscess?
   A. Conservative
   B. Antibiotics only
   C. Percutaneous drainage
   D. Surgery

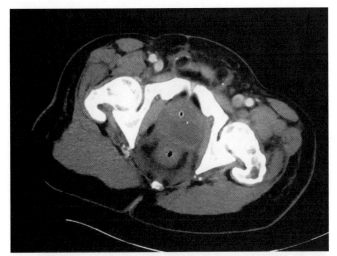

Fig. 98.1

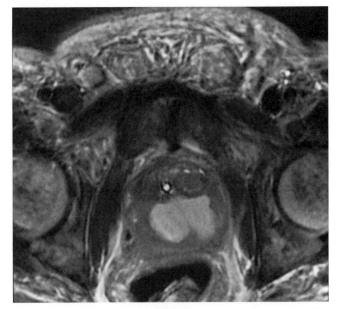

Fig. 98.2

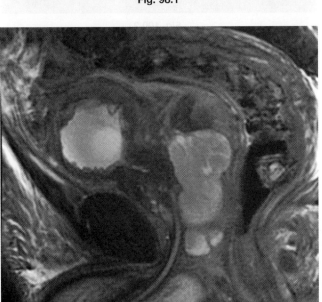

Fig. 98.3

Case 99 is online only and accessible at www.expertconsult.com.

Case 100

History: 29-year-old man presents with fever and dysuria.

1. The abnormality shown on the magnetic resonance imaging (MRI) is in the:
   A. Transitional zone
   B. Peripheral zone
   C. Seminal vesicles
   D. Rectum
2. The mostly likely diagnosis is:
   A. Prostatitis
   B. Prostatic abscess
   C. Prostate malignancy
   D. Rectal abscess
3. Prostate specific antigen (PSA) when used for biochemical screening of prostate cancer is most commonly considered abnormally elevated at the threshold of:
   A. 1 ng/mL
   B. 4 ng/mL
   C. 10 ng/mL
   D. 4 mg/mL
4. PSA can be falsely suppressed by which of the following medications?
   A. Tamsulosin
   B. Terazosin
   C. Doxazosin
   D. Finasteride

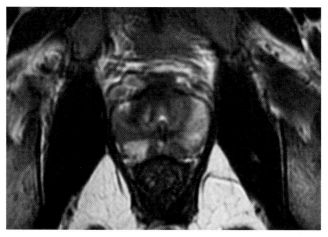

Fig. 100.1

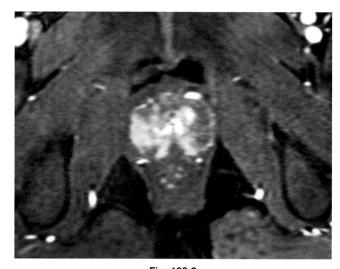

Fig. 100.2

Case 101

History: 64-year-old man presents with elevated serum prostate specific antigen (PSA).

1. On the provided images, a finding suspicious for prostate cancer is centered in the:
   A. Left transitional zone
   B. Right transitional zone
   C. Left peripheral zone
   D. Right peripheral zone
2. On the provided images, the most appropriate classification of the lesion according to Prostate Imaging Reporting and Data System (PI-RADS) v2.1, in terms of its likelihood to correlate with the presence of clinically significant prostate cancer, is:
   A. PI-RADS 1: very low
   B. PI-RADS 2: low
   C. PI-RADS 3: intermediate
   D. PI-RADS 4: high
   E. PI-RADS 5: very high
3. According to PI-RADS v2.1, which is the dominant signal sequence for characterization of a peripheral zone finding?
   A. T1 weighted imaging
   B. T2 weighted imaging
   C. Diffusion weighted imaging
   D. Dynamic contrast enhanced imaging
4. According to PI-RADS v2.1, which is the dominant signal sequence for characterization of a transitional zone finding?
   A. T1 weighted imaging
   B. T2 weighted imaging
   C. Diffusion weighted imaging
   D. Dynamic contrast enhanced imaging

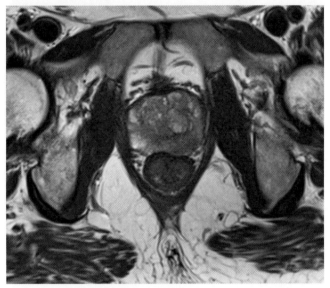

Fig. 101.1

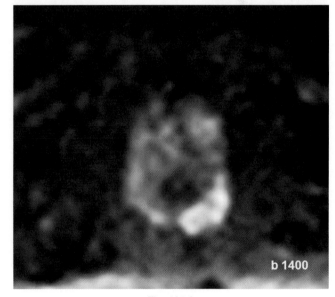

Fig. 101.2

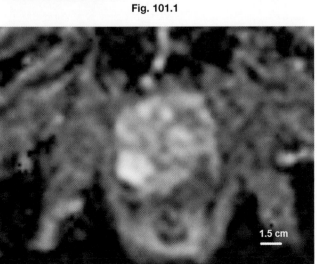

Fig. 101.3

Case 102

History: 54-year-old female post upper gastrointestinal endoscopy.

1. What should be included in the differential diagnosis of the imaging finding shown in Fig. 102.1? (Choose all that apply.)
   A. Gastric emphysema
   B. Normal air in the stomach
   C. Emphysematous gastritis
   D. Traumatic injury
2. Which findings help in differentiating between gastric emphysema and emphysematous gastritis?
   A. Presence of portal venous gas
   B. Presence of air in the adjacent draining vein
   C. Clinical features such as fever, acute abdominal pain, and vomiting
   D. Presence of mediastinal air

3. Which of the following are associated with higher risk for gastric emphysema? (Choose all that apply.)
   A. Gastric outlet obstruction
   B. Severe vomiting
   C. Endoscopy
   D. Portal vein thrombosis
4. Which of the following are associated with higher risk for emphysematous gastritis? (Choose all that apply.)
   A. Gastroduodenal surgery
   B. Diabetes
   C. Immunosuppression
   D. Abdominal surgery

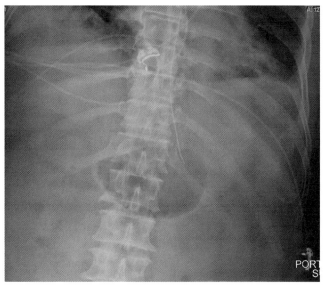

Fig. 102.1

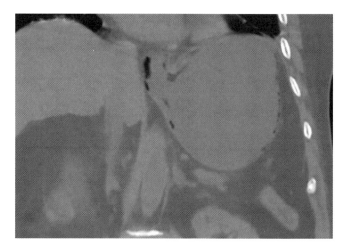

Fig. 102.2

Case 103

1. The device shown on this abdominal radiograph is a:
   A. Gastrostomy tube
   B. Medication pump device
   C. Gastric band
2. The device is:
   A. Appropriately positioned
   B. Malpositioned
3. The most pertinent measurement of this device is its:
   A. Length
   B. Short-axis diameter
   C. Kappa statistic
   D. Phi angle

4. The configuration of the device is associated with:
   A. Cessation of weight loss
   B. Posterior device slippage
   C. Gastroesophageal reflux
   D. All of these

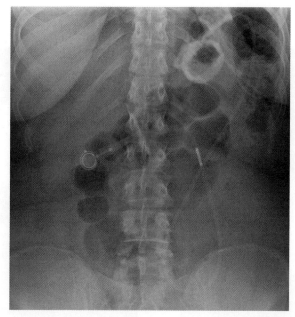

Fig. 103.1

Case 104

History: Patient presents for follow-up evaluation after prior bariatric surgery.

1. The respective positions in which these images were acquired are:
   A. Supine; prone
   B. Prone; left posterior oblique
   C. Prone; supine
   D. Right decubitus; supine
2. The prior surgery was:
   A. Sleeve gastrectomy
   B. Roux-en-Y gastric bypass
   C. Nissen fundoplication
   D. Esophagectomy
3. The abnormality shown is:
   A. Intraperitoneal contrast extravasation
   B. Anastomotic stricture
   C. Gastrocutaneous fistula
   D. Gastrogastric fistula
4. The main symptom of this imaging abnormality is:
   A. Weight regain
   B. Diffuse abdominal pain
   C. Bloating
   D. Weight loss, malaise

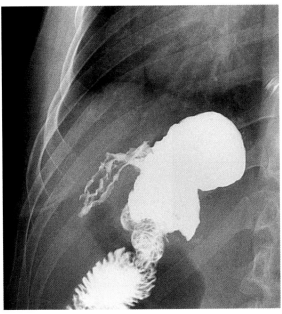

Fig. 104.1

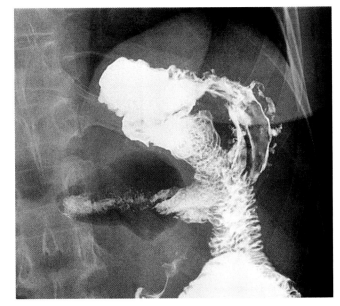

Fig. 104.2

Case 105

History: Patient with history of prior gastroesophageal surgery presents for follow-up evaluation.

1. The position in which these images were acquired is:
   A. Prone
   B. Prone, right anterior oblique
   C. Supine
   D. Left lateral decubitus
2. Of the following positions, the gastroesophageal junction is typically imaged without overlapping projection of vertebral bodies in:
   A. Upright, frontal
   B. Upright, left posterior oblique
   C. Prone
   D. Prone, right anterior oblique
   E. Both B and D

3. The prior surgery this patient underwent is most likely:
   A. Heller myotomy
   B. Sleeve gastrectomy
   C. Esophagectomy
   D. Nissen fundoplication
4. The images most likely represent:
   A. Normal postsurgical appearance
   B. Abnormal; recurrent hernia
   C. Abnormal; leak
   D. Abnormal; anastomotic ulcer

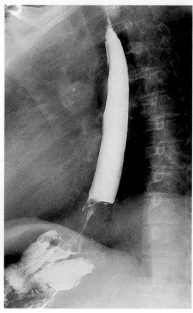

Fig. 105.1

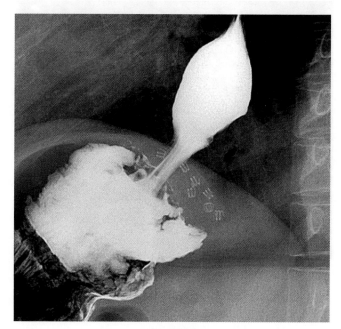

Fig. 105.2

Case 106 is online only and accessible at www.expertconsult.com.

Case 107

History: 54-year-old man with recurrent epigastric pain.

1. Which of the following should be included in the differential diagnosis of the imaging finding shown? (Choose all that apply.)
   A. Gastric carcinoma with liver metastases
   B. Gastrointestinal stromal tumor with liver metastases
   C. Gastric lymphoma with liver metastases
   D. Gastric tumor with liver cysts
2. Which of the following is the commonest location of gastrointestinal stromal tumors (GIST) in the abdomen?
   A. Esophagus
   B. Stomach
   C. Small bowel
   D. Colon

3. Which of the following is the most common imaging appearance of GIST on computed tomography (CT) scan?
   A. Large intraluminal mass
   B. Predominantly cystic mass
   C. Necrotic mass with air fluid level within it
   D. Exophytic extragastric mass
4. What is the most common route of metastasis in a GIST tumor?
   A. Lymphatic
   B. Hematogenous
   C. Peritoneal spread of disease
   D. Transdiaphragmatic

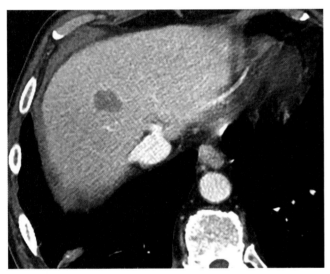

Fig. 107.1

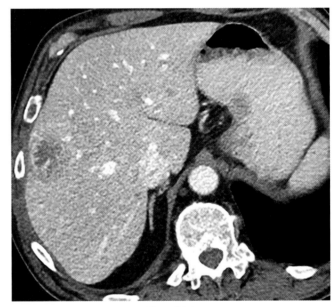

Fig. 107.2

Case 108

History: 68-year-old female with weight loss.

1. The appearance of the thickened small bowel in Fig. 108.1 is most characteristic for which pathology?
   A. Crohn's disease
   B. Lymphoma
   C. Infectious enteritis
   D. Radiation enteritis
2. Which of the following findings can help distinguish small bowel lymphoma from small bowel adenocarcinoma? (Choose all that apply.)
   A. Ileal involvement
   B. Lymphadenopathy
   C. Splenomegaly
   D. Concentric bowel wall thickening

3. What patient demographic is at highest risk for developing small bowel lymphoma?
   A. Acquired immunodeficiency syndrome (AIDS)
   B. Lupus
   C. Celiac disease
   D. Transplant recipients
4. Which of the following is a rare complication of lymphoma that can occur, especially in the setting of recent chemotherapy induction?
   A. Perforation
   B. Hemorrhage
   C. Obstruction
   D. Diarrhea

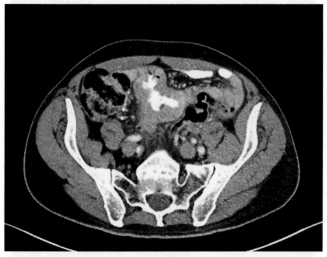

Fig. 108.1

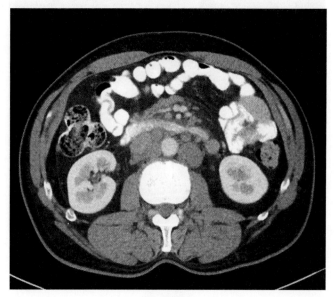

Fig. 108.2

Case 109

History: 46-year-old male with abdominal cramping and diarrhea.

1. What is the most common location of carcinoid tumors?
   A. Small bowel
   B. Colon
   C. Appendix
   D. Bronchi
2. What is the major hormone secreted by active carcinoid tumors?
   A. Serotonin
   B. Histamine
   C. 5-Hydroxyindoleacetic acid
   D. Epinephrine

3. Which of the following symptoms may occur in carcinoid syndrome? (Choose all that apply.)
   A. Flushing
   B. Wheezing
   C. Bronchospasm
   D. Diarrhea
4. Mesenteric fibrosis causes what characteristic appearance in the setting of metastatic carcinoid? (Choose all that apply.)
   A. Whirled appearance
   B. Comb sign
   C. Spokelike appearance
   D. Tethered small bowel

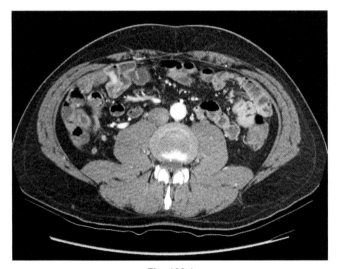

Fig. 109.1

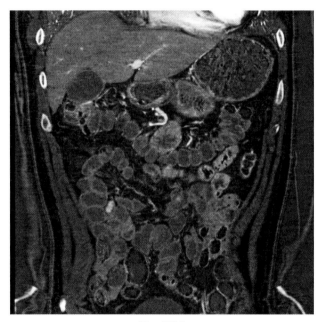

Fig. 109.2

Case 110

History: 52-year-old woman presents with symptomatic iron deficiency anemia.

1. Which of the following should be included in the differential diagnosis of the imaging finding shown? (Choose all that apply.)
   A. Small bowel lymphoma
   B. Gastrointestinal stromal tumor
   C. Carcinoid
   D. Leiomyosarcoma
2. Which of the following statements is true about gastrointestinal stromal tumors (GIST) in the abdomen?
   A. More common in females
   B. More common in males
   C. Most often diagnosed in the sixth or seventh decade of life
   D. Usually malignant

3. Which of the following are features suggesting response to imatinib therapy on computed tomography (CT) scan? (Choose all that apply.)
   A. Homogenously cystic appearance
   B. Resolution of enhancing components
   C. Decrease in size of tumor
   D. Development of an enhancing nodule within the treated tumor
4. What are the features that suggest malignancy in GIST on CT scan? (Choose all that apply.)
   A. Diameter >5 cm
   B. Ill-defined margins
   C. Central necrosis
   D. Invasion of surrounding structures

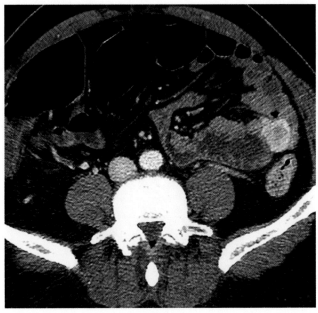

Fig. 110.1

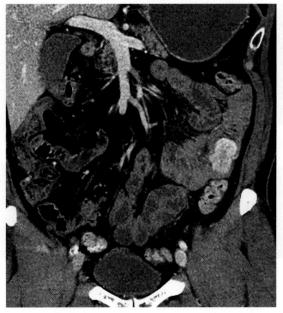

Fig. 110.2

Case 111

History: 67-year-old man with remote history of colectomy presents with severe abdominal pain.

1. Which of the following would be included in the differential diagnosis for the imaging findings presented?
   A. Acute mesenteric ischemia
   B. Small bowel obstruction
   C. Small bowel volvulus
   D. Normal bowel
2. What is the most common etiology for acute mesenteric ischemia?
   A. Bowel obstruction
   B. Infection
   C. Superior mesenteric artery occlusion
   D. Superior mesenteric vein occlusion
3. Which of the following is the commonest feature seen on computed tomography (CT) in acute mesenteric ischemia?
   A. Bowel wall thickening
   B. Bowel wall hyperenhancement
   C. Paper thin bowel wall
   D. Pneumatosis
4. Which of the following are reasons for bowel wall thickening seen on CT scan in acute mesenteric ischemia? (Choose all that apply.)
   A. Mural edema
   B. Hemorrhage
   C. Infection
   D. Mass development

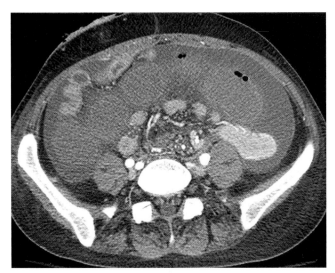

Fig. 111.1

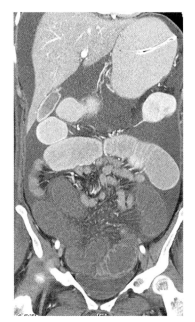

Fig. 111.2

Case 112

History: 54-year-old man presents with acute onset of left abdominal pain.

1. In the provided images, the most likely diagnosis is:
   A. Omental infarction
   B. Acute diverticulitis
   C. Peritoneal abscess
   D. Epiploic appendagitis
2. The most appropriate therapy is:
   A. Urgent laparotomy
   B. Lower endoscopy/sigmoidoscopy
   C. Pain management/nonsteroidal antiinflammatory drugs (NSAIDs)
   D. Intravenous antibiotics

3. The most common colonic distribution of this abnormality is:
   A. Rectosigmoid colon
   B. Descending colon
   C. Transverse colon
   D. Cecum/ascending colon
   E. C and D
4. The most common colonic distribution of omental infarction is:
   A. Rectosigmoid colon
   B. Descending colon
   C. Transverse colon
   D. Cecum/ascending colon
   E. C and D

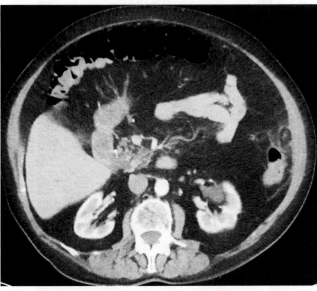

Fig. 112.1

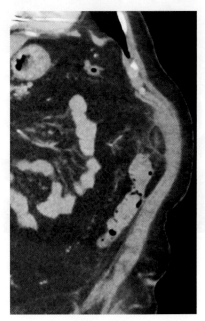

Fig. 112.2

Case 113

History: 52-year-old woman presents with intermittent right lower quadrant pain.

1. From the provided images, the most likely diagnosis is:
   A. Perforated appendicitis
   B. Cecal adenocarcinoma
   C. Appendiceal neuroendocrine tumor
   D. Appendiceal mucinous neoplasm
2. A pattern of disease extension associated with this diagnosis is:
   A. Lung metastases
   B. Brain metastases
   C. Bone metastases
   D. Pseudomyxoma peritonei

3. The next best step in the management of this patient is:
   A. Intravenous (IV) antibiotic therapy
   B. Percutaneous catheter drainage
   C. Surgical/oncologic consultation
   D. Trial of corticosteroid therapy
4. Appendiceal neuroendocrine tumor has the typical imaging appearance of:
   A. Small enhancing mass at the appendiceal tip
   B. Large enhancing mass at the cecal base
   C. Large cystic mass at the appendiceal tip
   D. Small cystic mass at the cecal base

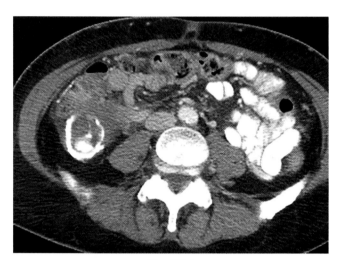

Fig. 113.1

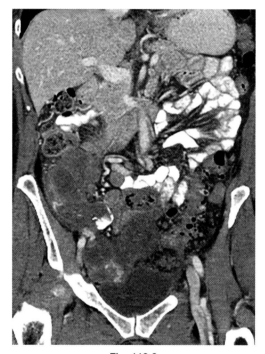

Fig. 113.2

Case 114

History: 45-year-old man was injured in a motor vehicle accident.

1. Which of the following should be included in the differential diagnosis of the dominant imaging finding on Fig. 114.1? (Choose all that apply.)
   A. Morgagni hernia
   B. Bochdalek hernia
   C. Spigelian hernia
   D. Diaphragmatic eventration
   E. Traumatic diaphragmatic hernia
2. What other abdominal or pelvic injuries are most commonly involved with this abnormality?
   A. Splenic laceration
   B. Aortic injuries
   C. Fractures
   D. Hollow organ perforation
3. What is the most commonly herniated organ in patients with traumatic diaphragmatic injury?
   A. Stomach
   B. Liver
   C. Spleen
   D. Colon
4. What is the most common sign of the diaphragmatic hernia on computed tomography (CT), including coronal and sagittal reformats?
   A. Abdominal viscera in the thorax
   B. Elevated hemidiaphragm
   C. Collar sign
   D. Discontinuity of the diaphragm

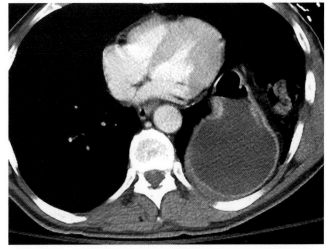

Fig. 114.2

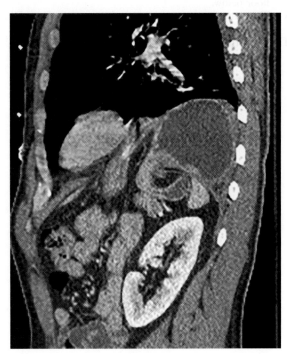

Fig. 114.3

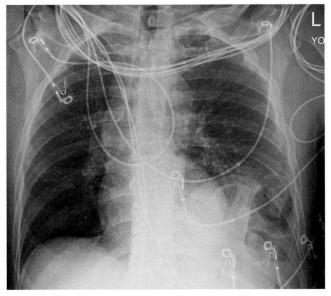

Fig. 114.1

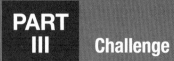

Case 115

This case has no associated history or images.

1. In a hospital's MRI suite, an area is designated for the intake of patients, including their pre-MRI interview and screening. Facilities in this area include toilets and change rooms; patient movement through this area is supervised by MR personnel. This description is of what MR zone?
   A. Zone I
   B. Zone II
   C. Zone III
   D. Zone IV

2. Which of the following statements accurately applies to MR Zone III?
   A. Free access by unscreened non-MR personnel or equipment can result in serious injury, or death.
   B. The extent of Zone III is limited to the area demarcated on the floor and does not apply to the floor above or the floor below.
   C. To ensure free passage in case of emergency, Zone III is to remain unlocked at all times.
   D. All of these are accurate.

3. Which of the following statements accurately applies to MR Zone IV?
   A. Represents physical space of the MR scanner magnet room
   B. By definition, always located within Zone III
   C. Should be clearly marked as being potentially hazardous due to the presence of very strong magnetic fields
   D. All of these

4. In the event of a medical emergency that occurs in the MR scanner magnet room, best practice is to:
   A. Alert the appropriate local resources, to initiate and carry out resuscitation in the MR scanner magnet room
   B. Immediately quench the magnet, then initiate and carry out resuscitation in the MR scanner magnet room
   C. MR personnel should initiate basic life support while the patient is removed from the scanner magnet room, to a magnetically safe location
   D. A or B, depending on the circumstances

Case 116

History: 28-year-old man with thalassemia.

1. Which of the following would be included in the differential diagnosis for the imaging findings in the liver in Figs. 116.1 and 116.2?
   A. Fatty infiltration
   B. Iron overload
   C. Wilson disease
   D. Amyloidosis
2. What are the techniques for iron quantification on magnetic resonance imaging (MRI)?
   A. Gradient recalled echo (GRE)
   B. T2 relaxometry
   C. Signal intensity ratio (SIR) imaging
   D. Fast spin echo (FSE) imaging

3. Which of the following are considered features of iron overload in the liver seen on MRI? (Choose all that apply.)
   A. Decreased liver attenuation on in-phase images
   B. Increased liver attenuation on in-phase images
   C. Low signal in the liver on T2 weighted images compared to spleen
   D. Hypointense liver compared to paraspinous muscle on GRE sequence
4. Which of the following diseases can cause increase in liver attenuation on nonenhanced computed tomography (CT)? (Choose all that apply.)
   A. Fatty infiltration
   B. Wilson disease
   C. Iron overload
   D. Amyloidosis

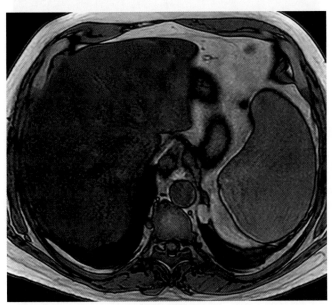

Fig. 116.1

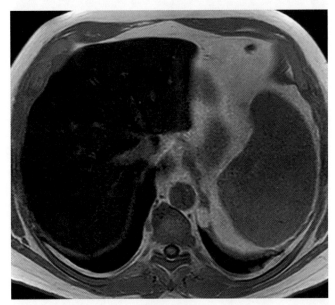

Fig. 116.2

Case 117

History: 58-year-old woman with history of liver transplantation 5 years ago due to hepatitis C and hepatoma. She presented for yearly routine ultrasound screening of her liver.

1. Which of the following would be included in the differential diagnosis for the imaging findings presented? (Choose all that apply.)
   A. Metastasis
   B. Posttransplant lymphoproliferative disease
   C. Inflammatory pseudotumor
   D. Abscess

2. Which particular modality is most useful for definitive diagnosis of this process?
   A. Computed tomography (CT)
   B. Magnetic resonance imaging (MRI)
   C. Ultrasound (US)
   D. Biopsy

3. What is the most common location of inflammatory pseudotumor (IPT)?
   A. Liver
   B. Lung
   C. Bowel
   D. Pancreas

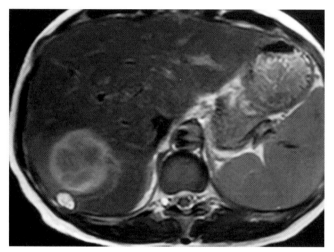

Fig. 117.1

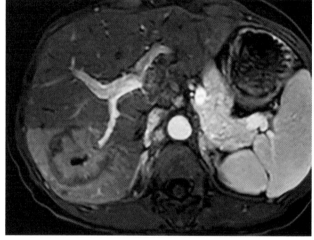

Fig. 117.2

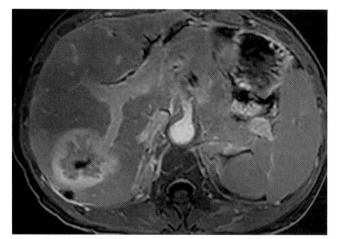

Fig. 117.3

Case 118 is online only and accessible at www.expertconsult.com.

Case 119

History: 36-year-old man with no prior history presents with incidentally detected liver lesion.

1. From the provided images, the most likely diagnosis is:
   A. Hemangioma
   B. Hepatocellular carcinoma
   C. Fibrolamellar hepatocellular carcinoma
   D. Liver abscess
2. Patients with the diagnosis depicted from the provided images are typically:
   A. Younger than 40 years of age; no history of hepatitis/cirrhosis
   B. Older than 40 years of age; no history of hepatitis/cirrhosis
   C. Younger than 40 years of age; history of hepatitis/cirrhosis
   D. Older than 40 years of age; history of hepatitis/cirrhosis

3. Patients with the diagnosis depicted from the provided images typically demonstrate:
   A. Normal serum alpha-fetoprotein
   B. Elevated serum alpha-fetoprotein, 2x upper limit of normal
   C. Elevated serum alpha-fetoprotein, 5x upper limit of normal
   D. Elevated serum alpha-fetoprotein, 10x upper limit of normal
4. Magnetic resonance imaging (MRI) is subsequently performed on this patient. Opposed phase imaging is:
   A. Expected to show intralesional fat
   B. Not expected to show intralesional fat

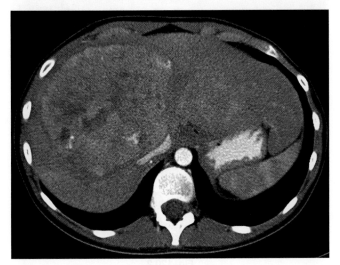

Fig. 119.1

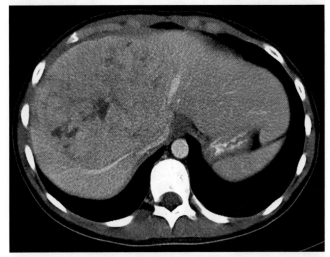

Fig. 119.2

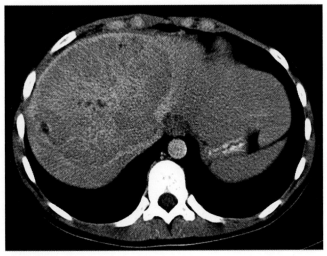

Fig. 119.3

Case 120

History: 71-year-old man with history of chronic left knee osteoarthritis presents with abdominal pain and fatigue.

1. From the provided images, what is the most likely diagnosis?
   A. Acute cholecystitis
   B. Spontaneous bacterial peritonitis
   C. Gastritis
   D. Perforated hollow viscus
2. This patient's condition is most likely to have been precipitated by which of the following risk factors?
   A. Nonsteroidal antiinflammatory drug (NSAID) therapy
   B. Corticosteroid therapy
   C. Zollinger-Ellison syndrome
   D. Smoking

3. The next best step in the management of this patient is:
   A. Sonographic examination of the abdomen
   B. Contrast enhanced abdominal magnetic resonance imaging (MRI)
   C. Corticosteroid therapy
   D. Surgical consultation
4. The most likely surgical intervention the patient will undergo is:
   A. Graham patch
   B. Whipple resection
   C. Nissen fundoplication
   D. Hartmann procedure

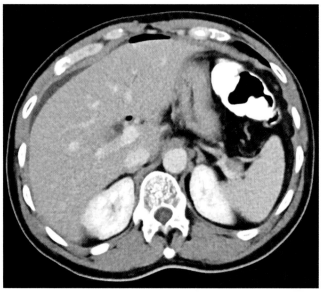

Fig. 120.1

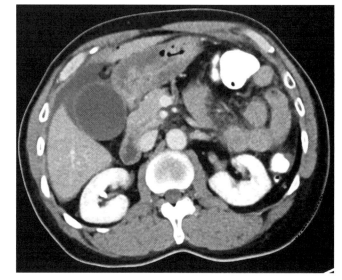

Fig. 120.2

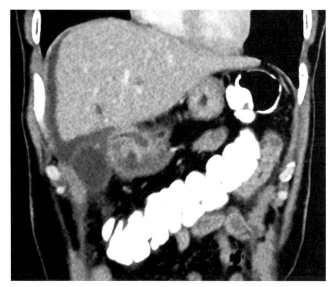

Fig. 120.3

Case 121

History: 50-year-old woman with epigastric pain and nausea.

1. Which of the following would be included in the differential diagnosis for the imaging findings presented? (Choose all that apply.)
   A. Biliary cystic tumor (BCT)
   B. Cystic primary liver tumor
   C. Cystic metastasis
   D. Simple cyst
2. Which of the following features on magnetic resonance imaging (MRI) can help differentiate between biliary cystadenoma and hemorrhagic cyst?
   A. Septation in the cyst
   B. High signal intensity in the cyst on T1 weighted images
   C. High signal intensity in the cyst on T2 weighted images
   D. Irregular and nodular wall

3. Which of the following is the preferred treatment for a suspected biliary cystadenoma (BCA)?
   A. Percutaneous aspiration
   B. Fenestration
   C. Ethanol injection
   D. Surgical resection
4. If aspiration of a biliary cystadenoma is undertaken, the fluid aspirated will have which of the following characteristics?
   A. Bile-tinged mucinous fluid
   B. Bloody aspirate
   C. Simple clear fluid
   D. Thick yellowish fluid

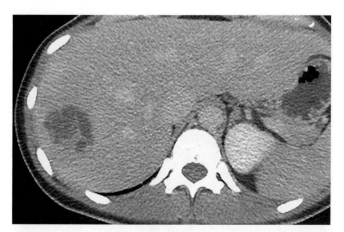

Fig. 121.1

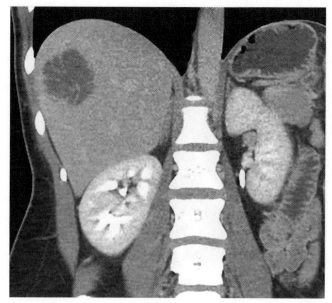

Fig. 121.2

Case 122

History: 65-year-old man 5 years post liver transplant with increasing bilirubin.

1. Which of the following would be included in the differential diagnosis for the imaging findings presented?
   A. Bilomas
   B. Biliary dilatation
   C. Cystic metastasis
   D. Malignant stricture
2. What is the most common etiology for late (>6 months) biliary complications in postorthotopic liver transplant patients?
   A. Stones
   B. Ampullary dysfunction
   C. Bile leak
   D. Strictures
3. Which of the following are considered features of malignant biliary stricture seen on magnetic resonance imaging (MRI)? (Choose all that apply.)
   A. Irregular stricture
   B. Asymmetric strictures with a shouldered margin
   C. Longer strictures (>30 mm)
   D. Smooth tapered margins
4. Which of the following are treatment options for biliary strictures in post–liver transplant patients? (Choose all that apply.)
   A. Endoscopic retrograde cholangiography (ERC)-guided therapy
   B. Percutaneous transhepatic cholangiography (PTC)-guided therapy
   C. Surgical revision
   D. Retransplantation

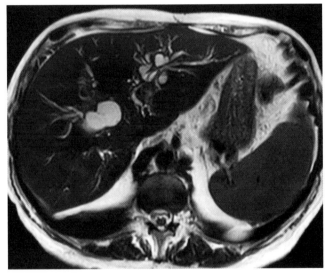

Fig. 122.1

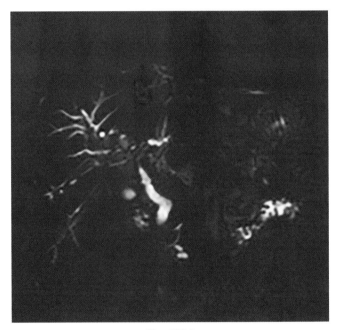

Fig. 122.2

Case 123

History: 53-year-old patient presenting with repeated episodes of abdominal pain.

1. Which of the following would be included in the differential diagnosis for the imaging findings presented? (Choose all that apply.)
   A. Lymphoma
   B. Gastrointestinal stromal tumor
   C. Adenocarcinoma
   D. Heterotopic pancreatic tissue
2. What is the most common location of heterotopic pancreatic tissue?
   A. Stomach
   B. Colon
   C. Spleen
   D. Mesentery

3. Which of the following statements about heterotopic pancreatic tissue is incorrect?
   A. 75% of cases of heterotopic pancreatic tissue are submucosal in location
   B. Most cases are asymptomatic
   C. The incidence of malignant transformation in these cases is high
   D. Diagnosis of heterotopic pancreas is easier in the lower gastrointestinal tract
4. What is the most definitive diagnostic test for heterotopic pancreas?
   A. Ultrasound
   B. Computed tomography (CT)
   C. Endoscopy
   D. Histopathology

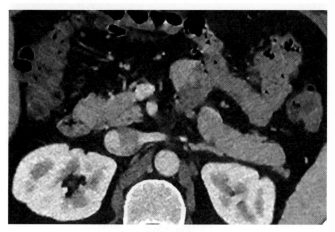

Fig. 123.1

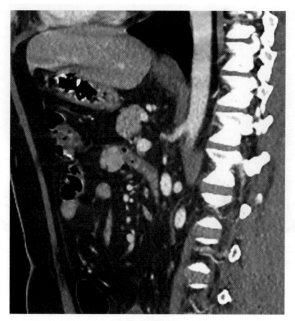

Fig. 123.2

Case 124

History: 36-year-old woman presents for evaluation of fainting episodes.

1. Which of the following would be included in the differential diagnosis for the imaging findings presented? (Choose all that apply.)
   A. Neuroendocrine tumor
   B. Metastases from renal cell carcinoma
   C. Adenocarcinoma
   D. Pancreatic cyst
2. Which modality has the highest sensitivity for detection of an insulinoma?
   A. Ultrasound with contrast
   B. Computed tomography (CT)
   C. Magnetic resonance imaging (MRI)
   D. ^{68}Ga-dotate positron emission tomography (PET)/CT

3. Which of the following statements about insulinoma is incorrect?
   A. 90% of insulinomas have been reported to be malignant
   B. 90% are solitary
   C. >90% occur at intrapancreatic sites
   D. 90% are <2 cm in diameter
4. Which of the following is the most common pancreatic neuroendocrine tumor?
   A. VIPoma
   B. Insulinoma
   C. Gastrinoma
   D. Nonfunctioning islet cell tumor

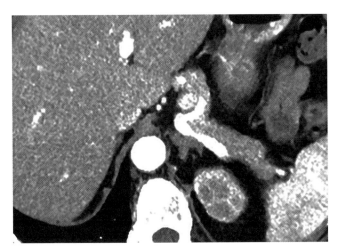

Fig. 124.1

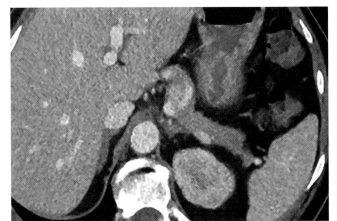

Fig. 124.2

Case 125

History: 65-year-old man presents with months-long history of abdominal pain; serum IgG4 levels are found to be mildly elevated.

1. In the provided images, the appearance of the pancreas and pancreatic duct, respectively, is:
   A. Normal; nondilated duct
   B. Normal; dilated duct
   C. Abnormally enlarged; nondilated duct
   D. Abnormally enlarged; dilated duct
2. In the provided magnetic resonance cholangiopancreatography (MRCP) image, the appearance of the biliary system is:
   A. Normal
   B. Abnormal; beaded appearance
   C. Abnormal; dilated
   D. Abnormal; cystic outpouching

3. From the provided history and images, the most likely diagnosis is:
   A. Pancreatic ductal adenocarcinoma
   B. Chronic pancreatitis
   C. Autoimmune pancreatitis
   D. Postpancreatitis pseudocyst
4. Comparing Figs. 125.1 and 125.2 (pretreatment) to Fig. 125.4 (posttreatment), the patient has undergone a course of medical therapy, most likely:
   A. Antibiotics
   B. Corticosteroids
   C. Targeted tyrosine kinase inhibitor therapy
   D. Intravenous immunoglobulin (IVIG) infusion

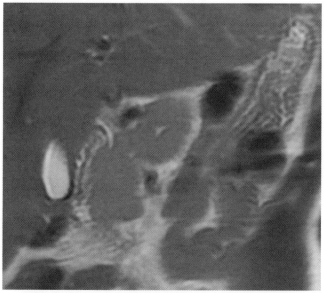

Fig. 125.1

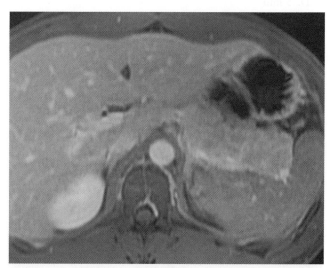

Fig. 125.2

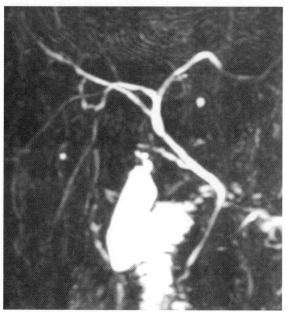

Fig. 125.3

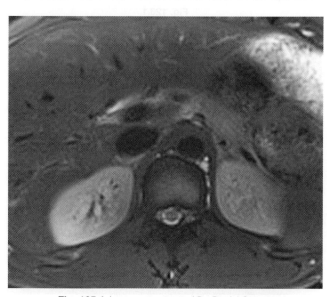

Fig. 125.4 Images courtesy of Dr. Daniel Souza.

Case 126

History: 73-year-old male with chronic abdominal pain and weight loss.

1. The magnetic resonance imaging (MRI) findings depicted in Figs. 126.1 through 126.3 are most concerning for what condition?
   A. Chronic pancreatitis
   B. Pancreatic ductal adenocarcinoma
   C. Intraductal papillary mucinous neoplasm (IPMN)
   D. Pancreas divisum
2. Dilation of the main pancreatic duct beyond what caliber becomes concerning for potential main duct IMPN?
   A. 3 mm
   B. 3.5 mm
   C. 4 mm
   D. 5 mm
3. Malignant degeneration should be suspected in patients with a dilated pancreatic duct and which additional abnormalities? (Choose all that apply.)
   A. New-onset diabetes
   B. Jaundice
   C. Acute pancreatitis
   D. Elevated serum CA 19-9
4. Which endoscopic finding is pathognomonic for main duct IPMN?
   A. Double bubble sign
   B. Bulging papilla
   C. Double duct sign
   D. Long common channel

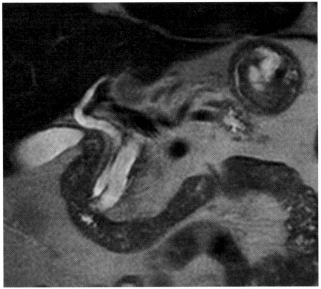

Fig. 126.1

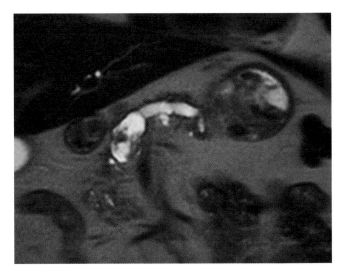

Fig. 126.2

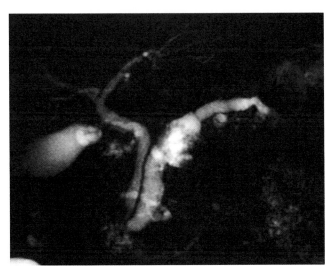

Fig. 126.3

Case 127

History: 78-year-old woman presents for evaluation of incidentally detected pancreatic mass.

1. From the provided images, what is the most likely diagnosis?
   A. Pseudocyst
   B. Serous cystadenoma
   C. Mucinous cystic neoplasm
   D. Intraductal papillary mucinous neoplasm
2. Which premalignant cystic pancreatic neoplasm occurs exclusively in women?
   A. Serous cystic neoplasm
   B. Mucinous cystic neoplasm
   C. Intraductal papillary mucinous neoplasm
   D. Cystic neuroendocrine tumor

3. Which cystic pancreatic neoplasm occurs in young female patients (teens and 20s)?
   A. Serous cystadenoma
   B. Mucinous cystic neoplasm
   C. Intraductal papillary mucinous neoplasm
   D. Solid pseudopapillary epithelial neoplasm
4. Thin peripheral rim enhancement with a solid mural nodule is a classic finding of which cystic pancreatic neoplasm?
   A. Serous cystadenoma
   B. Mucinous cystic neoplasm
   C. Solid pseudopapillary epithelial neoplasm
   D. Cystic neuroendocrine tumor

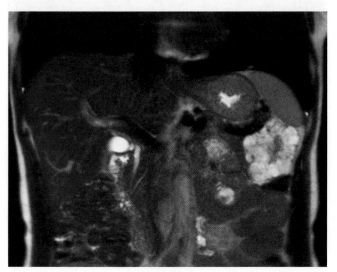

Fig. 127.1

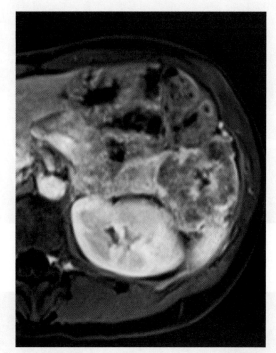

Fig. 127.2

Case 128

History: 48-year-old female with cough and shortness of breath.

1. What is the hallmark pathologic finding in sarcoidosis?
   A. Howell-Jolly bodies
   B. Noncaseating granulomas
   C. Reed-Sternberg cells
   D. Owl's eye
2. Which organ is typically involved in abdominal manifestations of sarcoidosis?
   A. Liver
   B. Spleen
   C. Kidneys
   D. Testicles

3. What is the typical appearance of sarcoidosis in the spleen on ultrasound?
   A. Small hyperechoic nodules in a normal-sized spleen
   B. Small hypoechoic nodules in a normal-sized spleen
   C. Small hyperechoic nodules in an enlarged spleen
   D. Large hypoechoic nodules in an enlarged spleen
4. Which imaging modality can be used to direct needle biopsy for tissue diagnosis?
   A. Ultrasound
   B. Sulfur colloid scan
   C. Positron emission tomography (PET)
   D. Magnetic resonance imaging (MRI)

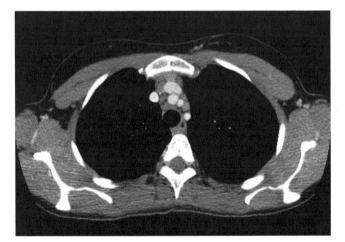

Fig. 128.1

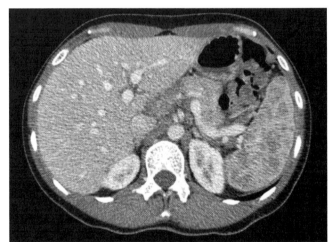

Fig. 128.2

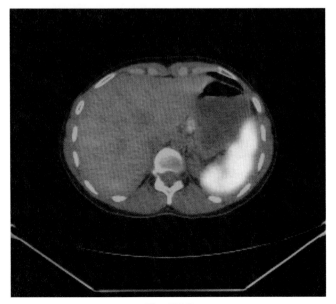

Fig. 128.3

Case 129

History: 47-year-old male with distant history of mononucleosis presented initially with acute left upper quadrant (LUQ) and left shoulder pain.

1. Which of the following would be included in the differential diagnosis for the imaging findings presented?
   A. Splenic rupture
   B. Splenic lymphoma
   C. Splenic abscess
   D. Splenic cyst
2. Which of the following are considered as diagnostic criteria for splenic rupture? (Choose all that apply.)
   A. No history of trauma or unusual effort, either prior to or on retrospect questioning after operation
   B. No evidence of disease that could involve the spleen
   C. Evidence of adhesions or scarring of the spleen to suggest trauma or previous rupture
   D. Rise in viral antibody titers

3. Which of the following are considered features of splenic rupture seen on computed tomography (CT)? (Choose all that apply.)
   A. Subcapsular hematoma
   B. Intraparenchymal hematoma
   C. Nonenhancement of the spleen
   D. Wedge-shaped areas of nonenhancement
4. Presence of splenic vascular injury is classified as which type of American Association for the Surgery of Trauma (AAST) grade injury?
   A. Grade I
   B. Grade II
   C. Grade III
   D. Grade IV

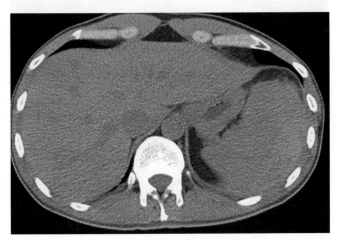

Fig. 129.1

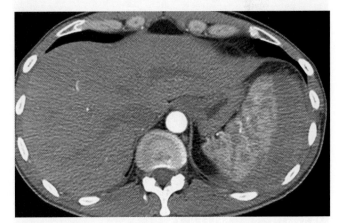

Fig. 129.2

Case 130

History: 40-year-old woman presents with left upper quadrant pain. There is no relevant travel history.

1. Based on the provided images, an appropriate differential diagnosis should NOT include:
   A. Splenic pseudocyst
   B. Splenic lymphangiomatosis
   C. Echinococcal disease
   D. Lymphoma
2. Based on the provided history and images, of the following choices, the most likely diagnosis is:
   A. Splenic abscesses
   B. Splenic lymphangiomatosis
   C. Echinococcal disease
   D. Lymphoma

3. Regarding splenic cysts, which of the following statements are true?
   A. Primary cysts are more prevalent than secondary cysts
   B. Secondary cysts are more prevalent than primary cysts
   C. Primary and secondary cysts require annual imaging follow-up
   D. None of these
4. Regarding echinococcal cysts, which of the following statements is true?
   A. Cysts may involve liver and/or spleen
   B. Cysts may have cyst-within-a-cyst appearance
   C. Water-lily sign is pathognomonic
   D. All of these are true

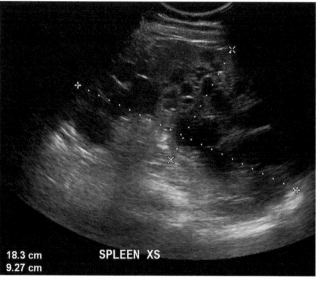

Fig. 130.1

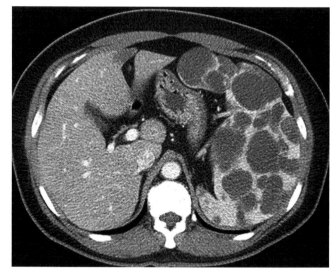

Fig. 130.2

Case 131

History: 42-year-old female with a history of recurrent abdominal pain.

1. What should be included in the differential diagnosis of the imaging finding shown? (Choose all that apply.)
   A. Adrenal metastasis
   B. Pheochromocytoma
   C. Renal cell carcinoma
   D. Adrenocortical carcinoma
2. The patient is found to have an elevated adrenocortical hormone level. Which of the following is the most likely diagnosis for this patient?
   A. Adrenal metastasis
   B. Pheochromocytoma
   C. Adrenal adenoma
   D. Adrenocortical carcinoma

3. Which of the following is correct regarding hormonally functional adrenocortical carcinoma?
   A. Less than 10% of cases of adrenocortical carcinomas produce excess hormones
   B. Hormonally active adrenocortical carcinomas are more common in adults than in children
   C. Hormonally active adrenocortical carcinomas tend to be smaller than nonfunctioning tumors at presentation
   D. Hormonally active adrenocortical carcinomas usually secrete only one class of steroid
4. In adult patients with hormonally functional adrenocortical carcinoma, which of the following is the most common clinical manifestation?
   A. Virilization
   B. Feminization
   C. Cushing syndrome
   D. Hyperaldosteronism

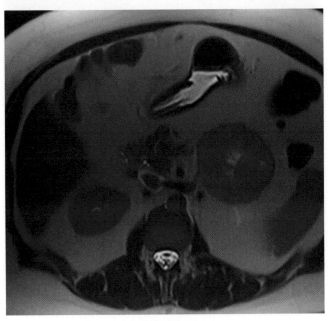

Fig. 131.1

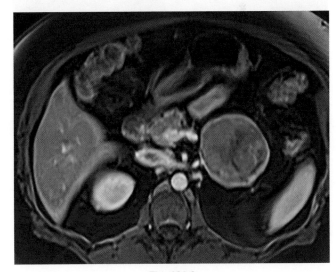

Fig. 131.2

Case 132

History: 28-year-old female with abdominal pain.

1. What should be included in the differential diagnosis of the imaging finding shown? (Choose all that apply.)
   A. Adrenal adenoma
   B. Adrenocortical carcinoma
   C. Lymph nodal mass
   D. Pheochromocytoma
2. Which of the following is the most common manifestation of Castleman disease?
   A. Retroperitoneal mass
   B. Mediastinal mass
   C. Multistation enhancing of notes
   D. Cervical lymphadenopathy
3. Which of the following is the classic imaging appearance of abdominal Castleman disease?
   A. Solitary nodal mass
   B. Infiltrative mass with extension into surrounding organs
   C. Matted lymph nodes without a dominant mass
   D. Large enhancing mass arising from the colon
4. Which of the following adrenal entities show intense enhancement after contrast administration? (Choose all that apply.)
   A. Pheochromocytoma
   B. Myelolipoma
   C. Adrenal cyst
   D. Adrenal adenoma

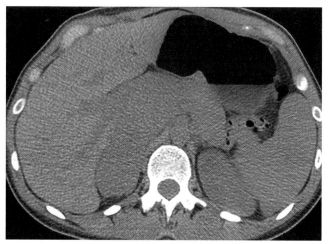

Fig. 132.1

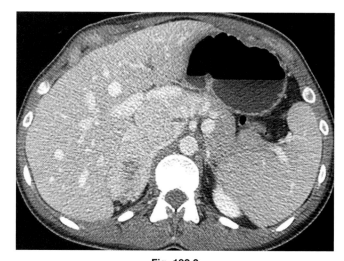

Fig. 132.2

Case 133

History: 62-year-old male with flank pain and leukocytosis.

1. What underlying condition is a risk factor for renal abscess?
   A. Hypertension
   B. Diabetes
   C. Hepatic steatosis
   D. Hypercholesterolemia
2. Which complication occurs if a renal abscess ruptures into the collecting system?
   A. Pyelonephritis
   B. Pyonephrosis
   C. Emphysematous pyelonephritis
   D. Pyelitis
3. What is the treatment for renal abscess? (Choose all that apply.)
   A. IV antibiotics
   B. Percutaneous drainage
   C. Conservative management
   D. Nephrectomy
4. Which characteristic on magnetic resonance imaging (MRI) can help distinguish renal abscess from a complex cyst?
   A. T2 hyperintensity
   B. Peripheral enhancement
   C. Internal septations
   D. Restricted diffusion

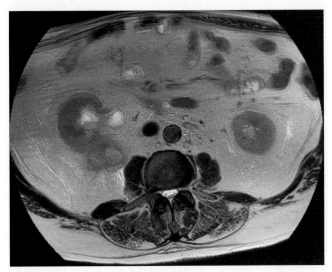

Fig. 133.1

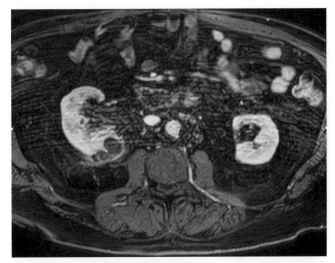

Fig. 133.2

Case 134

History: 67-year-old man with left flank pain.

1. Which of the following would be included in the differential diagnosis for the imaging findings presented?
   A. Simple cyst
   B. Hemorrhagic cyst
   C. Angiomyolipoma
   D. Renal cell carcinoma
2. What is the most common type of renal cell carcinoma (RCC) is commonly bilateral?
   A. Clear cell carcinoma
   B. Papillary RCC
   C. Medullary RCC
   D. Chromophobe RCC
3. Which of the following types of RCC appear hypovascular on computed tomography (CT)? (Choose all that apply.)
   A. Clear cell carcinoma
   B. Papillary RCC
   C. Medullary RCC
   D. Chromophobe RCC
4. Which of the following are familial syndrome, which can develop RCCs? (Choose all that apply.)
   A. Hereditary papillary RCC cancer syndrome
   B. Hereditary leiomyomatosis
   C. RCC syndrome
   D. Birt-Hogg-Dubé syndrome

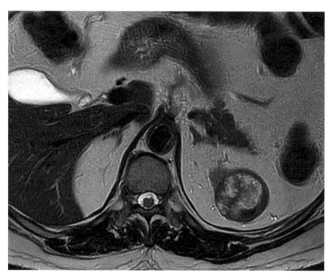

Fig. 134.1

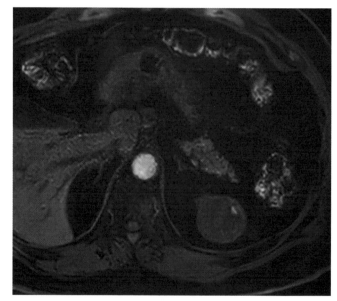

Fig. 134.2

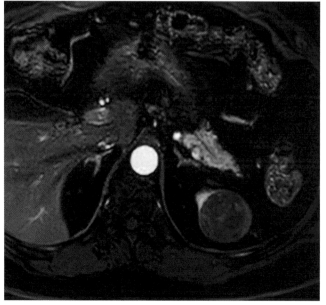

Fig. 134.3

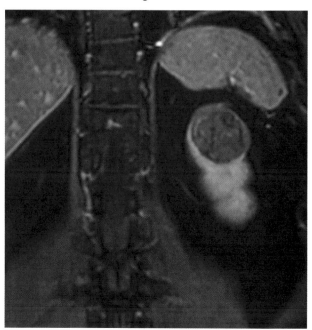

Fig. 134.4

Case 135

History: 45-year-old female with abdominal pain.

1. Which of the following Bosniak classifications is appropriate for the imaging findings presented?
   A. Bosniak I
   B. Bosniak II
   C. Bosniak IIF
   D. Bosniak III

2. What is the incidence of malignancy in Bosniak III cysts?
   A. 0%
   B. 5%
   C. 50%
   D. 100%

3. Homogenous masses markedly hyperintense at T1 weighted imaging at noncontrast MRI would be classified as which type of Bosniak cyst?
   A. I
   B. II
   C. IIF
   D. III

4. Presence of enhancing nodule >4 mm in size would be classified as which type of Bosniak cyst?
   A. I
   B. II
   C. III
   D. IV

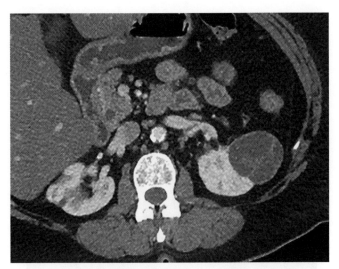

Fig. 135.1

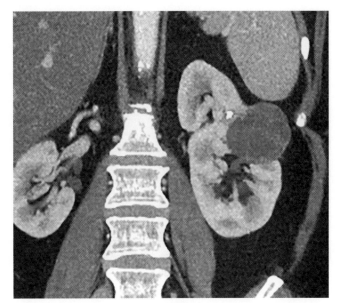

Fig. 135.2

Case 136

History: 67-year-old woman with hematuria.

1. Which of the following feature on magnetic resonance imaging (MRI) is considered to be muscle invasive (T2b) disease?
   A. Irregular mass within the bladder lumen
   B. Enhancement of the bladder mucosa
   C. Filling defect in the bladder lumen
   D. Loss of hypointense band on T2 weighted images
2. Which of the following features on computed tomography (CT) imaging is considered to be muscle invasive disease?
   A. Irregular mass within the bladder lumen
   B. Enhancement of the bladder mucosa
   C. Filling defect in the bladder lumen
   D. Retraction of outer bladder wall

3. What is the tumor stage in a patient with known bladder cancer and extension of the mass to the lateral pelvic wall?
   A. T1
   B. T2
   C. T3
   D. T4
4. What is the nodal stage in a patient with known bladder cancer and enlarged common iliac lymph nodes?
   A. N0
   B. N1
   C. N2
   D. N3

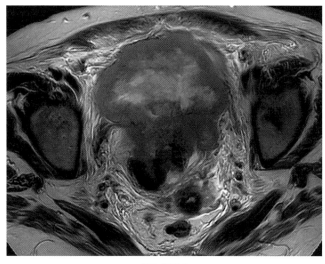

Fig. 136.1

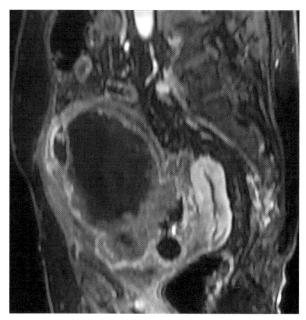

Fig. 136.2

Case 137 is online only and accessible at www.expertconsult.com.

Case 138

History: 30-year-old woman with constipation and dyschezia. She has history of infertility and endometriosis.

1. What should be included in the differential diagnosis of this rectal mass seen on magnetic resonance imaging (MRI)? (Choose all that apply.)
   A. Rectal adenocarcinoma
   B. Rectal gastrointestinal stromal tumor
   C. Rectal endometriosis
   D. Peritoneal metastatic deposit
2. What is the most common theory for the development of endometriosis?
   A. Iatrogenic theory, where intimate real implants are inadvertently injected during pelvic surgery or biopsy
   B. Metastatic theory, where endometriosis results from the metastatic implantation of endometrial tissue from retrograde menstruation
   C. Vascular theory, where endometriosis results from lymphatic or vascular spread of endometrial cells
   D. Metaplastic theory, related to the metaplastic differentiation of serosal surfaces or the remnants of müllerian tissue.
3. Which MRI sequence is the most sensitive for detection of small endometrial implants?
   A. T1 weighted with fat suppression
   B. T2 weighted with fat suppression
   C. T1 weighted without fat suppression
   D. T2 weighted without fat suppression
4. What is the commonest site for extraovarian involvement from endometriosis?
   A. Bladder
   B. Rectosigmoid colon
   C. Vagina
   D. Uterosacral ligaments

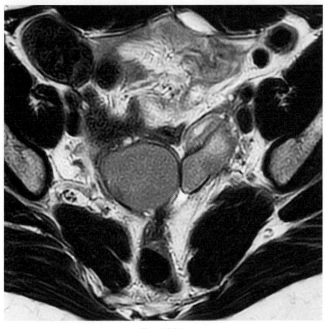

Fig. 138.1

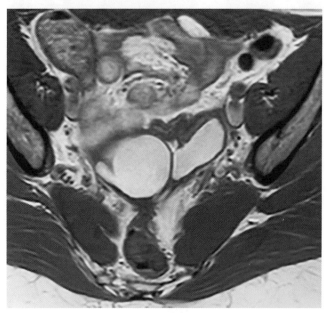

Fig. 138.2

Case 139

History: 42-year-old woman with pain and postcoital bleeding.

1. The International Federation of Gynecology and Obstetrics (FIGO) uses a surgical staging system for which of the following gynecologic malignancies? (Choose all that apply.)
   A. Cervical carcinoma
   B. Endometrial carcinoma
   C. Ovarian carcinoma
   D. Vulvar carcinoma
2. Cervical carcinoma that involves the lower one-third of the vagina is which FIGO stage?
   A. Stage I
   B. Stage II
   C. Stage III
   D. Stage IV
3. Cervical cancer that invades the mucosa of the bladder is which FIGO stage?
   A. Stage I
   B. Stage II
   C. Stage III
   D. Stage IV
4. As per the FIGO staging, cervical cancer that involves para-aortic lymph nodes is which stage?
   A. Stage I
   B. Stage II
   C. Stage III
   D. Stage IV

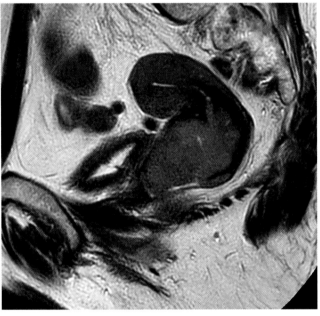

Fig. 139.1

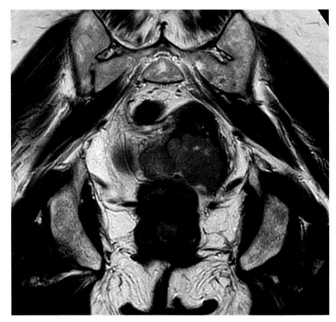

Fig. 139.2

Case 140

History: 68-year-old women presented with postmenopausal vaginal bleeding.

1. In standard clinical work, surgical staging of endometrial carcinoma includes which of the following? (Choose all that apply.)
   A. Bilateral salpingo-oophorectomy (BSO)
   B. Hysterectomy
   C. Node dissection
   D. Peritoneal washing and omental biopsy
2. Which of the following is the most accurate modality for local preoperative uterine staging of endometrial carcinoma?
   A. Ultrasound
   B. Computed tomography (CT)
   C. Hysterosalpingography
   D. Magnetic resonance imaging (MRI)

3. What is stage III endometrial carcinoma?
   A. Tumor confined to the corpus uteri
   B. Tumor invading the cervical stroma
   C. Local or regional spread of tumor
   D. Invasion of the bladder or bowel
4. What is the typical treatment approach to endometrial carcinoma stage II?
   A. Hormonal therapy
   B. Laparoscopic hysterectomy
   C. Vaginal brachytherapy
   D. Hysterectomy, BSO, and pelvic/paraaortic lymph node sampling

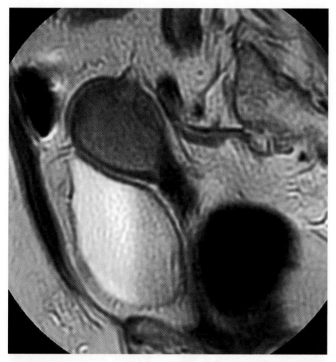

Fig. 140.1

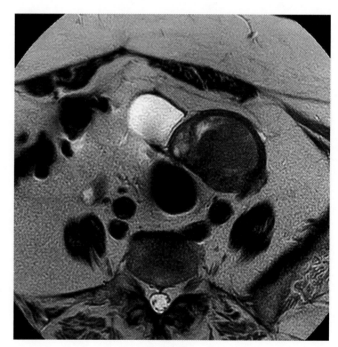

Fig. 140.2

Case 141

History: 56-year-old woman with known gastric adenocarcinoma with staging computed tomography (CT) scan.

1. Which of the following would be included in the differential diagnosis for the imaging findings presented? (Choose all that apply.)
   A. Primary ovarian tumors
   B. Ovarian metastases
   C. Lymph nodal masses
   D. Abscesses
2. Which of the following primary tumors can result in ovarian metastasis? (Choose all that apply.)
   A. Stomach
   B. Colon
   C. Breast
   D. Lymphoma
3. What is the commonest imaging feature of metastatic tumors to the ovary?
   A. Solid appearance
   B. Mixed cystic and solid appearance
   C. Unilaterality
   D. Bilaterality
4. What are the imaging features seen on CT scan in Krukenberg tumors? (Choose all that apply.)
   A. Oval masses that maintain the ovarian shape
   B. Solid or predominantly solid
   C. Strong enhancement after contrast administration
   D. Concomitant presence of primary tumor in another organ in the abdomen

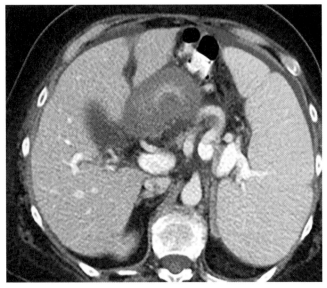

Fig. 141.1

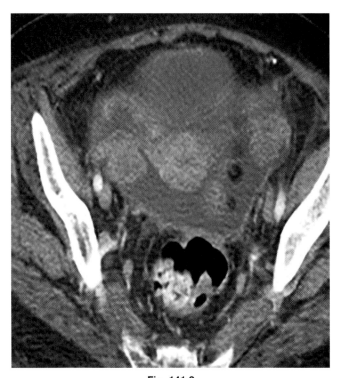

Fig. 141.2

Case 142

History: 65-year-old woman with bloating and pelvic pain.

1. Which of the following would be included in the differential diagnosis for the imaging findings presented? (Choose all that apply.)
   A. Endometrioid carcinoma
   B. High-grade serous carcinoma
   C. Mucinous carcinoma
   D. Mature teratoma
2. Extrapelvic metastasis of ovarian carcinoma most frequently occur by which of the following?
   A. Hematogenous spread
   B. Lymphatic transmission
   C. Intraperitoneal seeding
   D. Direct extension

3. Ovarian carcinoma with peritoneal implants outside the pelvis is considered which International Federation of Gynecology and Obstetrics (FIGO) stage?
   A. Stage I
   B. Stage II
   C. Stage III
   D. Stage IV
4. Ovarian carcinoma with metastatic lymph node seen in the paraaortic region at the level of the renal hilum is considered which FIGO stage?
   A. Stage I
   B. Stage II
   C. Stage III
   D. Stage IV

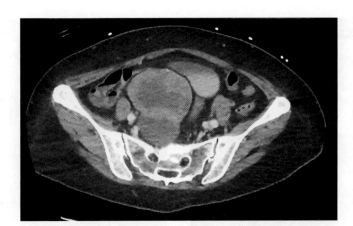

Fig. 142.1

Case 143

History: 45-year-old woman with increasing abdominal girth and palpable adnexal mass.

1. Which of the following would be included in the differential diagnosis for the imaging findings presented? (Choose all that apply.)
   A. Serous cystadenoma
   B. Mucinous cystadenoma
   C. Granulosa cell tumor
   D. Cystadenocarcinoma
2. Which imaging features listed on magnetic resonance imaging (MRI) increase the likelihood of a malignant ovarian lesion? (Choose all that apply.)
   A. Thick irregular wall
   B. Papillary projections
   C. Large soft tissue mass with necrosis
   D. Ascites

3. Which imaging features listed are more commonly seen in serous cystadenocarcinomas compared to mucinous cystadenocarcinomas?
   A. Unilaterality
   B. Peritoneal carcinomatosis
   C. Thick irregular wall
   D. Papillary projections
4. Which of the following are the common epithelial ovarian tumors seen? (Choose all that apply.)
   A. Serous tumors
   B. Mucinous tumors
   C. Endometrioid tumor
   D. Clear cell carcinomas

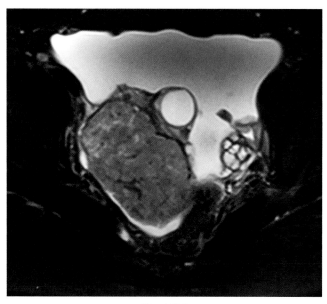

Fig. 143.1

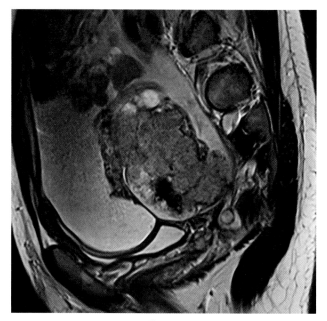

Fig. 143.2

Case 144

History: 65-year-old woman with abnormal postmenopausal bleeding.

1. Which of the following would be included in the differential diagnosis for the imaging findings presented? (Choose all that apply.)
   A. Mucinous cystadenoma
   B. Cystadenocarcinoma
   C. Granulosa cell tumor
   D. Steroid cell tumor
2. Which of the following represent ovarian tumors arising from primitive sex cord cells?
   A. Granulosa cell tumor
   B. Fibroma
   C. Fibrothecoma
   D. Thecoma
3. Which type of ovarian tumors show delayed enhancement after administration of gadolinium contrast on magnetic resonance imaging (MRI)?
   A. Granulosa cell tumor
   B. Sertoli-Leydig cell tumors
   C. Fibroma
   D. Sclerosing stromal tumor of the ovary
4. Which type of ovarian tumors can develop pleural effusion? (Choose all that apply.)
   A. Fibromas
   B. Mucinous adenocarcinoma
   C. Cystadenoma
   D. Granulosa cell tumor

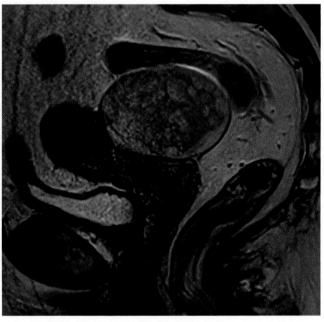

Fig. 144.1

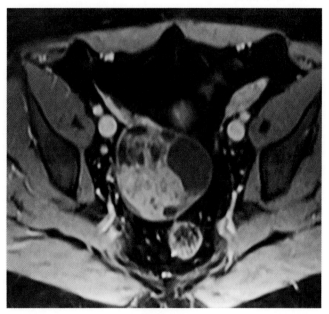

Fig. 144.2

Case 145 is online only and accessible at www.expertconsult.com.

Case 146

History: 27-year-old woman with history of prior cesarean section presents for evaluation of abdominal pain in the setting of new first-trimester pregnancy.

1. The earliest time at which a gestational sac in a normal intrauterine pregnancy is shown by transvaginal ultrasound is what time after the last menstrual period?
   A. 2–3 weeks
   B. 4–5 weeks
   C. 6–8 weeks
   D. 10–12 weeks
2. In a patient with a positive serum beta–human chorionic gonadotropin (β-HCG) test, nonvisualization of an intrauterine pregnancy may represent a diagnosis of:
   A. Very early intrauterine pregnancy
   B. Failed pregnancy
   C. Ectopic pregnancy
   D. All of these

3. The classic triad of symptoms of ectopic pregnancy are:
   A. Fever, headache, pelvic pain
   B. Pelvic pain, fever, vaginal bleeding
   C. Pelvic pain, vaginal bleeding, tender adnexal mass
   D. Pelvic pain, fever, tender adnexal mass
4. From the provided images, the most likely diagnosis is:
   A. Normal intrauterine pregnancy
   B. Cesarean section implantation of pregnancy
   C. Intraovarian (ectopic) pregnancy
   D. Cystic ovarian mass

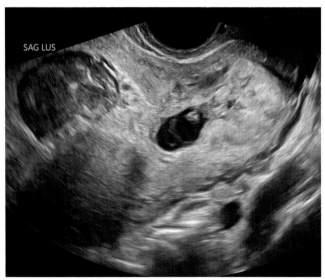

Fig. 146.1

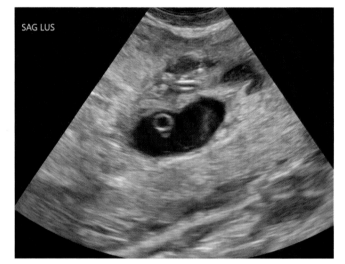

Fig. 146.2

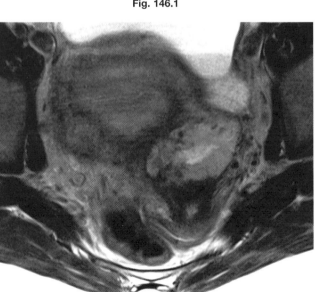

Fig. 146.3

Case 147

History: 34-year-old woman with history of fibroid uterus presents with worsening abdominal fullness and leg swelling.

1. On spin-echo magnetic resonance imaging (MRI), which statements related to flow voids are accurate?
   A. Flow voids are a finding of vascular patency
   B. Flow voids are a finding of vascular occlusion
   C. Result from protons moving out of plane, between radio-frequency pulses
   D. A and C
   E. None of these above
2. Which MR sequences are the most likely to demonstrate flow voids?
   A. T1 weighted
   B. T2 weighted
   C. PD weighted
   D. B and C
   E. All of these

3. From the provided images, appropriate differential considerations include:
   A. Malignant pelvic vascular invasion
   B. Intravascular leiomyomatosis
   C. Bland pelvic vein thrombosis
   D. A and B
   E. All of these
4. Which of the following represent malignant transformation of benign uterine leiomyoma?
   A. Metastasizing leiomyomatosis
   B. Intravascular leiomyomatosis
   C. A and B
   E. None of these

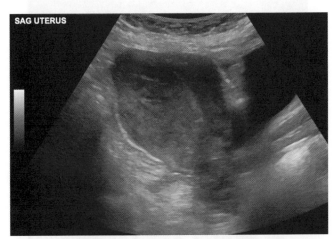

Fig. 147.1

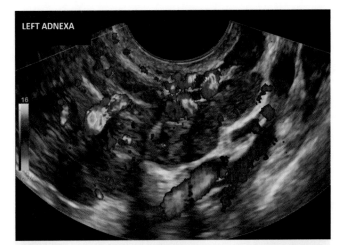

Fig. 147.2

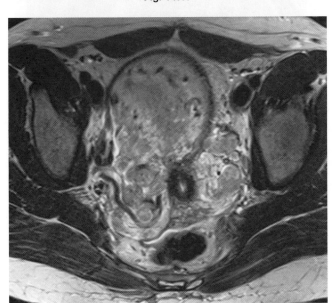

Fig. 147.3

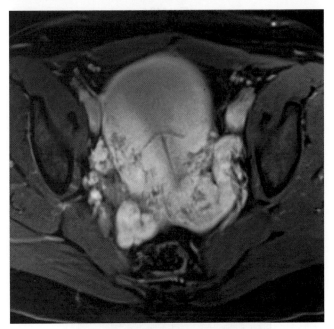

Fig. 147.4

Case 148

History: 28-year-old woman with history of prior cesarean section delivery presents for evaluation of pregnancy in the second trimester.

1. From the provided images, the most likely diagnosis is:
   A. Normal placentation
   B. Preeclampsia
   C. HELLP syndrome
   D. Invasive placentation
2. Which of the following are considered major risk factors of invasive placentation?
   A. Prior cesarean section
   B. Placenta previa
   C. Advanced maternal age
   D. Prior myomectomy
   E. A and B
   F. All of these

3. Placenta increta refers to:
   A. Chorionic villi attached to but not invading myometrium
   B. Chorionic villi partially invading myometrium
   C. Chorionic villi invades myometrium, and potentially beyond
   D. Is readily distinguished from placenta accreta by conventional imaging
4. Typical magnetic resonance (MR) features of invasive placentation include:
   A. Rounded or lumpy placental contour
   B. Uterine bulging
   C. T2 hyperintense intraplacental bands
   D. A and B
   E. All of these

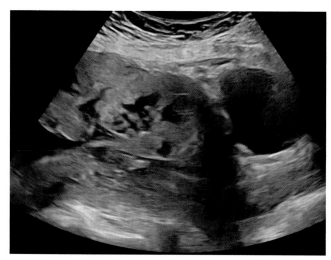

Fig. 148.1

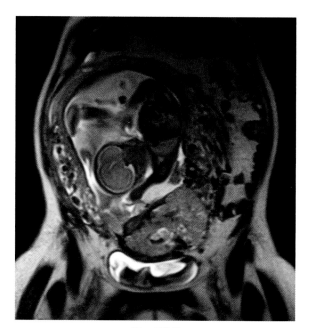

Fig. 148.2

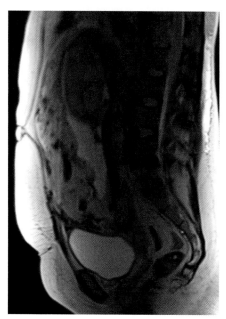

Fig. 148.3

Case 149

History: 47-year-old man with pain occurring during penetrative intercourse, after which he developed urethral bleeding.

1. Which of the following would be included in the differential diagnosis for the imaging findings presented? (Choose all that apply.)
   A. Peyronie disease
   B. Penile mass
   C. Penile fracture
   D. Urethral rupture
2. Which of the following is a common mechanism for penile fracture?
   A. Gunshot wound
   B. Stabbing wound
   C. Trauma to flaccid penis
   D. Trauma during coitus usually from thrusting the erect penis against the symphysis pubis or perineum

3. Which of the following is the preferred treatment for penile fracture?
   A. Compression bandages
   B. Surgical treatment
   C. Penis splint
   D. Fibrinolytic agents
4. Which of the following complications can be associated with penile fracture? (Choose all that apply.)
   A. Urethral injury
   B. Scrotal hematoma
   C. Prolonged erection
   D. Painful intercourse

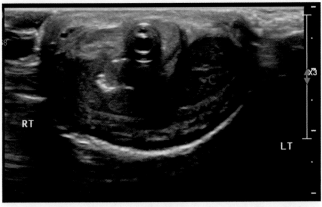

Fig. 149.1

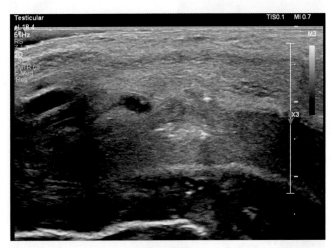

Fig. 149.2

Case 150

History: 56-year-old man with history of bladder carcinoma presented with new palpable masses in the penis.

1. Which of the following would be included in the differential diagnosis for the imaging findings presented? (Choose all that apply.)
   A. Metastases
   B. Penile carcinoma
   C. Abscesses
   D. Peyronie disease
2. From which organ do penile metastasis most often originate?
   A. Thyroid
   B. Lung
   C. Stomach
   D. Urinary bladder

3. What are the main prognostic factor(s) for patients with carcinoma of the penis? (Choose all that apply.)
   A. Location of the mass
   B. Degree of invasion of the mass
   C. Presence of metastatic lymph nodes
   D. Distant metastasis
4. What is the typical imaging appearance of primary carcinoma of the penis on magnetic resonance imaging (MRI)?
   A. Single T2 low-signal-intensity infiltrative mass compared to the corpus cavernosum
   B. Single T2 high-signal-intensity infiltrative mass compared to the corpus cavernosum
   C. Multiple T2 low-signal-intensity masses in the corpora cavernosum
   D. Multiple T2 high-signal-intensity masses in the corpora cavernosum

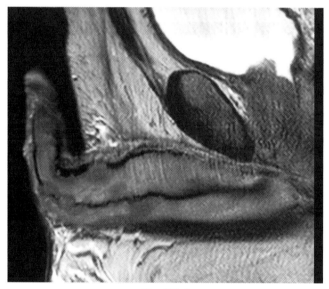

Fig. 150.1

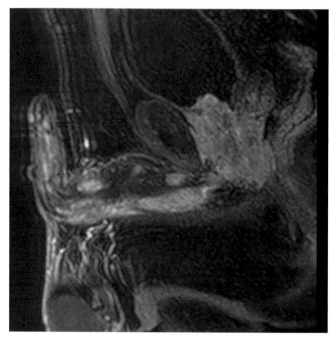

Fig. 150.2

Case 151 is online only and accessible at www.expertconsult.com.

Case 152

History: 67-year-old male with elevated prostate specific antigen (PSA).

1. Fig. 152.1 depicts what local tumor staging according to the TNM classification?
   A. T2
   B. T3a
   C. T3b
   D. T4
2. Fig. 152.2 demonstrates involvement of what structure that is critical for surgical planning?
   A. Rectum
   B. Neurovascular bundle
   C. Levator sling
   D. Bladder
3. Loss of the rectoprostatic angle is useful for detecting extra-prostatic extension of what type of prostate tumor?
   A. Posterior tumors
   B. Transition zone tumors
   C. Central zone tumors
   D. Anterior tumors
4. Which sign is the least specific for predicting extracapsular extension of tumor at magnetic resonance imaging (MRI)?
   A. Neurovascular bundle invasion
   B. Loss of the rectoprostatic angle
   C. Capsular bulge
   D. Broad capsular contact

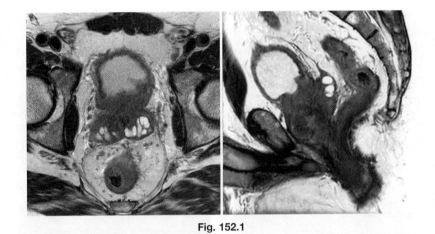

Fig. 152.1

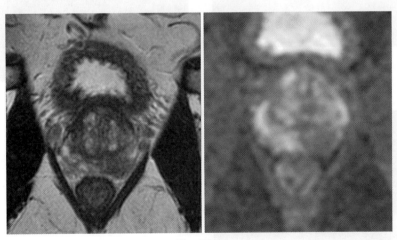

Fig. 152.2

Case 153

History: 70-year-old man presents with increasing prostate specific antigen (PSA), 2 years after radical prostatectomy for Gleason 4+3 prostate cancer.

1. Following radical prostatectomy, the most common site of local recurrence is:
   A. Vesicourethral anastomosis
   B. Lateral prostatectomy bed margin
   C. Superior prostatectomy bed margin (seminal vesicle)
   D. Bladder trigone
2. From the provided images, the most likely diagnosis is:
   A. Residual prostatic tissue
   B. Locally recurrent prostate cancer
   C. Postsurgical inflammatory change
   D. Postsurgical infection/abscess

3. In contrast to its adjunctive role in PI-RADS assessment, which of the following magnetic resonance imaging (MRI) sequences is of increased importance in the posttreatment assessment of prostate cancer?
   A. T2 weighted imaging
   B. T1 weighted imaging
   C. Diffusion weighted imaging
   D. Dynamic contrast enhanced imaging
4. Compared to its pretreatment appearance, the MRI appearance of a prostate in a patient who has undergone radiation therapy for prostate cancer is:
   A. Enlarged; increased T2 signal intensity
   B. Enlarged; decreased T2 signal intensity
   C. Atrophic; increased T2 signal intensity
   D. Atrophic; decreased T2 signal intensity

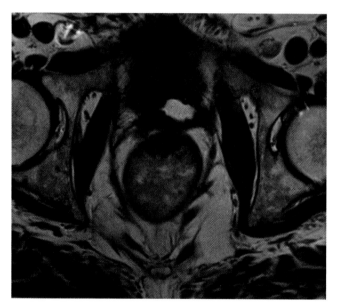

Fig. 153.1

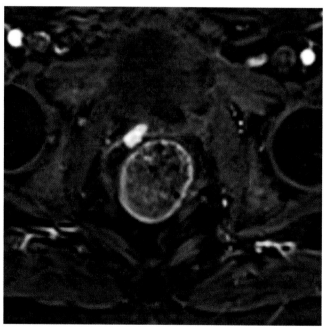

Fig. 153.2

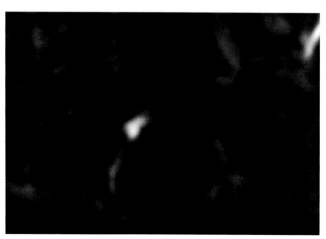

Fig. 153.3

Case 154

History: 75-year-old man with abdominal pain, significant loss of weight, and nausea.

1. Which of the following would be included in the differential diagnosis for the imaging findings presented? (Choose all that apply.)
   A. Gastric carcinoma
   B. Gastric lymphoma
   C. Gastrointestinal stromal tumor
   D. Gastric ulcer
2. Which part of the gastrointestinal tract is most commonly involved in lymphoma?
   A. Esophagus
   B. Stomach
   C. Small bowel
   D. Large bowel
3. What is not a common appearance of gastric lymphoma on computed tomography (CT)?
   A. Diffuse stomach wall thickening
   B. Stomach wall thickening
   C. Extension of the mass directly into the pancreas and spleen
   D. Enlarged surrounding lymph nodes
4. Which of the following is considered the gold standard for the diagnosis of primary gastric lymphoma?
   A. Esophagogastroduodenoscopy (EGD) with biopsy
   B. Computed tomography (CT)
   C. Magnetic resonance imaging (MRI)
   D. Positron emission tomography (PET)

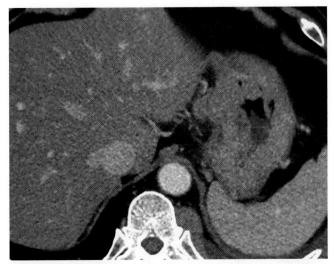

Fig. 154.1

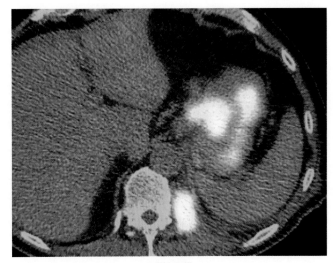

Fig. 154.2

Case 155

History: 53-year-old woman with known pancreatic adenocarcinoma with new pelvic masses seen on a staging computed tomography (CT) scan.

1. Which of the following would be included in the differential diagnosis for the imaging findings presented? (Choose all that apply.)
   A. Primary ovarian tumors
   B. Krukenberg tumors
   C. Lymph nodal masses
   D. Abscesses
2. Which of the following are the most common primary tumors that result in ovarian metastasis? (Choose all that apply.)
   A. Stomach
   B. Colon
   C. Liver
   D. Kidney

3. What percentage of ovarian tumors are represented by metastatic tumors to the ovary?
   A. 10%
   B. 25%
   C. 50%
   D. 75%
4. What imaging feature on CT scan favors Krukenberg tumors?
   A. Cystic appearance
   B. Solid appearance
   C. Presence of bilateral ovarian masses
   D. Concomitant presence of primary tumor in another organ in the abdomen

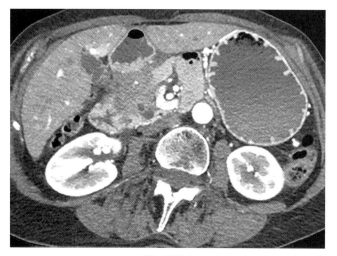

Fig. 155.1

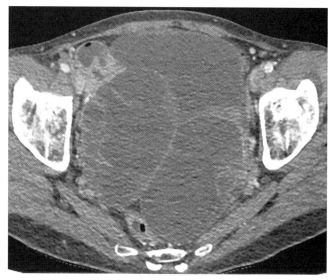

Fig. 155.2

Case 156

Case authored by Dr. Shanna Matalon
History: 31-year-old man presents with months-long abdominal pain, change in bowel habits.

1. From the provided images, the most likely diagnosis is:
   A. Ulcerative colitis with backwash ileitis
   B. Active inflammatory Crohn's disease
   C. Small bowel adenocarcinoma
   D. Salmonella infection
2. The most common distribution of this diagnosis is:
   A. Pancolonic
   B. Rectum only
   C. Terminal ileum
   D. Appendix
3. The imaging finding most SPECIFIC to this entity is:
   A. Vasa recta hyperemia
   B. Restricted diffusion
   C. Wall thickening
   D. Perienteric fat stranding
   E. Asymmetric wall hyperenhancement
4. A typical imaging finding of ulcerative colitis is:
   A. Transmural bowel wall involvement
   B. Skip lesions
   C. Presence of abscesses and/or fistulae
   D. Ahaustral colon (leadpipe colon)

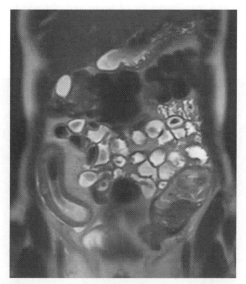

Fig. 156.1

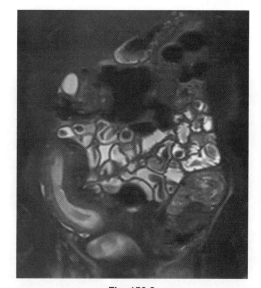

Fig. 156.2

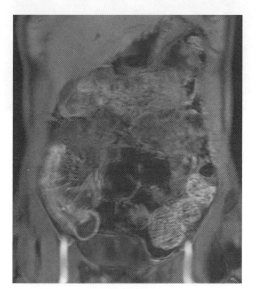

Fig. 156.3

Case 157 is online only and accessible at www.expertconsult.com.

Case 158

History: 34-year-old woman with history of allogeneic stem cell transplant 2 months prior for acute myelogenous leukemia presents with rash, vomiting, and diarrhea.

1. From the provided images, the imaging appearance suggests:
   A. Infectious enteritis
   B. Acute graft-versus-host disease
   C. Pseudomembranous colitis
   D. A and B
2. Typical manifestations of acute graft-versus-host disease are:
   A. Dermatitis
   B. Enterocolitis
   C. Cholestasis
   D. Meningitis
   E. A, B, and C
   F. A, B, C, and D

3. Typical abdominal imaging findings of acute graft-versus-host disease are:
   A. Diffuse, small bowel mucosal enhancement
   B. Fluid-filled small bowel
   C. Vasa recta engorgement
   D. Small bowel obstruction
   E. A, B, and C
   F. A, B, C, and D
4. Comparing acute and chronic graft-versus-host disease, which of the following statements is accurate?
   A. Clinical manifestations of acute and chronic forms are near identical
   B. The chronic form represents the prolonged form of the acute form
   C. Clinical manifestations of acute and chronic forms have minimal overlap
   D. A and B

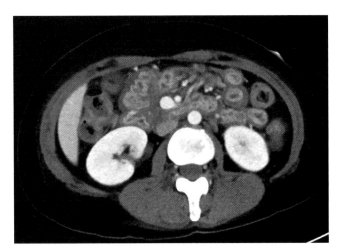

Fig. 158.1

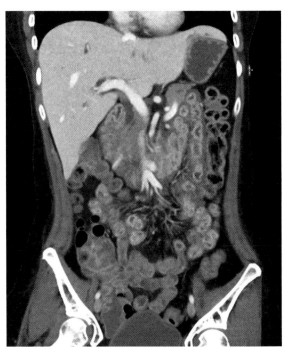

Fig. 158.2

Case 159

History: 37-year-old pregnant woman with history of gastric bypass surgery with acute abdominal pain.

1. Which of the following would be included in the differential diagnosis for the imaging findings presented?
   A. Gastric outlet obstruction
   B. Duodenal obstruction
   C. Stricture at the distal limb of Roux-en-Y
   D. Internal hernia
2. What is the most common type of internal hernia?
   A. Paraduodenal
   B. Pericecal
   C. Foramen of Winslow
   D. Transmesenteric and transmesocolic
3. Which of the following are considered features of internal hernia seen on computed tomography (CT)? (Choose all that apply.)
   A. Convergence of vessels and mesenteric fat at the hernia orifice
   B. Displacement of key mesenteric vessels
   C. Engorgement of mesenteric vessels
   D. Displacement of surrounding structures around the hernia sac
4. Which of the following statements is true regarding internal hernias? (Choose all that apply.)
   A. Nonenhanced scan is helpful to detect an increased bowel wall attenuation
   B. Contrast-enhanced scan is helpful for depicting mesenteric vessels
   C. Paraduodenal hernias are the least common type of internal hernias
   D. Cluster of small bowel loops in an abnormal location

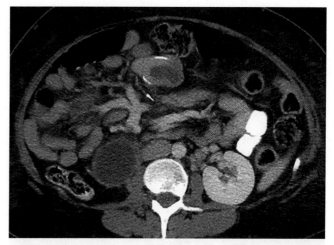

Fig. 159.2

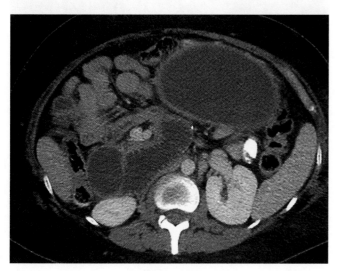

Fig. 159.1

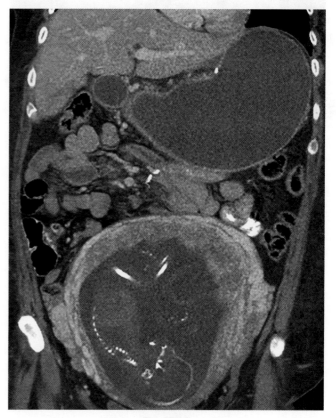

Fig. 159.3

Case 160

History: 67-year-old man with history of melanoma and acute abdominal pain, predominantly in the left midabdomen.

1. What is the diagnosis for the imaging findings presented?
   A. Small bowel obstruction
   B. Intussusception
   C. Bowel ischemia
   D. Internal hernia
2. What is the most common etiology for small bowel intussusception?
   A. Malignant neoplasm
   B. Transient
   C. Meckel diverticulum
   D. Postoperative adhesions
3. Which of the following are considered features of intussusception seen on computed tomography (CT)? (Choose all that apply.)
   A. Bowel obstruction
   B. Targetlike appearance
   C. Sausage-shaped appearance
   D. Coiled spring appearance

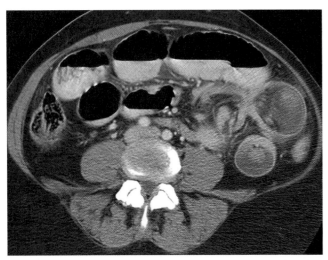

Fig. 160.1

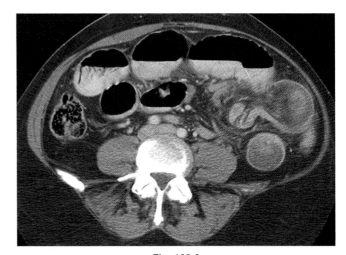

Fig. 160.2

Case 161

Case authored by Dr. Shanna Matalon
History: 47-year-old man with rectal mass on colonoscopy.

1. What is the most common location of this entity?
   A. Duodenum
   B. Rectum
   C. Cecum
   D. Stomach
2. What is the name of the condition when this entity is associated with uncontrolled watery diarrhea leading to fluid, protein, and electrolyte imbalance?
   A. McKittrick-Wheelock syndrome
   B. Bouveret syndrome
   C. Trousseau syndrome
   D. Rokitansky-Küster-Hauser syndrome
3. Which type of adenoma has the highest rate of malignant transformation?
   A. Tubular
   B. Tubulovillous
   C. Villous
4. The curved arrows on the images demonstrate:
   A. Vessels and desmoplastic response
   B. Extramural (T3) tumor

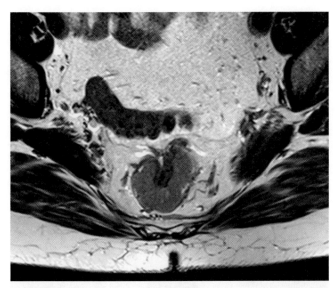

Fig. 161.1

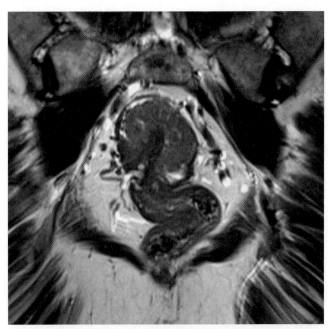

Fig. 161.2

Case 162

Case authored by Dr. Shanna Matalon

History: 60-year-old man with recent colonoscopy demonstrating biopsied rectal adenocarcinoma.

1. The outermost thin black line of the wall of the rectum on T2 weighted images represents the:
   A. Lamina propria
   B. Submucosa
   C. Muscularis propria
   D. Mesorectal fascia

2. If a tumor extends into the muscularis propria but not beyond the muscularis propria, the T stage is:
   A. T1
   B. T2
   C. T3
   D. T4a

3. Which T stage involves invasion of adjacent structures, such as a seminal vesical in men or uterus in women?
   A. T2
   B. T3
   C. T4a
   D. T4b

4. A patient is found to have a low anorectal junction tumor with pathology revealing squamous cell carcinoma. This should be staged as a:
   A. Rectal cancer regardless of where the tumor is located
   B. Anal cancer regardless of where the tumor is located
   C. Anal cancer if it mostly involves anal canal
   D. Rectal cancer if it mostly involves rectal wall

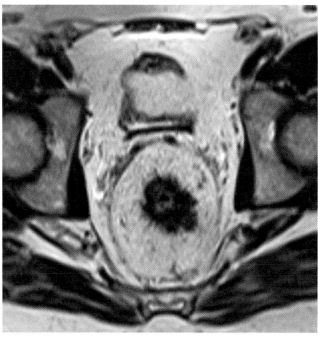

Fig. 162.1

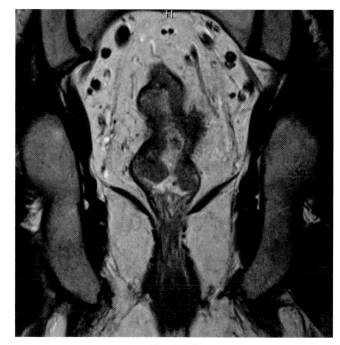

Fig. 162.2

Case 163

History: Two patients present for imaging evaluation of biopsied cervical adenocarcinoma, Patient A (Figs. 163.1 and 163.2) and Patient B (Figs. 163.3 and 163.4).

1. In which patient(s) is there evidence of parametrial extension?
   A. Patient A
   B. Patient B
   C. Both patients A and B
   D. Neither
2. From the provided images, there is evidence of:
   A. No parametrial extension
   B. Left parametrial extension
   C. Right parametrial extension
   D. Bilateral parametrial extension

3. How is cervical carcinoma staged?
   A. Clinically
   B. Ultrasound
   C. Positron emission tomography (PET)/computed tomography (CT)
   D. Magnetic resonance imaging (MRI)
4. Which findings should be reported as pertinent positives or negatives when dictating an MRI for cervical cancer staging? (Choose all that apply.)
   A. Tumor size
   B. Parametrial extension
   C. Vaginal invasion
   D. Hydronephrosis

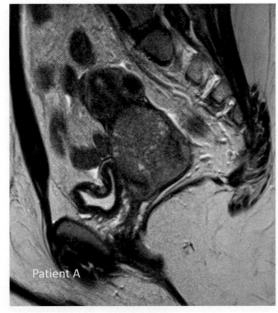

Fig. 163.1

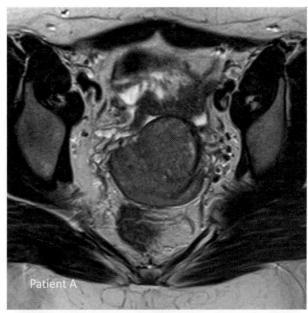

Fig. 163.2

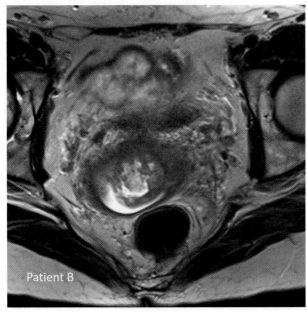

Fig. 163.3

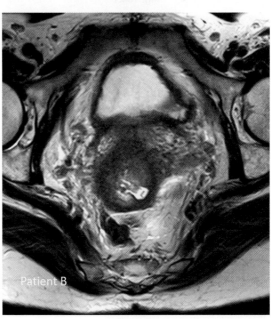

Fig. 163.4

Case 164

History: 34-year-old woman with history of Crohn's disease presents with perineal discomfort and painful bowel movements.

1. Figs. 164.1 through 164.4 demonstrate what process in this patient with the provided history?
   A. Rectal cancer
   B. Fistula-in-ano
   C. Rectocele
   D. Hemorrhoids
2. What is the Parks classification of the lesion shown on the magnetic resonance imaging (MRI)?
   A. Intersphincteric
   B. Transphincteric
   C. Suprasphincteric
   D. Extrasphincteric

3. Which is the least common type of fistula-in-ano?
   A. Intersphincteric
   B. Transphincteric
   C. Suprasphincteric
   D. Extrasphincteric
4. Which combination of MR findings best describes an active fistulous tract?
   A. T2 hypointense, enhancing
   B. T2 hypointense, not enhancing
   C. T2 hyperintense, enhancing
   D. T2 hyperintense, not enhancing

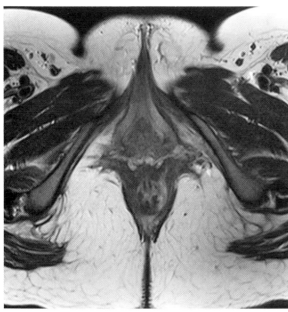
Fig. 164.1

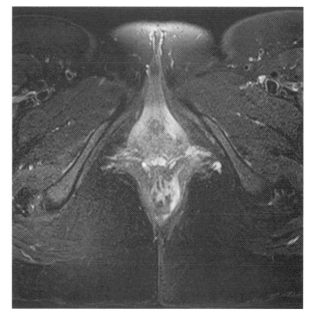
Fig. 164.2

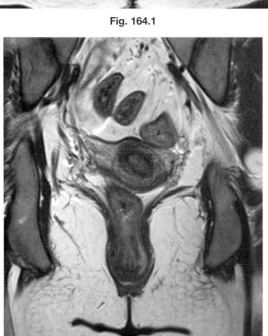
Fig. 164.3

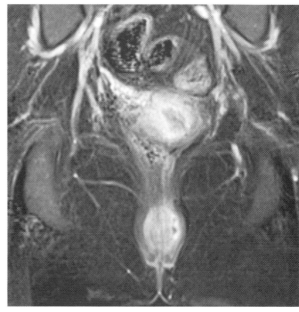
Fig. 164.4

Case 165

History: 24-year-old woman, in the second trimester of pregnancy, presents with abdominal pain and nausea.

1. From the provided images, the most likely diagnosis is:
   A. Normal; no acute pathology
   B. Obstructing renal stone
   C. Acute appendicitis
   D. Terminal ileitis of inflammatory bowel disease
2. Magnetic resonance imaging (MRI) features of acute appendicitis include:
   A. Appendiceal diameter >7 mm
   B. High luminal signal intensity on T2 weighted images
   C. Periappendiceal fat stranding and fluid
   D. All of these
3. Regarding MRI of pregnant patients, which of the following statements are true?
   A. Data have not conclusively documented deleterious effects of MRI exposure on the developing fetus
   B. Pregnant patients can undergo MRI scans in the first trimester of pregnancy, following appropriate risk-benefit analysis to the patient
   C. Pregnant patients can undergo MRI scans in the second and third trimesters of pregnancy, following appropriate risk-benefit analysis to the patient
   D. A and C
   E. A, B, and C
4. Regarding the use of MRI contrast agents in pregnant patients, which of the following statements is true?
   A. Gadolinium-based MRI contrast agents do not pass through the placental-fetal barrier
   B. Gadolinium is a pregnancy class C drug
   C. There are well-established fetal indications for the use of contrast enhanced MRI
   D. All of these

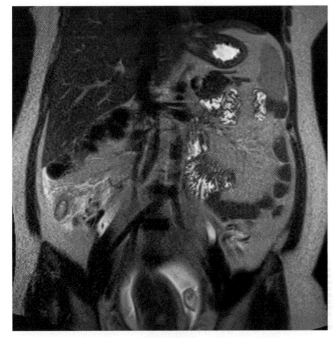

Fig. 165.2

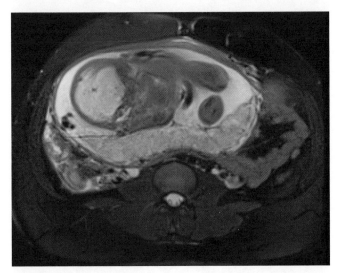

Fig. 165.1

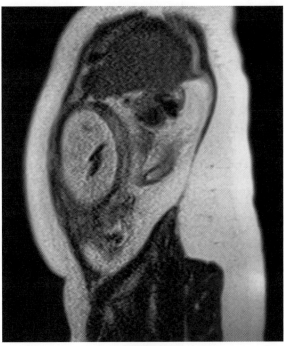

Fig. 165.3

Opening Round

CASE 1

Portal Venous Gas; Mesenteric Ischemia

1. A. In the liver, peripheral, linear, branching hypodensities represent portal venous gas. In contrast, pneumobilia, or air in the intrahepatic bile ducts, is typically represented by the finding of linear branching hypodensities in a central hepatic distribution.
2. E. Each of the listed etiologies is a potential cause of portal venous gas.
3. A. The figures demonstrate portal venous gas, and gas in mesenteric veins in the left hemiabdomen, likely secondary to mesenteric ischemia. There is neither pneumobilia nor diverticular abscess shown on the figures.
4. D. For the finding of portal venous gas in the setting of suspected mesenteric ischemia, surgical consultation is the next best step in management. There is no finding to indicate acute biliary obstruction, for which abdominal MRI/MRCP, and/or ERCP would be indicated. There is no abnormal dilatation of bowel loops for which nasogastric tube decompression would be indicated.

Comment

Portal Venous Gas
- A finding associated with a wide spectrum of abdominal diseases
- Portal vein formed at the confluence of the superior mesenteric vein and splenic vein
- Proposed mechanisms of portal venous gas include:
  - Translocation of gas, from bowel or abscess, into liver
  - Translocation of gas-forming bacteria into the portal venous system
- High morbidity and mortality associated with this finding as a result of the underlying etiologies that it signifies:
  - Bowel ischemia/necrosis: injury to bowel mucosa allows translocation of gas
  - Diverticulitis: either by septic thrombophlebitis or direct gas translocation from perforated bowel lumen
  - Inflammatory bowel disease
  - Intraabdominal abscess
  - Small bowel obstruction
  - Gastric ulcer
  - Iatrogenic
  - Idiopathic
  - Necrotizing enterocolitis (in neonates)

Imaging Appearance
- Radiography: branching lucency of the liver, extending peripherally
- US: echogenicity flow in the portal vein
- CT: branching lucency in the portal venous system, extending to within 2 cm of liver capsule
  - In contrast to pneumobilia, which is central to the liver because of the direction of bile flow

Management
- The finding of portal venous gas detected on CT, in the setting of bowel ischemia or necrosis, has been associated with high mortality (>50%), and emergent surgical consultation is indicated.
- In patients with intestinal obstruction, peptic ulcer disease, or inflammatory bowel disease, mortality is increased, though not to the same extent; heightened surveillance of the patient's condition may be indicated, with low threshold for operative management.
- However, portal venous gas may also be seen as a consequence of postsurgical or postprocedural states, without increased morbidity; consider watchful waiting if clinically appropriate.

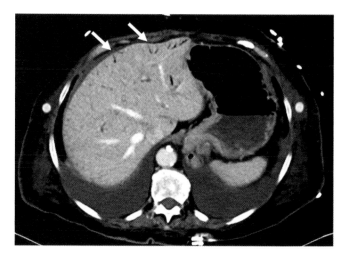

Fig. 1.1 Contrast-enhanced abdominal computed tomography (CT). In the liver, peripheral, linear, branching hypodensities *(straight arrows)* represent portal venous gas.

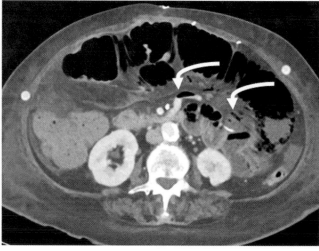

Fig. 1.2 Contrast-enhanced abdominal computed tomography (CT). Gas is shown in mesenteric veins in the left midabdomen *(curved arrows)*.

REFERENCES

Abbound, B., Hachem, J. E., Yazbeck, T., & Doumit, C. (2009). Hepatic portal venous gas: Pathophysiology, etiology, prognosis and treatment. *World Journal of Gastroenterology, 15*, 3585–3590.

Nelson, A. L., Millington, T. M., Sahani, D., Chung, R. T., Bauer, C., ... Hertl, M. (2009). Hepatic portal venous gas: The ABCs of management. *Archives of Surgery, 144*, 575–581.

CASE 2

Focal Nodular Hyperplasia

1. C. The lesion seen in the left hepatic lobe on this MRI shows isointense signal on T2 weighted imaging with arterial hyperenhancement, slight hyperintensity on portal venous phase, and uptake of contrast on the hepatobiliary phase with a central scar. These characteristics are most compatible with focal nodular hyperplasia. Hemangiomas are T2 hyperintense and do not take up contrast on the hepatobiliary phase. Hepatic adenomas can resemble focal nodular hyperplasia (FNH) but do not typically show a central scar. Hepatocellular carcinoma usually demonstrates mildly hyperintense T2 signal with washout on the portal venous phase and will not take up contrast on the hepatobiliary phase unless well differentiated.

2. D. Unlike hepatic adenoma, FNH is not associated with oral contraceptive usage. FNH and adenoma both occur most frequently in young women and are arterially enhancing liver lesions. Although contrast uptake on the hepatobiliary phase is a classic feature of FNH, it can also be seen with inflammatory adenoma.

3. A, B, C. FNH may occur in association with hepatic hemangioma, arteriovenous malformation, and hereditary hemorrhagic telangiectasia. It is not known to be associated with fibrolamellar hepatocellular carcinoma.

4. B. FNH is often isodense on CT and isointense on MRI on the unenhanced, portal venous, and equilibrium phases but is characteristically hypervascular on the arterial phase.

Comment

- Focal nodular hyperplasia (FNH) is the second most common benign tumor of the liver after hemangiomas.
- FNH is a hyperplasia of normal, nonneoplastic liver tissue that has an abnormal arrangement and is similar to a hamartomatous type of lesion.
- It is believed to develop as some type of response to a congenital vascular abnormality in the region.
- Histologically, the liver tissue is arranged in small nodules, with septa in between.
- Arterial vessels feed the nodules from a centrally located artery that is often within a central scar or septum. They do not have a portal venous supply. FNH contains Kupffer cells in most instances.
- Adenomas and FNH are similar in that they both occur in young women, although FNH also occurs in children and older patients. Unlike adenomas, FNH is not associated with the use of oral contraceptives. This tumor is rarely found in men.
- FNH must be differentiated from other hepatic tumors, such as adenomas, fibrolamellar hepatomas, and giant hemangiomas. All of these tumors are large vascular tumors that affect young women and often have a central scar.
- Focal nodular hyperplasia is usually found incidentally on imaging but can present with right upper quadrant pain in some patients due to mass effect.
- FNH may be associated with several benign conditions, such as hemangiomas, hereditary hemorrhagic telangiectasia, and arteriovenous malformations.

- Imaging findings of focal nodular hyperplasia:
  - US: variable appearance; often isoechoic to background liver. If visualized, may show a central scar with displacement of peripheral vasculature on color Doppler. On contrast-enhanced ultrasound, FNH will demonstrate enhancement in the early arterial phase, centrifugal filling on the late arterial phase, and persistent enhancement on the portal venous phase.
  - CT: FNH demonstrates avid arterial enhancement and is typically isodense to background liver on unenhanced, portal venous, and equilibrium phases. When present, a central scar usually shows delayed enhancement.
  - MRI: "stealth lesion." May be slightly T1 hypointense and slightly T2 hyperintense but characteristically isointense to the liver on all pulse sequences other than the arterial phase and hepatobiliary phase (when imaged with hepatocyte-specific contrast agents). May be difficult to distinguish from inflammatory adenoma.
  - Nuclear medicine: Due to the presence of Kupffer cells, FNH may take up ^{99m}Tc sulfur colloid.

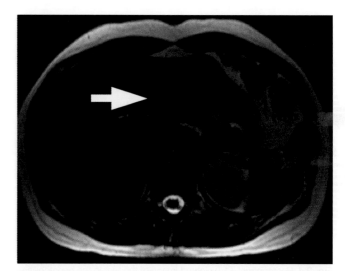

Fig. 2.1 T2 weighted magnetic resonance image without fat saturation demonstrating an isointense mass in the left hepatic lobe *(arrow)*.

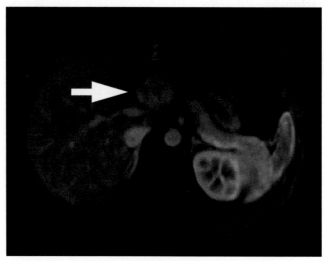

Fig. 2.2 Postcontrast T1 weighted image of the liver in the arterial phase shows a hypervascular mass in the left hepatic lobe *(arrow)*.

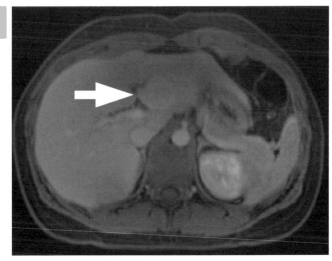

Fig. 2.3 Postcontrast T1 weighted image of the liver in the portal venous phase demonstrates slight residual hyperenhancement *(arrow)*.

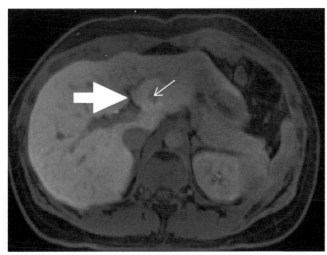

Fig. 2.4 Postcontrast T1-weighted image of the liver in the hepatobiliary phase at 20 minutes shows uptake of contrast in the mass *(large arrow)* with a nonenhancing central scar *(small arrow)*.

REFERENCES

Grazioli, L., Bondioni, M. P., Haradome, H., Motosugi, U., Tinti, R., … Frittoli, B. (2012). Hepatocellular adenoma and focal nodular hyperplasia: Value of gadoxetic acid-enhanced MR imaging in differential diagnosis. *Radiology, 262*(2), 520–529.

Hussain, S. M., Terkivatan, T., Zondervan, P. E., Lanjouw, E., de Rave, S., … Ijzermans, J. N. (2004). Focal nodular hyperplasia: Findings at state-of-the-art MR imaging, US, CT, and pathologic analysis. *Radiographics, 24*(1), 3–17.

McInnes, M. D., Hibbert, R. M., Inácio, J. R., & Schieda, N. (2015). Focal nodular hyperplasia and hepatocellular adenoma: Accuracy of gadoxetic acid-enhanced MR imaging—a systematic review. *Radiology, 277*(3), 927.

CASE 4

Hepatic Adenoma

1. A, B, C. Figures show an isointense mass in the left lobe of the liver with heterogenous enhancement on postcontrast images. This appearance can be seen in hepatic adenoma, hepatocellular

Case 3 is online only and accessible at www.expertconsult.com.

carcinoma, or focal nodular hyperplasia (FNH). This appearance is not seen in a typical hemangioma.
2. A, B. Oral contraceptive (OC) pills and obesity are recognized risk factors for development of hepatic adenomas.
3. B. Hepatic adenomas are relatively hyperintense to the liver on T1 weighted opposed phase images.
4. A, B, C, D. All of the responses are recognized treatment options for hepatic ademoma.

Comment

- Hepatic adenomas or hepatocellular adenomas are benign liver tumors with a predilection for hemorrhage.
- Hepatic adenomas are the most frequent tumors in young women on the oral contraceptive pill. Other situations in which they are found include:
  - Anabolic steroid use—typically in young men
  - Glycogen storage disease
  - Obesity
  - Metabolic syndrome
  - Diabetes mellitus
- Usually asymptomatic until they spontaneously rupture
- Usually solitary (70–80% cases) and large at the time of diagnosis (5–15 cm)
- Hepatic adenomatosis—when >10 in number
- Imaging appearance: usually round, well-defined pseudoencapsulated mass, occasional dystrophic calcification may be present; may appear heterogeneous due to hemorrhage, necrosis, fibrosis, and malignant transformation
  - US: homogeneous appearance, with somewhat variable echogenicity, which depends on the structural composition of the lesions as well as that of the surrounding liver
    - Color Doppler: may show perilesional sinusoids
    - Contrast-enhanced ultrasound: hypervascular in arterial phase with centripetal filling on portal venous and delayed phases
  - CT: HCA without complications are isodense with the surrounding liver on unenhanced CT, homogeneous blush of contrast enhancement on arterial phase and then fade to isodensity in the portal or delayed phase
  - MRI:
    - T1 weighted in-phase images: almost isointense or slightly hyperintense to the surrounding liver
    - T1 weighted opposed phase images: may become relatively hyperintense to the liver (due to decreased signal of the fatty liver) or hypointense as well as heterogeneous to the liver (due to decreased signal within the fatty lesion)
    - T2 fat suppressed images: slightly hyperintense or hypointense (depending mainly on whether the HCA is surrounded by fatty liver or the lesion itself contains abundant fat or fibrosis, respectively)
    - Postcontrast T1 weighted images: faint homogeneous enhancement (blush) in the arterial phase, and isointense in the delayed phase, without washout or capsular enhancement
    - Hepatocyte-specific postcontrast T1 weighted images: hypointense on hepatobiliary phase (20 minutes after injection)
- Complications:
  - Spontaneous rupture
  - Malignant transformation of HCA into hepatocellular carcinoma (HCC) has been described. Increase in size of the lesion at imaging, increased serum alpha-fetoprotein, and suspicious findings at fine-needle-aspiration biopsy are considered as signs of malignant transformation of HCA.
- Treatment:
  - Nonsurgical management with cessation of hormone therapy, serial radiologic examinations, and screening for

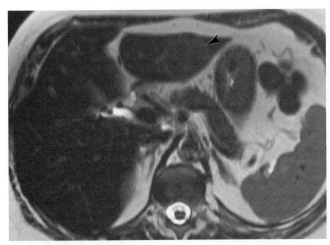

Fig. 4.1 Axial T2 weighted image from magnetic resonance imaging (MRI) shows a mildly hyperintense mass in the left lobe of the liver *(red arrow)*.

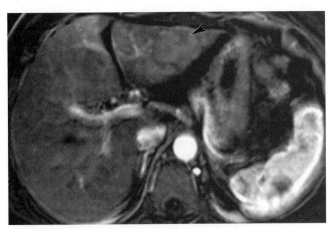

Fig. 4.2 Axial arterial phase postcontrast T1 weighted image from magnetic resonance imaging (MRI) shows mild hypervascularity within this mass *(red arrow)* in the left lobe of the liver.

elevated alpha-fetoprotein levels has been proposed for isolated small adenomas.

- Resection of adenomas can be considered due to the risk of rupture and hemorrhage.
- Hepatic arterial embolization can be effective for controlling acute hemorrhage in an adenoma.

REFERENCES

Grazioli, L., Federle, M. P., Brancatelli, G., Ichikawa, T., Olivetti, L., & Blachar, A. (2001). Hepatic adenomas: Imaging and pathologic findings. *Radiographics, 21,* 877–892; discussion 892–874.

Hussain, S. M., van den Bos, I. C., Dwarkasing, R. S., Kuiper, J. W., & den Hollander, J. (2006). Hepatocellular adenoma: findings at state-of-the-art magnetic resonance imaging, ultrasound, computed tomography and pathologic analysis. *European Radiology, 16,* 1873–1886.

CASE 5

Budd-Chiari

1. A, B, C. Cirrhosis, nutmeg liver, and carcinomatosis can give a heterogenous enhancement appearance on CT scan to the liver.

2. A. Chronic systemic venous congestion gives rise to the appearance of nutmeg liver, which is seen as in homogenous mottled appearance.

3. C. Caudate lobe enlargement in a patient with diffused mottled nutmeg liver on cross-sectional imaging suggests Budd-Chiari syndrome as the etiology.

4. A, B, C. A cyst would not have a hypervascular appearance on postcontrast imaging; however, metastasis, regenerative nodule, and hepatocellular carcinoma can appear hypervascular on postcontrast imaging.

Comment

- Consists of disorders causing hepatic venous obstruction either at the level of the hepatic veins (HV) or at the inferior vena cava (IVC) leading to an increase hepatic sinusoidal pressure and portal hypertension.
- Can occur at any age and is more common in women.
- Can be classified into acute form and chronic disease. Acute disease is commonly associated with the use of oral contraceptive pills, pregnancy, or underlying thrombotic disorder. Chronic disease is usually due to a membranous, fibrous obstruction of the IVC, HV, or both.
- Can also be classified into primary or secondary. Primary type is caused by HV of the obstruction originating from an endoluminal venous lesion such as a thrombus or membrane. Secondary form is caused by extrinsic compression or occlusion of the lumen due to material not originating from the venous system like malignant mass.
- Imaging findings: variable and depend on the stage of the disease
  - US: ascites, splenomegaly, and narrowing and lack of visualization or thrombosis of the hepatic veins. Color Doppler shows absent or monophasic flow in the hepatic veins; reverse flow in the hepatic veins, IVC, or both; and intrahepatic collateral pathways. Signs of portal hypertension are also seen.
  - CT:
    - In acute Budd-Chiari syndrome, morphologic features of the liver usually are normal, and occlusion of the hepatic veins with severe ascites is seen. The liver shows patchy decreased peripheral enhancement caused by portal and sinusoidal stasis and stronger enhancement of the central portion of the liver parenchyma. An inhomogenous mottled appearance contrasts the nutmeg liver. The thrombosed hepatic veins are hyperattenuating, and the IVC is compressed by the enlarged lobe. Ascites and splenomegaly are usually present.
    - Subacute or chronic syndrome: portosystemic and intrahepatic collateral vessels are often found. Contrast-enhanced CT shows regions of hypoperfusion liver parenchyma. Portal vein thrombosis can develop as a result of underlying thrombophilia and stagnation of portal flow caused by outflow block. Large intrahepatic collateral vessels can be seen.
    - Chronic syndrome multiple regenerative nodules are seen in addition to the other findings described earlier.
  - MRI:
    - T2 weighted images show heterogeneously increased signal intensity in the peripheral portion of the liver.
    - T2 weighted gradient recalled sequences show absence of flow in the hepatic veins and inferior vena cava.
    - T1 weighted sequences postcontrast administration show occlusion of the hepatic veins, IVC, or both.
    - Regenerative nodules are seen on the chronic phase, which are bright on T1 weighted MR images and strongly hypervascular after IV administration of

gadolinium contrast media. These regenerative nodules are isointense to hypointense relative to the liver on T2 weighted images.

- Treatment: therapeutic approach to Budd-Chiari syndrome is adapted to the disease severity. Surgical shunt (portocaval, mesocaval, or mesoatrial) can be created. Other treatments include placement of metallic stands in the IVC or hepatic vein, transjugular portosystemic shunt, and liver transplantation.

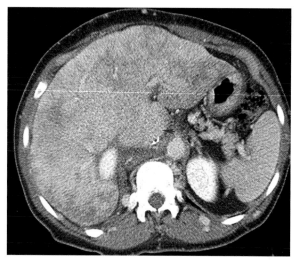

Fig. 5.1 Axial postcontrast computed tomography (CT) image showing an in-homogenous mottled appearance of the liver suggestive of nutmeg liver. Note enlargement of the caudate lobe *(red arrow)* and nonvisualization of the hepatic veins suggesting Budd-Chiari syndrome.

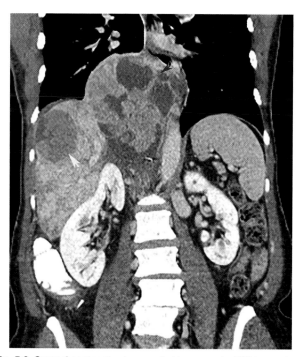

Fig. 5.2 Coronal postcontrast computed tomography (CT) image in the same patient. The inferior vena cava (IVC) was obstructed by large adrenocortical carcinoma *(red arrow)* arising from the right adrenal gland causing Budd-Chiari syndrome. Note metastasis in the right lobe of the liver *(yellow arrow)*.

REFERENCES

Brancatelli, G., Vilgrain, V., Federle, M. P., Hakime, A., Lagalla, R., ... Iannaccone, R. (2007). Budd-Chiari syndrome: Spectrum of imaging findings. *AJR. American Journal of Roentgenology, 188*(2), W168–W176. doi:10.2214/AJR.05.0168.

Mukund, A., & Gamanagatti, S. (2011). Imaging and interventions in Budd-Chiari syndrome. *World Journal of Radiology, 3*(7), 169–177. doi:10.4329/wjr.v3.i7.169.

CASE 7

Gallbladder Perforation

1. A, B, C. Figures shown could suggest hepatic abscess, gallbladder perforation, or hepatic cyst as an etiology.
2. C. Cholesterol pseudopolyps are the commonest polypoid lesion seen in the gallbladder accounting for 60% to 70% of lesions in some studies.
3. C. "Sonographic-hole" sign is the direct visualization of the gallbladder wall defect on ultrasound.
4. A, B, C, D. Complications from gallbladder perforation include bile leak and peritonitis, abscesses around the gallbladder fossa, intraperitoneal or intrahepatic abscess formation, intraperitoneal air, sepsis or septic shock, fistulae, and bowel obstruction.

Comment

- Background: uncommon and potentially life-threatening condition most commonly seen as a complication of acute cholecystitis
  - Incidence has dropped from between 2% and 15% to 0.8% and 3.2%.
  - May develop as early as 2 days after the onset of acute cholecystitis or up to several weeks later.
  - Typically seen in the setting of diseases such as cholecystitis, malignancy and corticosteroid use, and vascular compromise.
  - Medical diseases such as diabetes mellitus and atherosclerotic heart disease are also thought to be contributory.
  - Transcatheter arterial chemoembolization (TACE) or transcatheter arterial radio embolization (TARE) can lead to acute ischemic cholecystitis or radiation-induced cholecystitis and progress to perforation.
  - Gallbladder perforation can be seen in 2% of patients with blunt abdominal trauma.
- Clinical manifestations: clinical differentiation from uncomplicated acute cholecystitis is often difficult, leading to a delay in diagnosis, higher incidence of complications, and poor outcomes.
  - Should be suspected in patients who become toxic or have sudden clinical deterioration for unexplained reasons.
  - Complications from gallbladder perforation include bile leak and peritonitis, abscesses around the gallbladder fossa, intraperitoneal or intrahepatic abscess formation, intraperitoneal air, sepsis or septic shock, fistulae, and bowel obstruction.
  - Mortality rate as high as 42% has been reported.
- Classification: Neimeier in 1934 proposal classification for gallbladder perforation as follows:
  - Type I: acute free perforation of the gallbladder into the peritoneal cavity without protective adhesions
  - Type II: subacute perforation surrounded by a pericholecystic abscess walled off by adhesions
  - Type III: chronic perforation with presence of communication between the gallbladder and a viscus
- Imaging:
  - US: usually the initial method of investigation in patients with suspected acute cholecystitis. A very specific sign of

---

Case 6 is online only and accessible at www.expertconsult.com.

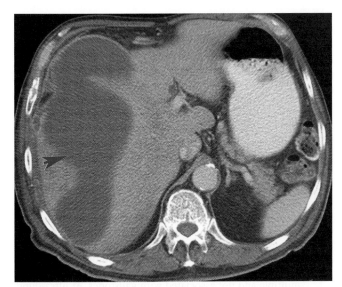

Fig. 7.1 Axial post contrast computed tomography image shows a large lobulated fluid collection in the right lobe of the liver *(red arrow)* with the gallbladder seen anteriorly with communication between the gallbladder and the fluid collection.

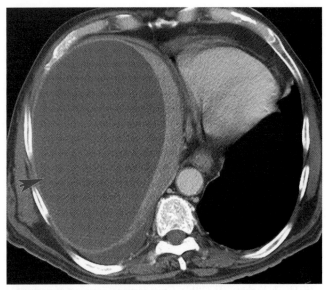

Fig. 7.3 Axial post contrast computed tomography image shows a large lobulated fluid collection in the right lobe of the liver *(red arrow)*.

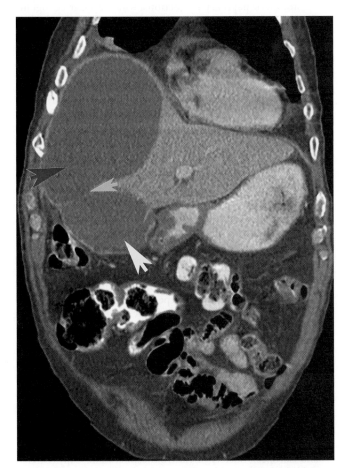

Fig. 7.2 Coronal post contrast image shows a large fluid collection in the right lobe of the liver *(red arrow)* with communication *(green arrow)* seen between this fluid collection and the gallbladder seen inferiorly *(yellow arrow)*.

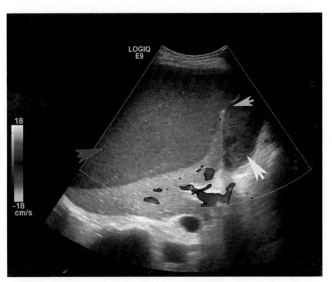

Fig. 7.4 Ultrasound image shows the large fluid collection in the right lobe of the liver *(red arrow)* with the gallbladder seen filled with sludge *(yellow arrow)* and a communication *(green arrow)* between the gallbladder and the fluid collection in the liver consistent with gallbladder perforation.

gallbladder perforation that can be seen on ultrasound is the "sonographic-hole" sign, which is the direct visualization of the gallbladder wall defect.

- CT: interruption of the gallbladder wall and extraluminal radiopaque gallstones can be seen along with mesenteric or omental fat streaking.
  - Subacute gallbladder perforations are usually contained by a pericholecystic abscess, which is seen as complex echogenic pericholecystic fluid collections in the presence of a thickened hypoechoic edematous gallbladder wall and cholelithiasis.
  - In chronic perforations there is formation of cholecysto-enteric fistula secondary to chronic inflammation of the gallbladder and its proximity to the intestine. Air can then pass from the intestine into the gallbladder and biliary tree, causing pneumobilia, and gallstones can pass through to the bowel, causing obstruction (gallstone ileus).

- MRI:
  - On contrast-enhanced T1 weighted MR images, pericholecystic or intrahepatic abscesses appear as fluid collections with rim enhancement.
- For traumatic gallbladder (GB) rupture, imaging findings on CT and MR include a collapsed GB despite prolonged fast (which would distend the GB); disruption of the GB wall; intraluminal hemorrhage (hemobilia); complex pericholecystic fluid collections; omental or mesenteric fat streaking; and thickened and edematous GB wall.
- Management: gallbladder perforation is initially treated by percutaneous cholecystostomy, and patients typically require intravenous antibiotics, volume resuscitation, and close monitoring with eventual cholecystectomy.

REFERENCES

Morris, B. S., Balpande, P. R., Morani, A. C., Chaudhary, R. K., Maheshwari, M., & Raut, A. A. (2007). The CT appearances of gallbladder perforation. *The British Journal of Radiology*, 80(959), 898–901. doi:10.1259/bjr/28510614.

Seyal, A. R., Parekh, K., Gonzalez-Guindalini, F. D., Nikolaidis, P., Miller, F. H., & Yaghmai, V. (2014). Cross-sectional imaging of perforated gallbladder. *Abdominal Imaging*, 39(4), 853–874. doi:10.1007/s00261-014-0121-1.

CASE 9

Gallbladder Polyp

1. A, B. Small polyps can be seen as echogenic lesions within the gallbladder lumen without shadowing, and adherent calculi in large patients can be seen as similar lesions as well.
2. C. Cholesterol pseudopolyps are the commonest polypoid lesion seen in the gallbladder, accounting for 60% to 70% of lesions in some studies.
3. C, D. Patients with primary sclerosing cholangitis (PSC) and females with Indian ethnicity have a higher incidence of gallbladder carcinoma. In patients with PSC, a substantial number (60%) of gallbladder polyps are malignant.
4. D. In most guidelines, cholecystectomy is recommended for gallbladder polyps >10 mm in size.

Comment

- Background: gallbladder polyp is an elevation of the gallbladder mucosa that protrudes into the gallbladder lumen.
  - Estimated prevalence is approximately 5% of the global population, but only 5% of these are considered to be true gallbladder polyps.
  - Commonly detected on ultrasound scans of the abdomen and incidental findings, a small number of patients with gallbladder polyps may be symptomatic and present with acute cholecystitis due to polyp obstructing the cystic duct or cholangitis due to fragments of the polyp breaking off and traveling down into the bile duct.
- Imaging: ultrasound is the best imaging choice and is often able to separate cholesterol polyps from those requiring treatment. Computed tomography (CT), positron emission tomography (PET)/CT, and magnetic resonance imaging (MRI) may also depict large polypoid lesions within the gallbladder, with MRI having the best sensitivity for depiction of vascular and bile duct invasion.
  - General features of gallbladder polyps include:
    - Small size
      - Cholesterol polyps are the most frequent; >90% are <10 mm and most of these are <5 mm in size.
      - Adenomas or malignant lesions tend to be larger.

Case 8 is online only and accessible at www.expertconsult.com.

- Echogenicity varies with size:
  - Small polyps are echogenic but nonshadowing
  - Larger cholesterol polyps tend to be hypoechoic
- Morphology
  - Small polyps may be adherent to the wall and smooth
  - Larger lesions tend to be regulated and in outline
- Mimics of gallbladder polyps: adherent gallstones and gallbladder sludge may be immobile and mimic true gallbladder polyps.
- Classification of gallbladder polyps: gallbladder polyps can be divided into pseudopolyps and true gallbladder polyps.
  - Pseudopolyps are more common than true polyps and include hyperplastic noninflammatory conditions such as cholesterol pseudopolyps and adenomyosis and inflammatory pseudopolyps. They do not have malignant potential.
  - Cholesterol polyps: cholesterol pseudopolyps are the commonest polypoid lesion seen in the gallbladder, accounting for 60% to 70% of lesions in some studies. It predominantly occurs in middle-aged women. They are typically multiple and not associated with gallstones. At ultrasound, cholesterol polyps appear as small round, smoothly contoured, intraluminal lesions that are attached to the wall. The stock is readily seen, and appearance gives rise to the "ball on the wall" sign.
  - Adenomyomatosis: accounts for ~25% of all polypoid lesions in the gallbladder. On ultrasound imaging, the diverticula seen in adenomyomatosis contains sludge, stones, or papillary projections, which appear echogenic with multiple acoustic interfaces creating twinkling artifact.
  - Inflammatory polyps: are present in 10% of all gallbladder polyps and are usually multiple and small, measuring <10 mm in diameter. They typically occur secondary to gallstones and chronic inflammation and start to be due to mucosal irritation, which leads to formation of granulation and fibrous tissue. On ultrasound they appear to be isoechoic or hypoechoic with a nonspecific appearance.
- True gallbladder polyps can be benign or malignant; benign polyps are most commonly adenomas while malignant polyps are usually adenocarcinomas. Other rare types include mesenchymal tumors, lymphomas, and metastasis.
  - Gallbladder adenomas are rare occurring in 0.15% of cholecystectomy specimens and accounting for 47% of all gallbladder polyps. The most frequently seen in patients with primary sclerosing cholangitis (PSC) and gastrointestinal polyposis syndromes such as Puetz-Jegher and Gardner syndromes.
    - On ultrasound imaging, gallbladder adenomas may vary in size, have a sessile or pedunculated appearance, demonstrate internal vascularity at color Doppler, and are typically solitary.
    - At CT and MR imaging, gallbladder adenomas typically demonstrate enhancement similar to that of adenocarcinoma. Adenomas cannot be reliably differentiated from polypoid gallbladder carcinoma at imaging.
- Management: in 2017 joint guidelines between the European Society of Gastrointestinal and Abdominal Radiology (ESGAR), European Association for Endoscopic Surgery and Other Interventional Techniques (EAES), International Society of Digestive Surgery—European Federation (EFISDS), and European Society of Gastrointestinal Endoscopy (ESGE) published and provided the most up-to-date and comprehensive guidance.
  - According to these guidelines:
    - Polyp >10 mm has an increased risk of malignancy, and cholecystectomy is recommended.

- Polyp <10 mm:
  - Symptoms attribute it to gallbladder: cholecystectomy suggested if no other cause for the symptoms is determined
  - If the patient has risk factors for gallbladder malignancy, which include >50 years of age, primary sclerosing cholangitis, Indian ethnicity, sessile polyp (including focal wall thickening >4 mm)
- Polyp <6 mm:
  - Follow-up ultrasound at 6 months, then yearly for 5 years
  - An increase in size ≥2 mm: consider cholecystectomy
- Polyp >6 mm: consider cholecystectomy
- No risk factors for gallbladder malignancy:
  - Polyp <6 mm: follow-up ultrasound at 1, 3, and 5 years
  - Polyp >6 mm:
    - Follow-up ultrasound at 6 months, then yearly for 5 years
    - An increase in size ≥2 mm: consider cholecystectomy

REFERENCES

McCain, R. S., Diamond, A., Jones, C., & Coleman, H. G. (2018). Current practices and future prospects for the management of gallbladder polyps: A topical review. *World Journal of Gastroenterology*, *24*, 2844–2852.

Mellnick, V. M., Menias, C. O., Sandrasegaran, K., Hara, A. M., Kielar, A. Z., … Brunt, E. M. (2015). Polypoid lesions of the gallbladder: Disease spectrum with pathologic correlation—erratum. *Radiographics*, *35*, 1316.

CASE 10
Acute Pancreatitis

1. A, B, C, D. Alcohol and gallstones are the two most common causes of acute pancreatitis (AP). Several other etiologies may cause AP, including endoscopic retrograde cholangiopancreatography (ERCP), trauma, medications, penetrating peptic ulcer, hypertriglyceridemia, and scorpion bite. Although controversial, pancreas divisum is also considered a cause of recurrent acute pancreatitis.

2. C. Four weeks is the time cutoff for naming fluid collections either acute peripancreatic fluid collection (<4 weeks) or pseudocyst (>4 weeks) in the setting of acute edematous interstitial pancreatitis and either acute necrotizing collection (<4 weeks) or walled-off necrosis (>4 weeks) in the setting of necrotizing pancreatitis.

3. B. The pancreas is usually poorly visualized on ultrasound due to suboptimal acoustic windows. Pancreatic edema, necrosis, or calcifications related to underlying chronic pancreatitis may be encountered but are not primarily evaluated by ultrasound. The main role of ultrasound is to identify gallstones as the potential cause of acute pancreatitis. Biliary dilation should be described if present.

4. A. Elevation of lipase (or amylase) more than three times the upper limit of normal is a major criterion for establishing a diagnosis of acute pancreatitis. Bilirubin, international normalized ratio (INR), and aspartate aminotransferase (AST) are markers of hepatic function.

Comment

- Acute pancreatitis (AP) is a relatively common inflammatory condition in which, for various reasons, autodigestion of the gland occurs, resulting in pancreatic and peripancreatic edema.
- Acute pancreatitis is diagnosed by meeting two of three criteria:
  - Acute onset of severe persistent epigastric pain
  - Lipase/amylase elevation more than three times the upper limit of normal
  - Characteristic imaging features on computed tomography (CT), magnetic resonance imaging (MRI), or ultrasound
- Imaging is only necessary if the first two criteria are not fulfilled. Ideally, imaging should not be performed until at least 48 to 72 hours after onset of symptoms, to detect complications and guide management.
- In addition to epigastric pain, sometimes radiating to the back, nausea, tachycardia, tachypnea, and often fever are common symptoms of acute pancreatitis. Occasionally the patient may be hypotensive, especially in severe hemorrhagic pancreatitis. Commonly taught but rarely seen physical exam findings of hemorrhagic AP include the Cullen sign (periumbilic bruising) and the Grey-Turner sign (flank bruising).
- The most common causes of acute pancreatitis are alcohol abuse and gallstones. However, other causes include endoscopic retrograde cholangiopancreatography (ERCP), trauma, certain medications, penetrating peptic ulcers, and pancreatic divisum.
- Complications related to the biliary and vascular system may occur. Inflammation involving the pancreatic head can result in narrowing of the distal common bile duct with upstream

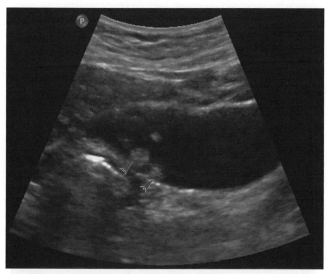

Fig. 9.1 Sagittal B-mode ultrasound image showing multiple soft tissue nodular masses *(red arrows)* in the gallbladder lumen consistent with gallbladder polyps.

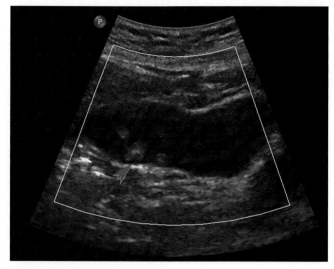

Fig. 9.2 Sagittal power Doppler ultrasound image showing minimal vascularity within the largest gallbladder polyp *(red arrow)*.

dilation. Splenic artery or gastroduodenal artery pseudoaneurysms can occur as a result of inflammation and enzymatic activity weakening a point in the artery wall. Although this complication is unusual, it constitutes a danger to the patient of sudden life-threatening bleeding.

- There are two major types of acute pancreatitis as defined by the 2012 Revised Atlanta Classification:
  - Interstitial edematous pancreatitis (90–95% of AP cases)
  - Necrotizing pancreatitis
- Pancreatitis fluid collections are defined by the type of AP and length of symptom duration:
  - Interstitial edematous pancreatitis
    - Acute peripancreatic fluid collection (APFC) <4 weeks
    - Pseudocysts >4 weeks
  - Necrotizing pancreatitis
    - Acute necrotic collection (ANC) <4 weeks
    - Walled-off necrosis (WON) after weeks
- The role of imaging in AP is to clarify the diagnosis in the setting of a confusing clinical presentation, assess severity of disease, identify complications, and detect potential causes.
- Imaging findings of acute pancreatitis:
  - US: the main role of ultrasound in imaging AP is to identify cholelithiasis as a potential cause and assess for any potential vascular complications. The pancreas is normally very difficult to adequately characterize sonographically due to poor acoustic windows. If the pancreas is visible in the setting of AP, it usually demonstrates gland enlargement with loss of parenchymal echogenicity.
  - CT: the CT appearance of AP is variable depending on the severity of disease and potential associated complications. The gland may be focally or diffusely enlarged with variable attenuation. Edema can be difficult to distinguish from necrosis, particularly in the first 24 to 48 hours of disease onset. There is often peripancreatic fat stranding. Hemorrhage may be present. CT offers high spatial resolution to detect vascular complications such as venous thrombosis or mesenteric arterial pseudoaneurysm.
  - MRI: is not typically used as a first-line tool for assessing AP. It can be used to characterize underlying etiologies such as choledocholithiasis and chronic pancreatitis. It may help guide endoscopic planning in some cases.

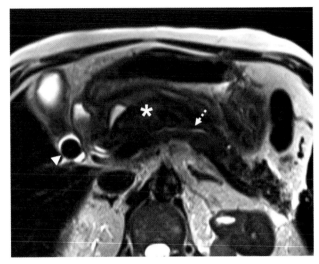

Fig. 10.2 Axial T2 weighted image demonstrates T2 hypointense signal in the expanded pancreatic neck and body *(asterisk);* the main pancreatic duct is nondilated *(dashed arrow).* A gallstone is shown in the gallbladder neck *(arrowhead).*

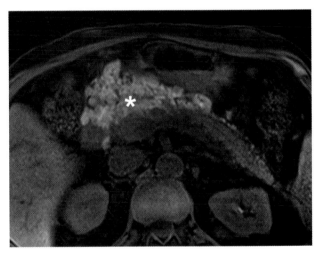

Fig. 10.3 Axial T1 fat-saturated image demonstrates T1 hyperintense signal at the pancreatic neck and body *(asterisk),* indicating hemorrhagic pancreatitis.

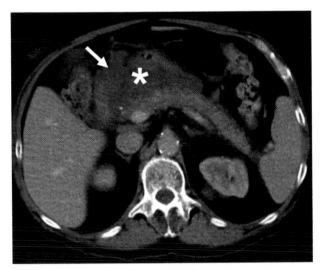

Fig. 10.1 Axial computed tomography (CT) image demonstrates hypoenhancing, expanded contour of the pancreatic head and neck *(asterisk),* with peripancreatic inflammatory fat stranding *(straight arrow).*

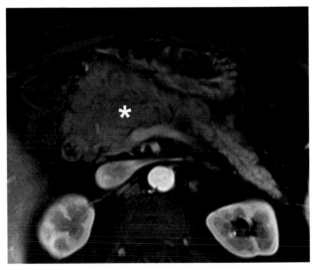

Fig. 10.4 Axial T1 fat-saturated postcontrast image redemonstrates the area of hemorrhagic pancreatitis as seen in Fig. 10.3.

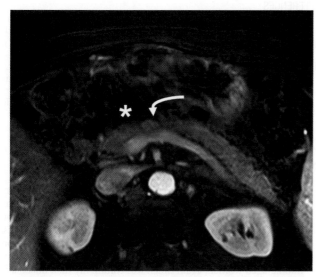

Fig. 10.5 At the pancreatic neck/body junction, subtraction postcontrast image showing focal nonenhancement of the pancreas *(curved arrow)*, representing necrotizing pancreatitis.

REFERENCES

Foster, B. R., Jensen, K. K., Bakis, G., Shaaban, A. M., & Coakley, F. V. (2016). Revised Atlanta classification for acute pancreatitis: A pictorial essay. *Radiographics, 36*(3), 675–687.

Thoeni, R. F. (2012). The revised Atlanta classification of acute pancreatitis: Its importance for the radiologist and its effect on treatment. *Radiology, 262*(3), 751–764.

CASE 11

Chronic Pancreatitis

1. D. Although alcohol is the most common cause of chronic pancreatitis in developed countries, malnutrition is overall the most common cause worldwide. Gallstones and hypertriglyceridemia are common causes of acute pancreatitis.

2. D. Magnetic resonance imaging (MRI) offers the best evaluation for parenchymal and ductal changes of chronic pancreatitis, particularly after the administration of secretin. MRI offers characterization of both early and late imaging manifestations. Computed tomography (CT) better demonstrates parenchymal and intraductal calcifications and can show complications of chronic pancreatitis, such as pseudocysts, pseudoaneurysm, and mesenteric venous thrombosis. Ultrasound and fluoroscopy can identify secondary complications of chronic pancreatitis, such as biliary obstruction and duodenal narrowing, but are not first-line imaging modalities for chronic pancreatitis.

3. D. Intraductal stones are the most specific finding for diagnosis of chronic pancreatitis. Pancreatic atrophy is nonspecific and can be seen in the normal process of aging. Pancreatic enlargement can be seen in the early stage of autoimmune pancreatitis ("sausage pancreas"). Main duct dilation can be seen in a number of settings, including ductal adenocarcinoma and main duct intraductal papillary mucinous neoplasm.

4. B. Delayed progressive enhancement is a characteristic pattern of fibrosis, which is seen in the pancreatic parenchyma in patients with chronic pancreatitis. Inflammation, acinar atrophy, and ductal sclerosis are all histologic findings of chronic pancreatitis but are not specifically characterized on postcontrast imaging.

Comment

- Chronic pancreatitis is a chronic inflammatory condition resulting in progressive, irreversible structural damage to the pancreas.
- It has a variable natural course with no specific treatment or preventive measures. Pancreatic enzyme replacement therapy can be considered in the setting of malabsorption.
- The most common cause of chronic pancreatitis in developed countries is alcohol, but worldwide it is malnutrition.
- Diagnosis of chronic pancreatitis is based on clinical history, exocrine function testing, and cross-sectional imaging.
- Clinical manifestations include abdominal pain, acute pancreatitis, exocrine and/or endocrine insufficiency, and pancreatic cancer. There is thought that patients with chronic pancreatitis are also at increased risk for developing type II diabetes mellitus.
- The pathologic manifestations of chronic pancreatitis include damage to the acinar cells, main pancreatic duct, and side branches resulting in acinar cell atrophy and fibrosis/sclerosis of the parenchyma and duct. This, in turn, results in pancreatic ductal dilation with possible stricture and intraductal stones.
- Imaging findings of chronic pancreatitis:
  - US: The pancreas may appear atrophic, potentially with parenchymal calcifications. The parenchyma may be hyperechoic due to underlying fibrosis. Pseudocysts and/or pseudoaneurysms may be present.
  - CT: The hallmark of chronic pancreatitis on CT is the presence of parenchymal calcifications, either punctate (<3 mm) or coarse (≥3 mm). Intraductal calcifications are the most specific finding of chronic pancreatitis. Calcifications are usually seen with alcohol-related chronic pancreatitis, but not other causes. The pancreas may demonstrate atrophy and abnormal shape or contour. Ductal dilation is a characteristic finding.
  - MRI: Chronic pancreatitis can be characterized by early and late stages on MRI. Early findings include loss of normal hyperintense signal of fat-saturated T1 weighted images, decreased and delayed enhancement on dynamic contrast-enhanced imaging, and dilated side branches. Late findings include parenchymal atrophy or enlargement and irregular dilation of the main pancreatic duct with chain-of-lakes appearance due to side branch ectasia. Intraductal calcifications may be present. Functional assessment of the pancreas can also be performed by administration of secretin, which evaluates the exocrine function of the pancreas.

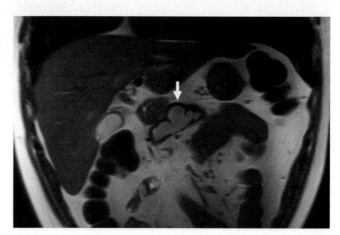

Fig. 11.1 Coronal T2 weighted image showing cystic dilatation of the main pancreatic duct *(arrow)*.

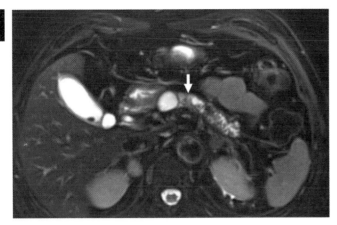

Fig. 11.2 Axial T2 weighted fat-suppressed image redemonstrates cystic dilatation of the main pancreatic duct *(arrow)*.

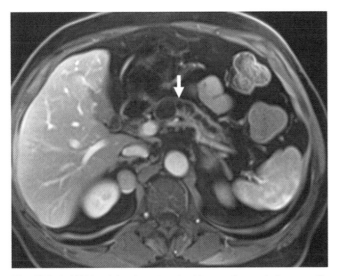

Fig. 11.3 Axial T1 weighted postcontrast image demonstrates smooth enhancement of the duct *(arrow)*.

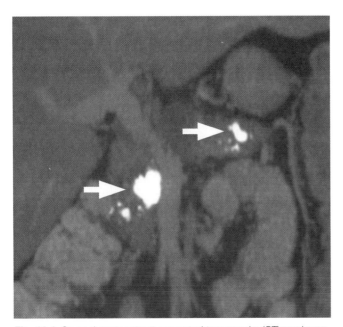

Fig. 11.4 Coronal postcontrast computed tomography (CT) maximum intensity projection (MIP) image shows coarse calcifications of the pancreatic head and tail *(arrows)*, indicating chronic pancreatitis.

REFERENCES

Hansen, T. M., Nilsson, M., Gram, M., & Frøkjær, J. B. (2013). Morphological and functional evalution of chronic pancreatitis with magnetic resonance imaging. *World Journal of Gastroenterology, 19*(42), 7241–7246.

Tirkes, T., Shah, Z. K., Takahashi, N., Grajo, J. R., Chang, S. T., ... Venkatesh, S. K. (2019). Reporting standards for chronic pancreatitis by using CT, MRI, and MR cholangiopancreatography: The consortium for the study of chronic pancreatitis, diabetes, and pancreatic cancer. *Radiology, 290*(1), 207–215.

CASE 12

Pancreatic Cancer

1. B. Pancreatic ductal adenocarcinoma accounts for the vast majority of pancreatic neoplasms. It is characterized by a low attenuation mass with desmoplastic reaction and abrupt cutoff of the upstream main pancreatic duct. It portends a very poor prognosis. Neuroendocrine tumor of the pancreas is much less common than ductal adenocarcinoma. Mucinous cystic neoplasm occurs in middle-aged women, again much less commonly than ductal adenocarcinoma. Metastatic disease to the pancreas can occur but is much less common than primary pancreatic neoplasms.

2. A, B, C, D. A family history of pancreatic cancer, cigarette smoking, chronic pancreatitis, and obesity are all risk factors for the development of pancreatic ductal adenocarcinoma. Pancreatic intraepithelial neoplasia, intraductal papillary mucinous neoplasm, and mucinous cystic neoplasm represent precursor lesions for pancreatic cancer development.

3. A. Abdominal pain is the most common presentation of pancreatic ductal adenocarcinoma. Painless jaundice can also occur, but pain is a prevailing symptom in most instances. Early satiety and weight loss are common. Endocrine and/or exocrine disorder of the pancreas may also manifest, particularly in the background of chronic pancreatitis or development of new diabetes mellitus.

4. B. Computed tomography (CT) is the workhorse modality for local and distant staging of pancreatic ductal adenocarcinoma. It offers the highest spatial resolution for evaluating anatomic relationship to the critical mesenteric vessels and offers evaluation for distant spread (i.e., to the lungs and peritoneal cavity). Magnetic resonance imaging (MRI) is utilized by some institutions as the primary staging modality for pancreatic cancer. Ultrasound may be the first modality utilized in the identification of pancreatic cancer but does not allow for adequate staging. Positron emission tomography (PET) scan may be used as a problem-solving tool when evaluating for recurrent disease.

Comment

- Pancreatic cancer comprises approximately 20% to 25% of all deaths related to gastrointestinal malignancy.
- Pancreatic ductal adenocarcinoma (PDAC) accounts for the overwhelming majority of all pancreatic neoplasms (~90%). PDAC is a very aggressive cancer resulting in poor prognosis and high morbidity. Despite representing only the 12th most common type of cancer in the United States, PDAC is the 4th most common cause of cancer-related death.
- Ductal adenocarcinoma is primarily a disease that afflicts the elderly, mostly after the age of 60 years.
- Risk factors for the development of PDAC include smoking, chronic pancreatitis, obesity, family history, a diet rich in animal fats and protein, and certain hereditary syndromes (i.e., hereditary nonpolyposis colorectal cancer [HNPCC]).
- Despite the classic teaching of patient presentation with "painless jaundice," abdominal pain is the most common presentation of patients with pancreatic ductal adenocarcinoma. Patients frequently exhibit weight loss. Other classic presentations may include new-onset diabetes mellitus, Courvoisier gallbladder (painless jaundice with marked gallbladder distention), and Trousseau syndrome (migratory thrombophlebitis).

- PDAC arises from pancreatic ductal epithelium. Pancreatic intraepithelial neoplasia, intraductal papillary mucinous neoplasm (IPMN, particularly main duct IPMN), and mucinous cystic neoplasm (MCN) have been identified as precursor lesions for pancreatic carcinoma.
- PDAC most commonly arises in the head or uncinate process of the pancreas, with up to one-third occurring in the body or tail.
- The only cure for PDAC is complete surgical excision (either via Whipple procedure or distal pancreatectomy). However, most patients are unresectable at the time of presentation. Furthermore, most patients who undergo complete excision will experience recurrence with a grim prognosis.
- Imaging findings of pancreatic cancer:
  - US: Nonspecific findings. May demonstrate hypoechoic mass with ductal dilation (i.e., double duct sign).
  - CT: Mainstay modality for pancreatic cancer characterization and staging. Multiphase imaging should include pancreatic phase and portal venous phase to allow for adequate staging. PDAC is usually hypodense with a lower degree of enhancement than normal pancreatic parenchyma and surrounding desmoplastic reaction. Abrupt cutoff of the main

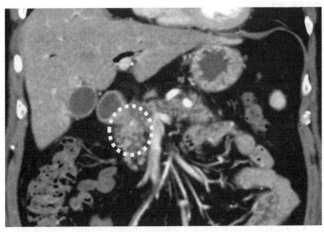

Fig. 12.3 Coronal contrast-enhanced CT image shows an enhancing mass in the pancreatic head *(dashed circle)*.

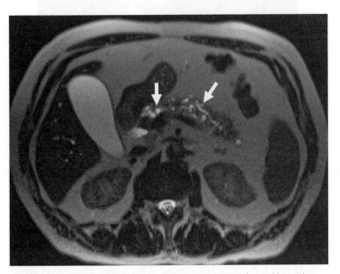

Fig. 12.1 Axial T2 weighted image demonstrates main and branch pancreatic ductal dilatation *(arrows)*.

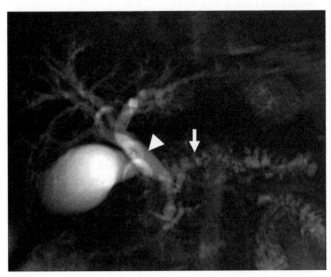

Fig. 12.2 Two-dimensional T2 weighted MRCP image demonstrates intrahepatic and extrahepatic biliary ductal dilatation *(arrowhead)*, in addition to pancreatic ductal dilatation *(arrow)*.

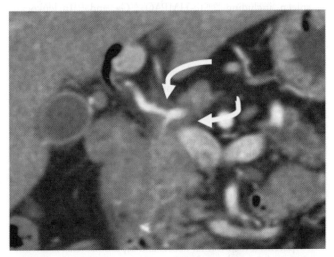

Fig. 12.4 Coronal contrast-enhanced CT image shows hypoenhancing soft tissue encasing the common hepatic artery *(curved arrows)*, indicating perivascular involvement by pancreatic adenocarcinoma.

pancreatic duct upstream from the tumor +/− parenchymal atrophy is a hallmark finding. Staging assessment should include description of the tumor's relationship to the superior mesenteric artery (SMA), superior mesenteric vein (SMV), portal vein, celiac axis, and hepatic artery as well as discussion of potential distant metastatic disease (e.g., liver, lung, omentum).
- MRI: Ideal for detection of subtle pancreatic mass that may be occult on CT. Used by some institutions as primary modality for local PDAC staging. Ideal for characterization of the pancreatic duct.

REFERENCES

Bowman, A. W., & Bolan, C. W. (2019). MRI evaluation of pancreatic ductal adenocarcinoma: Diagnosis, mimics, and staging. *Abdominal Radiology (New York), 44*(3), 936–949.

Lu, D. S., Reber, H. A., Krasny, R. N., Kadell, B. M., & Sayre. J. (1997). Local staging of pancreatic cancer: criteria for unresectability of major vessels as revealed by pancreatic-phase, thin-section helical CT. *AJR. American Journal of Roentgenology, 168*(6), 1439–1443.

Morgan, D. E., Waggoner, C. N., Canon, C. L., Lockhart, M. E., Fineberg, N. S., ... Posey, J. A. (2010). Resectability of pancreatic adenocarcinoma in patients with locally advanced disease downstaged by preoperative therapy: A challenge for MDCT. *AJR. American Journal of Roentgenology, 194*(3), 615–622.

CASE 13

Splenic Abscess

1. A. Immunosuppression has led to an increase in the incidence of splenic abscess. This most commonly occurs in the setting of chemotherapy use, longer survival of patients with leukemia and acquired immunodeficiency syndrome (AIDS), and following organ transplant. Hematologic or direct extension of infection can also cause splenic abscess. Sequelae of trauma or infarct are also culprits.
2. D. Air is uncommonly seen in splenic abscess, either on ultrasound or computed tomography (CT). However, it is pathognomonic when present. Peripheral enhancement is a later sign of infection that can occur once a capsule forms in the inflammation process. Low attenuation and internal septations are both nonspecific.
3. C. Fungal infections are usually multifocal and smaller than pyogenic abscesses (<2 cm). They typically do not demonstrate peripheral enhancement on CT or magnetic resonance imaging (MRI). Candidiasis is a common infecting organism.
4. A. Several nuclear medicine agents can be used to image the spleen, including ^{99m}Tc-HMPAO, ^{67}Ga, and ^{111}In leukocyte scans. Lymphoma is gallium positive and therefore cannot differentiate splenic abscess.

Comment

- Splenic abscess most commonly occurs in the setting of immunosuppression (i.e., chemotherapy, leukemia, AIDS, transplant).
- It can also occur in general states of sepsis, direct extension of infection (e.g., pancreatitis), as a result of trauma or infarct, or septic emboli from endocarditis.
- Splenic abscess is uncommon and typically presents with nonspecific symptoms, such as fever, rigors/chills, and vomiting.
- Left upper tenderness may be present. It is usually caused by an opportunistic bacterial, viral, or parasitic infection.
- Imaging findings of splenic abscess:
  - US: variable appearance, hypoechoic to hyperechoic with potential for internal debris and septations. Gas is uncommon but can be seen.
  - CT: most common imaging modality. Low-attenuation splenic lesion that can demonstrate peripheral enhancement (capsule). Can be nonspecific as many other splenic

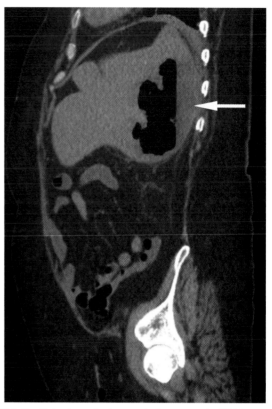

Fig. 13.2 Sagittal reformatted computed tomography (CT) image of the same patient confirming intrasplenic location of the abscess.

lesions have similar low attenuation. Left-sided pleural effusion and/or ascites may be present.
  - MRI: variable, but typically T1 hypointense and T2 hyperintense +/− peripheral/perilesional enhancement.

REFERENCES

Elsayes, K. M., Narra, V. R., Mukundan, G., Lewis, J. S., Menias, C. O., & Heiken J. P. (2005). MR imaging of the spleen: Spectrum of abnormalities. *Radiographics*, 25(4), 967–972.

Karlo, C. A., Stolzmann, P., Do, R. K., & Alkadhi, H. (2013). Computed tomography of the spleen: How to interpret the hypodense lesion. *Insights Into Imaging*, 4(1), 65–76.

CASE 15

Splenic Gamna-Gandy Bodies

1. B. Gamna-Gandy bodies are siderotic nodules that deposit in the spleen, most commonly in association with portal hypertension. They can also be seen with paroxysmal nocturnal hemoglobinuria (PNH). They are not associated with lymphoma or melanoma.
2. B. Gamna-Gandy bodies are typically seen as numerous tiny (subcentimeter) nodules of similar size and shape throughout the spleen. They are not solitary and not large.
3. D. The appearance of Gamna-Gandy bodies on imaging and pathologic evaluation is related to microhemorrhage with resultant hemosiderin deposition. Melanin can cause hyperintense T1 signal in the spleen with metastatic melanoma. Gamna-Gandy bodies do not enhance, thus their appearance is not related to gadolinium or iodine deposition.

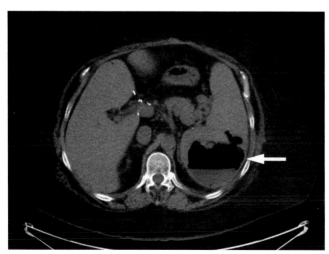

Fig. 13.1 Axial unenhanced computed tomography (CT) of the upper abdomen demonstrating a large fluid collection with air-fluid level *(arrow)* in the spleen.

Case 14 is online only and accessible at www.expertconsult.com.

4. C. Gamna-Gandy bodies are classically demonstrated on magnetic resonance imaging (MRI) with chemical shift imaging (in-phase and out-of-phase T1 weighted gradient echo sequences), in which signal blooming is typical on out-of-phase images. Although Gamna-Gandy bodies are hypointense on T2 weighted images and thus low B-value diffusion weighted images, they are more classically depicted on chemical shift imaging.

Comment

- Gamna-Gandy bodies are siderotic nodules found in the spleen, most commonly in the setting of portal hypertension. Less commonly, they can also occur in association with portal or splenic vein thrombosis, paroxysmal nocturnal hemoglobinuria (PNH), sickle cell anemia, and hemolytic anemias (among others).
- Pathologically, Gamna-Gandy bodies are characterized by numerous subcentimeter well-circumscribed nodules of similar size throughout the spleen.
- Microhemorrhage deposition in the spleen results in hemosiderin deposition, which accounts for the characteristic findings on chemical shift imaging with magnetic resonance imaging (MRI) as described later.
- Imaging findings of Gamna-Gandy bodies:
  - US: numerous tiny echogenic foci without posterior shadowing

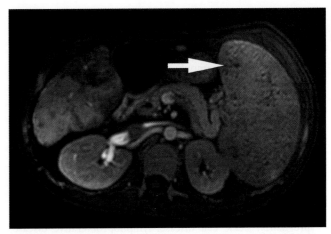

Fig. 15.3 Postcontrast T1 weighted image demonstrating that these siderotic nodules *(arrow)* do not enhance.

- CT: usually not visible as discrete nodules. Can sometimes show high attenuation due to calcium deposition that can be seen with Gamna-Gandy bodies.
- MRI: hypointense on gradient echo sequences and very hypointense on T2 weighted images. The classic appearance is blooming on in-phase T1 weighted images when compared to out-of-phase T1 weighted images due to the paramagnetic effect of hemosiderin. This is a type of susceptibility artifact in which a paramagnetic substance affects the local magnetic field (depicted as more prominent and hypointense signal on in-phase images).

REFERENCES
Dobritz, M., NöMayr, A., Bautz, W., & Fellner, F. A. (2002). Gamna-Gandy bodies of the spleen detected with MR imaging: A case report. *Magnetic Resonance Imaging, 19*(9), 1249–1251.
Minami, M., Itai, Y., Ohtomo, K. Ohnishi, S., Niki, T., … Kokubo, T. (1989). Siderotic nodules in the spleen: MR imaging of portal hypertension. *Radiology, 172*(3), 681–684.

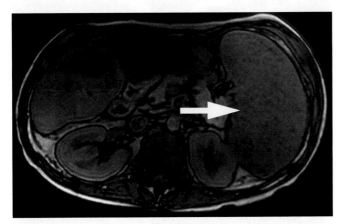

Fig. 15.1 Opposed-phase T1 weighted gradient echo image of the abdomen demonstrating small hypointense nodules within the spleen *(arrow)*.

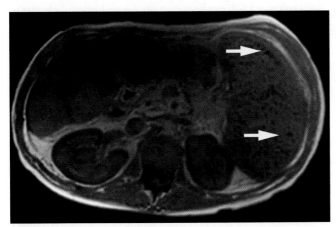

Fig. 15.2 In-phase T1 weighted gradient echo image shows blooming within the tiny nodules *(arrows)* throughout the spleen due to iron deposition within these Gamna-Gandy bodies.

CASE 16
Wandering Spleen

1. C. Wandering spleen occurs when the spleen migrates from the left upper quadrant to the lower abdomen or pelvis due to a congenital or acquired abnormality of the suspensory ligaments that normally affix the spleen to its usual anatomic position. It is not due to an underlying internal hernia or malrotation.
2. C. The typical management of wandering spleen involves surgical detorsion with splenopexy. This is first attempted laparoscopically. If splenic infarction is present, splenectomy may be necessary. Delay of surgery for conservative measures may increase risk of torsion and infarct.
3. A, B, C, D. Any condition associated with splenomegaly may contribute to acquired laxity of the suspensory ligaments and therefore be present in the setting of wandering spleen. These include infectious, neoplastic, or inflammatory conditions such as mononucleosis, lymphoma, and sickle cell disease. The spleen is also enlarged in pregnancy.
4. B. Technetium labeled sulfur colloid is taken up by the reticuloendothelial cells of the liver, spleen, and bone marrow. As such, an enlarged spleen in the lower abdomen/pelvis can easily be identified on a sulfur colloid scan.

Comment

- Wandering spleen is an unusual condition in which the spleen migrates from the left upper quadrant to the lower abdomen/pelvis. It is most commonly seen in young adults, particularly multiparous women.
- Wandering spleen may be asymptomatic or can present as a painful abdominal mass. When complicated by torsion or other conditions such as bowel obstruction or acute pancreatitis, wandering spleen can present as an acute abdomen.
- The cause of wandering spleen is due to an underlying abnormality of the suspensory ligaments that normally keep the spleen affixed to its mesentery in the left upper quadrant. This may be due to a congenital absence or abnormal development of the suspensory ligaments or an acquired laxity of the ligaments due to various reasons for splenomegaly (i.e., pregnancy, sickle cell disease, lymphoproliferative disease, mononucleosis).
- Twisting of the abnormally long vascular pedicle seen in wandering spleen can result in torsion and splenic infarction.

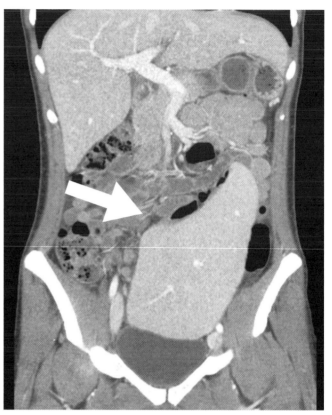

Fig. 16.3 Coronal reformatted computed tomography (CT) showing the longitudinal span of the enlarged spleen *(arrow)* with location in the the pelvis.

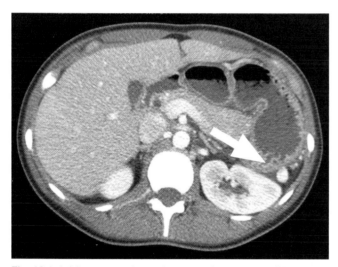

Fig. 16.1 Axial contrast-enhanced computed tomography (CT) of the upper abdomen shows no spleen in the splenic fossa within the left upper quadrant *(arrow)*.

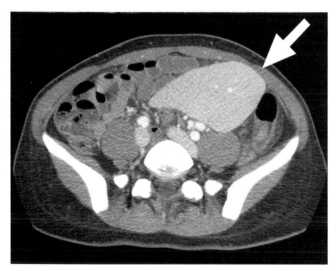

Fig. 16.2 Axial contrast-enhanced computed tomography (CT) image of the lower abdomen demonstrating an enlarged spleen located within the lower abdomen *(arrow)*.

- Managed surgically, typically with laparoscopic detorsion and splenopexy. Splenectomy may be necessary if infarction is present.
- Imaging findings of wandering spleen:
  - US: absence of the spleen in the left upper quadrant. Splenic mobility in wandering spleen can be demonstrated with the patient in the right lateral decubitus position. Doppler evaluation can help evaluate for splenic torsion or infarct.
  - CT: malpositioned spleen in the lower abdomen or pelvis with "whirl sign" of elongated vascular pedicle. Contrast-enhanced CT can help evaluate for end-organ ischemia in the setting of torsion.
  - MRI: enlarged spleen in the lower abdomen or pelvis. Can evaluate for ischemia or infarct as on CT.
  - Nuclear medicine: technetium sulfur colloid scan can identify the abnormally positioned and enlarged spleen.

REFERENCE

Reisner, D. C., & Burgan, C. M. (2018). Wandering spleen: An overview. *Current Problems in Diagnostic Radiology*, *47*(1), 68–70.

CASE 17

Splenic Laceration

1. B. The spleen is the most commonly injured organ in the abdomen following blunt trauma, followed by the liver. Injury to the adrenal glands may also occur, particularly the right adrenal gland in association with traumatic liver injury. Pancreatic injury occurs in <10% of blunt trauma cases.

2. A. Patients undergoing splenectomy are at risk for infection due to encapsulated bacteria. For this reason, postsplenectomy patients receive pneumococcal, meningococcal, and *Haemophilus influenzae* vaccinations. These patients are not at increased risk for other bacterial, viral, or fungal infections.

3. C. Computed tomography (CT) is the best imaging modality to identify and characterize acute traumatic injury to the spleen and other abdominal organs. Ultrasound may be utilized (focused assessment with sonography for trauma = FAST) to evaluate for hemoperitoneum but is not useful for grading laceration or subcapsular hematoma. Plain radiography is utilized to quickly and portably detect hollow viscus perforation in the setting of trauma. Magnetic resonance imaging (MRI) is not utilized due to exam time, lack of immediate availability, and cost.

4. C. The portal venous phase is the best phase for evaluating traumatic injury to the spleen because the spleen homogeneously enhances during this time. The normal heterogeneous enhancement of the spleen in the arterial phase can be mistaken for injury. Noncontrast CT is useful for detecting hemorrhage and potential laceration but cannot detect active bleeding. A 3-minute delay can be used to identify pooling of extravasated blood but is not routinely utilized in a typical trauma CT protocol.

Comment

- The spleen is the most commonly injured organ in the abdomen in the setting of blunt trauma, with an incidence of 25% to 50%.
- Historically, the treatment of choice for splenic injury was surgical, commonly splenectomy. However, splenectomy is associated with a lifelong risk for potentially fatal sepsis due to encapsulated bacteria.
- This has led to an evolution in the management of splenic injuries to appropriately triage patients toward operative versus nonoperative management. Currently, nonoperative management of isolated blunt splenic injury is considered the standard of care for hemodynamically unstable patients. Some patients who are hemodynamically unstable proceed directly to surgical exploration. Splenic artery embolization is commonly utilized for treating high-grade injuries in both hemodynamically stable and unstable patients.
- Patients who are hemodynamically stable routinely receive a computed tomography (CT) examination.
- The degree of splenic injury is assigned a grade, commonly according to the American Association for the Surgery of Trauma (AAST) grading scale. The grade will determine whether the patient will or will not require intervention and the need for continued evaluation of the spleen.
- Grading depends on size, depth, and number of lacerations and hematomas as well as the amount of extravasation and whether there is continued bleeding.
- AAST splenic injury scale (revised in 2018):
  - Grade I
    - Parenchymal laceration <1 cm in depth
    - Subcapsular hematoma <10% of surface area
    - Capsular tear
  - Grade II
    - Parenchymal laceration 1 to 3 cm in depth
    - Subcapsular hematoma 10% to 50% of surface area
    - Intraparenchymal hematoma <5 cm
  - Grade III
    - Parenchymal laceration >3 cm in depth
    - Subcapsular hematoma >50% of surface area
    - Ruptured subcapsular or intraparenchymal hematoma >5 cm
  - Grade IV
    - Parenchymal laceration involving segmental or hilar vessels producing >25% devascularization

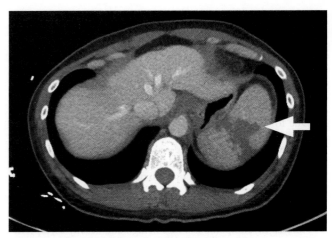

Fig. 17.1 Axial postcontrast computed tomography (CT) of the upper abdomen in the portal venous phase demonstrates a branching linear hypodense abnormality within the spleen *(arrow),* compatible with a laceration.

- Any injury with splenic vascular injury or active bleeding confined within the splenic capsule
  - Grade V
    - Any injury with splenic vascular injury with active bleeding extending into the peritoneum
    - Shattered spleen
- Imaging findings of splenic laceration:
  - CT: arterial and portal venous phase imaging is recommended for evaluation of blunt or penetrating trauma to the abdomen. The splenic parenchyma is best evaluated in the portal venous phase while vascular injury is best assessed on the arterial phase. Lacerations are areas of linear or branching low attenuation in a geographic pattern. Subcapsular hematomas are low-attenuation fluid collections that distort the splenic capsule. Active hemorrhage demonstrates a blush of contrast on the arterial phase with pooling on the venous phase. Traumatic pseudoaneurysms are also hyperdense on the arterial phase but follow the blood pool on dynamic imaging.

REFERENCES

Kozar, R. A., Crandall, M., Shanmuganathan, K., Zarzaur, B. L., Coburn, M., ... Cribari, C. (2018). Organ injury scaling 2018 update: Spleen, liver, and kidney. *The Journal of Trauma and Acute Care Surgery, 85*(6), 1119–1122.

Madoff, D. C., Denys, A., Wallace, M. J., Murthy, R., Gupta, S., ... Pillsbury, E. P. (2005). Splenic arterial interventions: Anatomy, indications, technical considerations, and potential complications. *Radiographics, 25*(Suppl. 1), S191–S211.

CASE 18

Adrenal Myelolipoma

1. C, D. The presence of macroscopic fat in the lesion (e.g., <-30 Hounsfield units [HU] on computed tomography [CT]) in the tumor originating from the adrenal gland is diagnostic of myelolipoma. The lesion does not have wedge-shaped defect with the adjacent kidney to suggest a renal origin of the mass, and hence renal angiomyolipoma is unlikely. Colonic carcinoma metastases do not have fat within them, hence it is unlikely. Lipid-rich adenoma can be characterized on noncontrast CT as low-density lesion with CT attenuation values between -10 and 10 HU, but usually it does not show a large amount of macroscopic fat.

2. A. Macroscopic fat in an adrenal mass is virtually pathognomonic for myelolipoma. Most myelolipomas are incidentalomas

and nonfunctioning. If diagnosis is established by computed tomography (CT) or magnetic resonance imaging (MRI), then further workup is usually not necessary.

3. D. Adrenal myelolipomas are usually asymptomatic and are discovered incidentally. However, they may present with flank pain or discomfort due to mass effect or hemorrhage.

4. C. Intracytoplasmic fat can be seen in metastases from renal cell carcinoma, hepatocellular carcinoma, and liposarcoma. Due to the presence of microscopic intracellular fat in these lesions, a signal drop similar to adrenal adenoma can be seen on chemical shift magnetic resonance imaging (MRI). Lung cancer, colonic carcinoma, and melanoma may metastasize to adrenal glands; however, they do not contain intracellular fat.

Comment

- Adrenal myelolipoma is a rare benign and usually asymptomatic tumor of the adrenal gland characterized by the presence of mature adipocytes.
- Incidence of adrenal myelolipoma is estimated to be 0.1% to 0.2% of autopsies.
- Myelolipomas can occur at extraadrenal sites, most commonly in the retroperitoneum.
- Most are asymptomatic and discovered incidentally on imaging studies. Can rarely cause symptoms such as abdominal and flank pain due to mass effect from large size or intratumoral or retroperitoneal hemorrhage.
- Most are <5 cm at presentation, but tumors >20 cm have been reported.
- May be variable amount of fat within the adrenal myelolipoma, ranging from only a few small regions of fat in a predominantly soft tissue density mass to nearly entirely composed of fatty tissue as seen in this case. Detection of macroscopic fat within an adrenal mass on imaging is virtually diagnostic of a myelolipoma.
- CT: appears as a fat-containing lesion, usually well circumscribed; however, masses that are mostly fat may be difficult to separate from the surrounding retroperitoneal fat.
  - Some may be heterogenous in attenuation due to the presence of mixed adipose and myeloid tissue.
  - The macroscopic fatty component is low density on CT, usually <-30 HU and often as low as -100 HU.
  - Calcifications can be seen in 25% to 30% of cases particularly when prior hemorrhage has occurred.

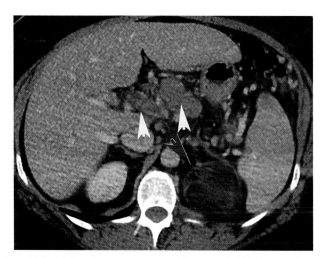

Fig. 18.1 Axial postcontrast computed tomography (CT) image shows a predominantly fat-containing mass *(red arrow)* arising from the left adrenal gland. This was consistent with a myelolipoma. Note enlarged lymph nodes *(yellow arrow)* at the porta from colonic carcinoma.

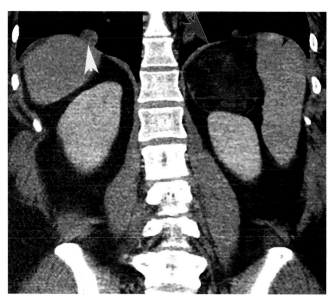

Fig. 18.2 Coronal postcontrast computed tomography (CT) image shows a predominantly fat-containing mass *(red arrow)* arising from the left adrenal gland. This was consistent with a myelolipoma. Note lung metastases *(yellow arrow)* in this patient from colonic carcinoma.

- Intratumoral hemorrhage may modify the classic appearance of the tumor.
- MRI: macroscopic fat component appears hyperintense on T1 weighted imaging and hypointense on frequency selective fat-suppressed sequences.
- US: myelolipoma is generally seen as a suprarenal mass of increased echogenicity. A hypoechoic component may be seen in the presence of myeloid elements.
- If the diagnosis of myelolipoma is established by characteristic imaging features, further workup is usually not required. Typically conservatively managed; if the patient is symptomatic, surgical removal may be indicated.

REFERENCES

Albano, D., Agnello, F., Midiri, F., Bruno, A., Alongi, P., ... Toia, P. (2019). Imaging features of adrenal masses. *Insights Into Imaging, 10*, 1.

Caoili, E. M., Korobkin, M., Francis, I. R., Cohan, R. H., Platt, J. F., ... Dunnick, N. R. (2002). Adrenal masses: Characterization with combined unenhanced and delayed enhanced CT. *Radiology, 222*, 629–633.

Kenney, P. J., Wagner, B. J., Rao, P., & Heffess, C. S. (1998). Myelolipoma: CT and pathologic features. *Radiology, 208*, 87–95.

CASE 20

Lipid-Poor Adrenal Adenoma

1. A, B, C. Computed tomography (CT) images show a well-circumscribed left adrenal mass of homogenous attenuation (23 HU on unenhanced CT), which enhances contrast administration. This may be consistent with a pheochromocytoma or adrenal metastasis; however, in a young 30-year-old patient this is most likely to represent a lipid-poor adrenal adenoma. There is no macroscopic fat (typically <-38 HU) to suggest myelolipoma.

2. B. Attenuation value <10 HU at unenhanced CT is used to characterize an adrenal nodule as an adenoma.

3. B. Absolute washout is calculated with the equation (Post HU – Delayed HU)/(Post HU – Pre HU), and relative

---

Case 19 is online only and accessible at www.expertconsult.com.

washout is calculated with the equation (Post HU – Delayed HU)/Post HU. 60% or greater absolute washout and 40% or greater relative washout are used for the diagnosis of adrenal adenoma with a high sensitivity and specificity.

4. B. Some hypervascular adrenal masses, including pheochromocytomas and metastasis from renal cell carcinoma and hepatocellular carcinoma, show rapid washout of contrast, and their absolute or relative washout characteristics can overlap with those of lipid-poor adenomas. Adrenal hematoma without underlying mass does not enhance.

Comment

- Introduction: incidental adrenal nodules are detected in approximately 4% to 5% of patients undergoing computed tomography (CT) examinations.
  - The prevalence of adrenal incidentalomas increases with age, and benign adenomas are the most common adrenal nodule encountered in the general population.
  - Adrenal adenoma is the most common adrenal tumor.
  - Most adenomas are nonfunctioning, so these lesions are detected incidentally on routine imaging for unrelated reasons.
  - Presence of ipsilateral or contralateral adrenocortical atrophy is strongly suggestive of a functioning adenoma.
- Imaging:
  - CT diagnosis of adrenal adenoma: characterization of adrenal masses on CT can be performed with or without the use of iodinated contrast material.
  - Unenhanced CT characterization of adrenal nodules relies on detection of intracytoplasmic lipid found within the adrenal adenomas, which decreases their attenuation to <10 HU. This has a sensitivity of 71% and specificity of 98% for adenoma characterization.
  - Analysis of histogram from pixel mapping can provide a higher sensitivity than attenuation measurement on unenhanced CT. Using a threshold of >10% negative pixel presence achieves a sensitivity of 84% to 91% and specificity of 100% for adenoma characterization.
  - Virtual unenhanced images obtained from the dual-energy CT (DECT) have not been shown to have a high sensitivity and specificity at the present time for characterization of adrenal adenomas based only on the attenuation values from the unenhanced images.
  - Approximately 10% to 40% of adrenal adenomas have CT attenuation value >10 HU on unenhanced CT and are called lipid-poor adenomas. They may not be differentiated from other adrenal masses on unenhanced CT.
  - Adrenal adenomas demonstrate rapid enhancement and washout of contrast material on CT, and the degree of washout can be calculated to characterize adrenal adenomas.
    - Absolute washout is calculated as (Postcontrast HU – Delayed HU)/(Postcontrast HU – Precontrast HU) × 100.
    - Relative washout is calculated as (Postcontrast HU – Delayed HU)/Postcontrast HU × 100.
    - The threshold for absolute and relative washout are 60% and 40%, respectively, for diagnosis of adrenal adenoma.
- Pitfalls: many false-positive lesions may show adenoma-like enhancement, which includes hyperplasia, pheochromocytoma, and hypervascular metastasis. Therefore, for patients suspected to have these tumors, careful follow-up or biochemical screening to exclude pheochromocytoma may be required.
- Management: for adrenal adenomas found incidentally, no further workup is generally required. For equivocal findings, further workup, including MRI, biopsy, positron emission tomography (PET) scan, or follow-up imaging, can be performed based on the clinical scenarios. Pheochromocytoma should be excluded by clinical and laboratory assessment before biopsy to avoid potentially life-threatening hemorrhage and hypertensive crisis.

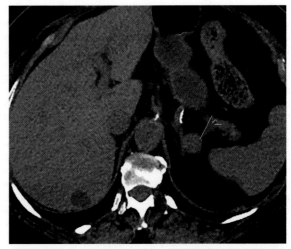

Fig. 20.1 Axial noncontrast computed tomography (CT) shows round homogenous left adrenal mass that measures 25 HU *(arrow)*.

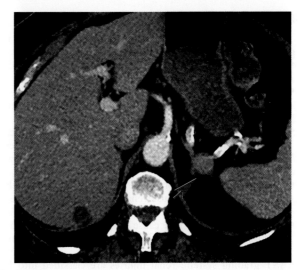

Fig. 20.2 Axial venous phase postcontrast computed tomography (CT) at 60 seconds after intravenous contrast administration shows enhancement of the left adrenal mass that measures 85 HU *(arrow)*.

REFERENCE
Park, J. J., Park, B. K., & Kim, C. K. (2016). Adrenal imaging for adenoma characterization: Imaging features, diagnostic accuracies and differential diagnoses. *The British Journal of Radiology, 89*(1062), 20151018.

CASE 21

Deep Renal Laceration With Active Bleeding

1. B, D. Computed tomography (CT) images show deep renal lacerations and amorphous hyperattenuating foci in a large perinephric hematoma, representing active bleeding. Pseudoaneurysm is a round or ovoid, well-circumscribed lesion, which demonstrates enhancement synchronous to the blood pool and does not change its size and shape on later phase.

2. D. Computed tomography (CT) protocol for major trauma usually includes a single phase typically acquired in the late cortical medullary or early nephrographic phase. However, when vascular examination is necessary, dual-phase CT is performed during the arterial and nephrographic phases. Early examination allows for accurate evaluation of the vasculature, and delayed 5-minute imaging can help in evaluation of the renal collecting system injuries. Intravenous urography is no

longer the preferred imaging modality, although it may still be used when the patient is rushed straight to the operating room or CT is unavailable. Noncontrast CT scan is usually not preferred for evaluation of trauma, since it does not give adequate information about the vasculature and intraabdominal organs.

3. C. Renal lacerations >1 cm in depth without collecting system injury are classified as grade III. The AAST grading system does not describe active bleeding or pseudoaneurysm in the grades because it is a surgical grading system based on the appearance of the kidney and surgery.

4. B. Absolute indications for surgery include life-threatening hemorrhage or expanding or pulsatile retroperitoneal hematoma (most often from severe vascular pedicles injury), complete ureteral pelvic junction avulsion, and polytrauma patients in shock. Renal contusion and subsegmental renal infarction are treated conservatively. Free fluid in the abdomen or retroperitoneum is not by itself an indication for surgery. However, it may represent a more serious injury such as collecting system or vascular pedicle injury. In such a case, the appropriate procedural management must be pursued.

Comment

- The kidney is the most commonly involved organ of the genitourinary system during trauma.
  - Renal trauma can be an isolated injury, but in 80% to 95% of cases there are concomitant injuries as well.
  - Renal trauma affects predominantly men, 72% to 93% of cases, and is more frequently seen in the young population with a mean age range from 31 to 38 years.
  - Blunt renal trauma is the most common mechanism for renal injury and accounts for 71% to 95% of renal trauma cases.
- Major elements that cause the trauma are deceleration and acceleration forces.
  - Deceleration forces on renal pedicle and ureteropelvic junction (UPJ) may cause renal injury such as rupture or thrombosis.
  - Acceleration forces may cause collision of the kidney in its surrounding elements, such as the ribs and spine, and cause parenchymal and vascular injury.
- AAST grading system: renal injuries are classified into five main categories by the AAST grading system.
  - Grade I (~80% of injuries): hematuria with normal urologic findings, renal contusions, and nonexpanding subcapsular hematomas
  - Grade II: nonexpanding perirenal hematomas and superficial (<1 cm in depth) cortical lacerations
  - Grade III: deep (>1 cm) renal lacerations without collecting system injury
  - Grade IV: deep renal lacerations extending into the collecting system, injuries involving the main renal artery or vein with contained hematoma, thrombosis of segmental renal artery without parenchymal laceration
  - Grade V: shattered kidney, ureteropelvic junction avulsion, complete avulsion of the vascular pedicle or thrombosis of the main renal artery or vein
- Imaging technique: computed tomography (CT) is the primary modality for imaging of suspected renal injuries.
  - CT for renal trauma may include four phases: precontrast, postcontrast arterial (35-second postintravenous injection), postcontrast nephrogenic/portal venous (75-second postintravenous injection), and delayed (5–10-min postintravenous injection); however, a dual-phase CT can also be performed during the arterial and nephrographic phases.
  - Early imaging will demonstrate optimal vascular enhancement and helps evaluate for vascular injury and presence of active bleeding. Delayed (5 minutes) imaging is necessary to evaluate for renal collecting system injuries and to detect contrast extravasation from the collecting system.
  - Renal injury with active hemorrhage: active arterial extravasation is typically seen as amorphous hyperattenuating foci isodense to adjacent enhanced vascular structures on CT. This hyperattenuating focus often increases and accumulates on later phases in the presence of active bleeding.
- Management of major renal injuries:
  - Absolute indications for renal intervention include hemodynamic instability and unresponsiveness to aggressive resuscitation due to renal hemorrhage, grade V vascular injury, and an expanding or pulsatile perirenal hematoma found during laparotomy performed for associated injuries.

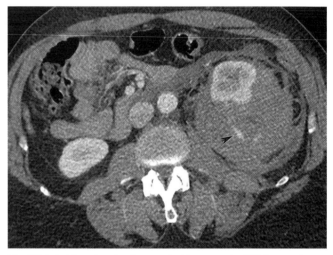

Fig. 21.1 Axial postcontrast computed tomography (CT) image showing a large perirenal hematoma surrounding the left kidney with an area of active extravasation *(red arrow)*.

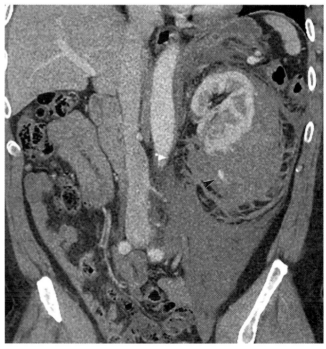

Fig. 21.2 Coronal reformat from a postcontrast computed tomography (CT) shows a large perirenal hematoma around the left kidney with an area of active extravasation *(red arrow)*.

- Relative indications for renal exploration include a large laceration of the renal pelvis, avulsion of the UPJ, coexisting bowel or pancreatic injuries, persistent urinary leakage, and postinjury urinoma or perinephric abscess with failed percutaneous or endoscopic management.
- Nonoperative management includes observation with supportive care, bed rest with vital signs, and laboratory test monitoring and reimaging when there is any deterioration, with the use of minimally invasive procedures (angioembolization or ureteral stenting) if indicated.

REFERENCES

Erlich, T., & Kitrey, N. D. (2018). Renal trauma: The current best practice. *Therapeutic Advances in Urology, 10*, 295–303.

Ramchandani, P., & Buckler, P. M. (2009). Imaging of genitourinary trauma. *AJR. American Journal of Roentgenology, 192*, 1514–1523.

Srinivasa, R. N., Akbar, S. A., Jafri, S. Z., & Howells, G. A. (2009). Genitourinary trauma: A pictorial essay. *Emergency Radiology, 16*, 21–33.

CASE 22

Acute Obstructing Ureteral Calculus

1. A, B, C, D. Ultrasound and computed tomography (CT) image shows hydronephrosis in the left kidney. This can be seen with any etiology causing obstruction of the ureter, including retroperitoneal fibrosis, calculus at the ureterovesicular junction, or a recently passed calculus. A large retroperitoneal hematoma compressing on the ureter may also cause hydronephrosis in the kidney.
2. C. Computed tomography (CT) is known to be the most sensitive exam for detection of urinary calculi with 99% of renal tract calculi seen on a noncontrast CT.
3. A, C, D. Imaging studies may show direct finding (obstructive calculus) as well as indirect findings (hydronephrosis, hydroureter to the level of the obstructing stone, perinephric/periuretral edema, and swollen kidney). Renal atrophy can be seen in chronic urinary obstruction but is not associated with acute obstruction.
4. C. Almost all urinary stones are seen as high attenuation focus on CT; however, indinavir stones in patients with human immunodeficiency virus (HIV) infection receiving indinavir (antiretroviral drug) may not be visible on CT.

Comment

- Urolithiasis is most commonly seen in patients between 30 and 60 years of age.
- Approximately 5% of women and 12% of men have renal calculi.
- The commonest stone is calcium oxalate. The more common composition of stones includes:
  - Calcium oxalate +/− calcium phosphate (75%)
  - Struvite (triple phosphate) (15%)
  - Pure calcium phosphate (5–7%)
  - Uric acid (5–8%)
  - Cystine (1%)
  - Lithogenic medications (1%)
- Although some renal stones remain asymptomatic, most will result in pain. Hematuria is also commonly seen. Some patients may present with complication of obstructive pyelonephritis.
- Imaging:
  - Plain radiograph: calcium containing stones are radiopaque. Lucent stones include uric acid, cystine, medication stones (indinavir is best known), and pure matrix stones.
  - US: is frequently the first investigation of the urinary tract but is not as sensitive as CT to identify stones.

- Features include:
  - Echogenic foci
  - Acoustic shadowing
  - Twinkle artifact on color Doppler
  - Decreased or absent ureter jets on the side of obstruction
  - Significantly higher renal resistive index in obstructed kidney
- CT: almost all stones are opaque on CT but vary in density. Average Hounsfield units (HU) are as follows:
  - Calcium oxalate +/− calcium phosphate: 400 to 600 HU
  - Struvite (triple phospohate): variable but usually opaque
  - Pure calcium phosphate: 400 to 600 HU
  - Uric acid: 100 to 200 HU
  - Cystine: opaque
- Radiolucent stones seen include medication stones (protease inhibitor [indinavor]) and pure matric stones. These are usually undetectable on noncontrast CT. They can be seen on the delayed phase as a filling defect in the ureter.
- Primary findings: direct visualization of the calculus within the urinary tract
  - Soft tissue rim sign refers to a realm of soft tissue attenuation surrounding the ureteral calculus representing ureteral edema resulting from mucosal irritation obstruction.
  - Comet tail sign refers to tapering soft tissue attenuation adjacent to a phlebolith representing the noncalcified portion of a pelvic vein and is not seen with ureteral calculus.
- Secondary findings: imaging science of obstruction or infection, which includes hydronephrosis, perinephric edema, and periureteral edema
- Treatment:
  - Calcium stones: small ones can be ignored if patients maintain good state of hydration. Bladder stones may be treated with extracorporeal shockwave lithotripsy (ESWL) or percutaneous nephrostomy.
  - Struvite stones: are usually large (staghorn calculi) and are treated by surgical removal since they result from infection.
  - Uric acid stones: are usually the result of low urinary pH and hydration, and elevation of the urinary pH is usually sufficient.
  - Cystine stones: may be difficult to treat and shatter with ESWL. Hydration and alkalinization are usually the first-line therapy.

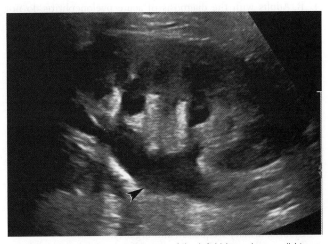

Fig. 22.1 Coronal ultrasound image of the left kidney shows mild to moderate hydronephrosis (*arrow*) with hydroureter.

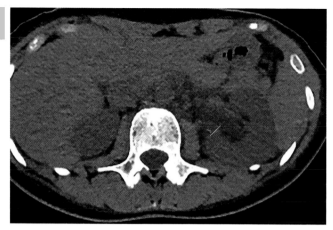

Fig. 22.2 Axial noncontrast computed tomography (CT) image shows mild to moderate hydronephrosis in the left kidney.

REFERENCES

Cheng, P. M., Moin, P., Dunn, M. D., Boswell, W. D., & Duddalwar, V. A. (2012). What the radiologist needs to know about urolithiasis: Part 1—pathogenesis, types, assessment, and variant anatomy. *AJR. American Journal of Roentgenology, 198,* W540–W547.

Cheng, P. M., Moin, P., Dunn, M. D., Boswell, W. D., & Duddalwar, V. A. (2012). What the radiologist needs to know about urolithiasis: Part 2—CT findings, reporting, and treatment. *AJR. American Journal of Roentgenology, 198,* W548–W554.

CASE 23

Acute Pyelonephritis

1. B, C, D. Wedge-shaped areas of decreased perfusion and striated nephrogram are typical computed tomography (CT) findings of acute pyelonephritis. Renal contusion is seen as an ill-defined area of decreased attenuation on CT and is one of the causes of striated nephrogram—the less likely in this case on the basis of clinical history and bilateral renal involvement. Renal lymphoma can present as multiple solid adrenal masses or diffuse infiltrative masses.
2. A, B. Striated nephrogram can be seen with acute high-grade obstruction and acute renal vein thrombosis; however, it is not seen with hypertension or renal lymphoma.
3. C. Hematogenous spread of infection from another source is less common in asymptomatic young patients and is usually seen in immunocompromised patients.
4. B. Adults with the diagnosis of acute pyelonephritis do not typically need any imaging, and diagnosis is made on the basis of clinical and laboratory findings.

Comment

- Acute pyelonephritis is usually diagnosed based on clinical symptoms and laboratory data without imaging examinations. Imaging studies are useful when the diagnosis of acute pyelonephritis cannot be made clinically and when possible complications need to be assessed. Imaging studies are also useful to assess underlying anatomic abnormality, including calculus or urinary tract obstruction that may prevent rapid therapeutic response or require further management.
- Classic symptoms include an abrupt onset of chills, fever, and unilateral or bilateral flank pain with costovertebral tenderness. These "upper tract signs" are often accompanied by dysuria, urinary frequency, and urgency.
- It is usually caused by ascending infection of the urinary tract from urinary blockade. Hematogenous spread of infection

from another source is less common and is usually seen in immunocompromised patients.
- Imaging findings:
  - Ultrasonography is often used as a first-line diagnostic tool to evaluate the urinary tract in patients with symptoms of pyelonephritis.
    - Focal or global areas of decreased and occasionally increased echogenicity and obligation of the cortical medullary differentiation are seen on ultrasound. Color and power Doppler ultrasound may show associated hypoperfusion.
    - Particulate matter/debris in the collecting system
  - CT: contrast-enhanced CT is considered the best imaging study to detect acute nephritis and its complications.
    - Imaging findings include ill-defined, wedge-shaped lesions of decreased attenuation and striated nephrogram, which is seen as linear bands of alternating hyperattenuation and hyperattenuation oriented parallel to the axis of the tubules and collecting ducts.
  - Striated nephrogram can be seen in a number of conditions, including the following:
    - Unilateral striated nephrogram:
      - Acute ureteric obstruction
      - Acute pyelonephritis
      - Acute renal vein thrombosis
      - Acute radiation therapy to the kidney
      - Acutely following renal contusion
    - Bilateral striated nephrograms
      - Autosomal recessive polycystic kidney disease
      - Acute pyelonephritis
      - Acute tubular obstruction
      - Acute tubular necrosis
      - Hypotension
  - Thickening of the pelvicalyceal wall, obligation of renal sinus and perinephric fat, and thickening of renal fascia may also be seen.
  - Associated nonenhancing fluid collections may indicate development of abscess.
- Management: treatment antibiotics are usually effective; however, when patients do not respond to appropriate antibiotic therapy within the first 72 hours, abscess should be suspected and imaging study may be required.

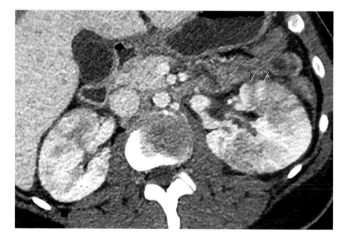

Fig. 23.1 Axial contrast-enhanced computed tomography (CT) image showing linear bands of alternating hyperattenuation and hypoattenuation *(red arrows)* in bilateral kidney suggesting a "striated nephrogram." This is consistent with bilateral acute pyelonephritis.

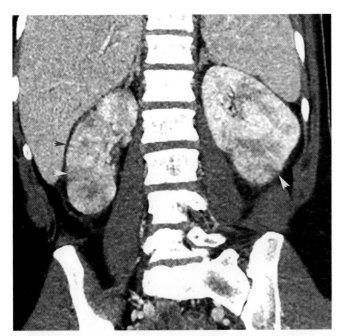

Fig. 23.2 Coronal reformat from a contrast-enhanced computed tomography (CT) image showing linear bands of alternating hyperattenuation and hypoattenuation *(red arrows)* in bilateral kidneys suggesting a "straited nephrogram" and areas of hypoperfusion *(yellow arrow)* consistent with bilateral acute pyelonephritis.

REFERENCES

Craig, W. D., Wagner, B. J., & Travis, M. D. (2008). Pyelonephritis: Radiologic-pathologic review. *Radiographics, 28*, 255–277.

Das, C. J., Ahmad, Z., Sharma, S., & Gupta, A. K. (2014). Multimodality imaging of renal inflammatory lesions. *World Journal of Radiology, 6*, 865–873.

CASE 24

Horseshoe Kidney

1. D. Horseshoe kidney is typically associated with fusion at the lower poles by an isthmus, which is most commonly composed of functioning parenchymal tissue. Rarely, the isthmus may be composed of nonfunctioning fibrous tissue. Fusion at the upper poles or interpolar kidneys is not common.
2. D. The isthmus at the lower pole of the horseshoe kidney typically gets caught on the inferior mesenteric artery during cranial migration, which prevents the kidney from rising to its normal level in the retroperitoneum. It does not get caught on the celiac axis or superior mesenteric artery because it usually cannot ascend that far cranially. Variant renal artery anatomy is common with horseshoe kidney.
3. A, B, C, D. Patients with horseshoe are more susceptible to many conditions, including renal stones, renal tumors (Wilms, transitional cell carcinoma, carcinoid), hydronephrosis (due to uteropelvic junction [UPJ] obstruction), and polyureteritis cystica. They are also more prone to recurrent infection and injury from blunt trauma.
4. B. Horseshoe kidney can be seen with multiple different chromosomal abnormalities, including Down syndrome, Turner syndrome, and Edwards syndrome. However, it is most commonly associated with Turner syndrome. Sixty percent of females with Turner syndrome have horseshoe kidneys.

Comment

- Horseshoe kidney is the most common renal fusion anomaly, occurring in 1 of 400 live births. There is a 2:1 male predilection.

- Horseshoe kidney results from abnormal contact of the metanephric blastema and usually presents as fusion of the lower poles with a connecting isthmus, which is typically composed of functional renal tissue.
- A horseshoe kidney is usually located in the lower abdomen because the isthmus prevents cranial migration beyond the level of the inferior mesenteric artery. The renal pelvis is oriented anteriorly while calyces are oriented more posteriorly than normal. Variant renal arterial and venous anatomy is common.
- Usually an asymptomatic condition, discovered incidentally at imaging.

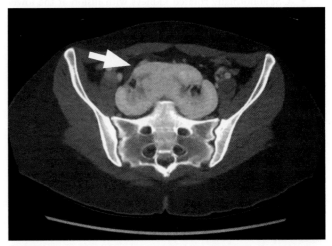

Fig. 24.1 Axial postcontrast CT of the lower abdomen demonstrates kidneys with fused inferior poles *(arrow)* at the level of the inferior mesenteric artery, compatible with a horseshoe kidney.

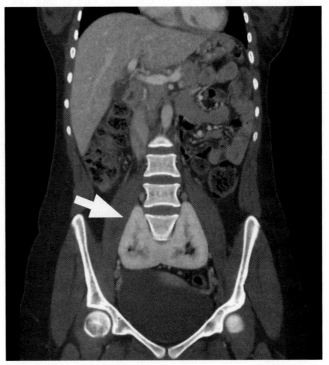

Fig. 24.2 Coronal reformatted postcontrast CT image redemonstrating the horseshoe kidney with fusion of the inferior right and left lower poles.

- However, patients with horseshoe kidney are more prone to urolithiasis, recurrent urinary tract infection, hydronephrosis (UPJ obstruction), polyureteritis cystica, renovascular hypertension, and renal malignancy (Wilms tumor, urothelial carcinoma, renal carcinoid). Renal injury from blunt trauma is also more common due to positioning adjacent to the vertebral bodies.
- Horseshoe kidney may also be associated with cardiovascular, gastrointestinal, and musculoskeletal anomalies as well as chromosomal abnormalities (i.e., Turner syndrome).
- Management is usually not necessary for incidentally detected cases of horseshoe kidney. Individual management depends on cases of underlying trauma, infection, etc.
- Imaging findings of horseshoe kidney:
  - US: abnormally rotated kidneys with fusion at the lower pole. If not correctly identified, the isthmus anterior to the aorta and inferior to the intefior mesenteric artery (IMA) may be mistaken for retroperitoneal soft tissue or adenopathy.
  - CT: fused kidneys located in the lower midline abdomen. Multiphase imaging can be utilized to assess for variant renal arterial and vascular anatomy as well as a potential duplicated collecting system.
  - MRI: same as on CT. Delineating the anatomy is critical for cases of surgical planning.

REFERENCE
Taghavi, K., Kirkpatrick, J., & Mirjalili, S. A. (2016). The horseshoe kidney: Surgical anatomy and embryology. *Journal of Pediatric Urology*, *12*(5), 275–280.

CASE 25

Crossed Fused Ectopia

1. D. An abnormal-appearing kidney actually represents two fused kidneys located in the right lower quadrant. The ureters and the bladder are in the normal position on each side of the midline. These findings are consistent with crossed fused renal ectopia.
2. B. Usually the ureter draining the upper kidney enters the bladder on the same side and the ureter draining the lower kidney crosses a midline to enter the bladder on the contralateral side in its normal position.
3. D. Patients with crossed fused renal ectopia are usually symptom free but are most susceptible to urinary tract infections, urolithiasis, and hydronephrosis in patients with normal kidneys.
4. A. Crossed fused ectopia is thought to occur in the first trimester at around 4 to 8 weeks of fetal development.

Comment

- Crossed fused renal ectopia refers to an anomaly where the kidneys are fused and located on the same side of the midline. The ectopic kidney is located on the opposite side of the midline from its ureteral orifice. The ureteral insertion in the bladder is normal without ectopy, and cystoscopy reveals a normal trigone.
- More common in males (2:1) than females, and left-to-right ectopia is three times more common than right-to-left ectopia
- Results from abnormal renal ascent in embryogenesis with the fusion of the kidneys within the pelvis.
- Thought to occur in the first trimester at around 4 to 8 weeks of fetal development.
- Subclassified into six types in decreasing order of frequency as follows:
  - Type A: inferior crossed fusion
  - Type B: sigmoid kidney
  - Type C: lump kidney

- Type D: disc kidney
- Type E: L-shaped kidney
- Type F: superiorly crossed fused
- Patients are usually asymptomatic but are more susceptible to trauma, hydronephrosis, ureteropelvic junction obstruction, the flux, urinary tract infection, and stone formation.

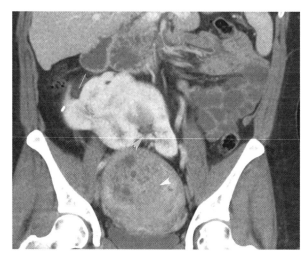

Fig. 25.1 Coronal reformat from a postcontrast computed tomography (CT) scan shows the kidneys are fused on the right side of the midline. The renal pelvis of the upper kidney is pointed upward *(red arrow)* while the pelvis of the lower kidneys points downward *(green arrow)*. Note incidentally seen large fibroid in the pelvis *(yellow arrow)*.

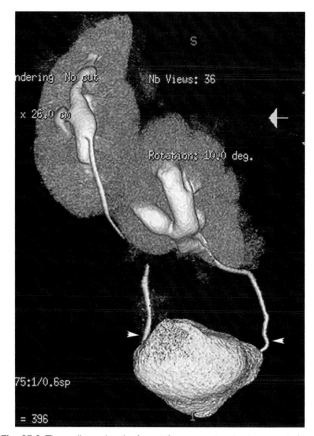

Fig. 25.2 Three-dimensional reformat from a postcontrast computed tomography (CT) scan shows the kidneys are fused on the right side of the midline. Note the normal insertion of the ureters *(arrow)* into the bladder.

- Imaging: empty renal fossae seen on one side with fused renal parenchyma with two collecting systems on the contralateral side. Usually the ureter draining the upper kidney enters the bladder on the same side and the ureter draining the lower kidney crosses a midline to enter the bladder on the contralateral side in its normal position. Vascular supply to the ectopic kidney is usually anomalous.
  - Ultrasound: there may be a characteristic anterior or posterior "notch" between the two fused kidneys
  - CT: the parenchymal band joining the two kidneys can be better visualized on CT scan.

REFERENCES

Singer, A., Simmons, M. Z., & Maldjian, P. D. (2007). Spectrum of congenital renal anomalies presenting in adulthood. *Clinical Imaging, 32*(3), 183–191. doi:10.1016/j.clinimag.2007.12.001.

Solanki, S., Bhatnagar, V., Gupta, A. K., & Kumar, R. (2013). Crossed fused renal ectopia: Challenges in diagnosis and management. *Journal of Indian Association of Pediatric Surgeons, 18*(1), 7–10. doi:10.4103/0971-9261.107006.

CASE 27

Renal Stone

1. D. The radiograph demonstrates a rounded radiodense structure projecting over the right lower pole kidney, a renal stone.
2. C. Calcium-based stones (i.e., oxalate and phosphate) are dense on radiography. Struvite stones are variable but also usually radiopaque. Uric acid stones are the lowest of the listed compositions in attenuation and may be lucent on plain radiography.
3. A. Most stones have at least some form of calcium, usually calcium oxalate (~75% of stone). Calcium phosphate is a common component of stones, but pure calcium phosphate stones are relatively uncommon (~5–7%). Struvite stones account for 15% of stones while uric acid stones comprise 5% to 8% of cases.
4. B. Ureteral stones >5 mm may require invasive urologic management as they are less likely to pass spontaneously or with the aid of medications. Stones most commonly obstruct at the ureteropelvic junction, ureterovesical junction, or in the ureter as it passes over the iliac vasculature.

Comment

- Renal stones are commonly encountered abnormalities, occurring in approximately 5% to 10% of the general population.
- Some renal stones are asymptomatic, whereas others will present with pain (renal colic), hematuria, or urinary tract obstruction.
- Risk factors for developing renal stones include:
  - Low fluid intake
  - Urinary tract infections
  - Urinary tract malformations (i.e., duplicated collecting system, horseshoe kidney)
  - Metabolic abnormality (i.e., hypercalciuria, hyperoxaluria, hyperuricosuria)
  - Urinary tract diversion
- Calcium oxalate stones comprise the vast majority of nephrolithiasis composition (~75%). Other stones include calcium phosphate, struvite, uric acid, and cystine stones.
  - Calcium stones
    - Most stones contain some degree of calcium, usually calcium oxalate +/− calcium phosphate
    - High in attenuation on CT (600–1200 HU)
    - Certain medications predispose (i.e., loop diuretics)
  - Struvite stones
    - Form in the setting of infection with urease-producing bacteria (i.e., *Proteus, Klebsiella*)
    - Form the majority of staghorn calculi, which form a cast of the renal pelvis and pyramids
  - Uric acid stones
    - Usually no identifiable cause
    - Lower in attenuation than calcium stones (200–400 HU)
    - May be treated medically with allopurinol
- Complications of renal stones can include recurrent urinary tract infection (UTI)/pyelonephritis, urinary obstruction (leading to impaired renal function if chronic), forniceal rupture, and potentially squamous metaplasia/carcinoma.
- Indications for treatment may include size >5 mm, long duration of symptoms, infection/sepsis, solitary kidney, and failed conservative management.
- Sensitivity for renal stone detection varies by imaging modality:
  - KUB: 57%
  - US: 84%
  - MRI: 82%
  - CT: 95%
- Imaging findings of renal stones:
  - Plain radiograph: radiopaque structures overlying the kidneys, ureters, or bladder. Stones that are radiolucent on radiography may be radiopaque on CT (i.e., uric acid stones).

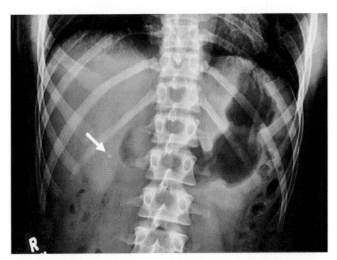

Fig. 27.1 Frontal abdominal radiograph demonstrates a round radiodensity projecting to the right lower pole kidney, a renal stone *(arrow)*.

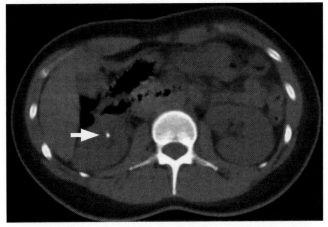

Fig. 27.2 Axial noncontrast computed tomography (CT) image shows the correlative position of the renal stone *(arrow)*.

Case 26 is online only and accessible at www.expertconsult.com.

- US: usually first-line imaging for investing the kidneys and bladder. Insensitive for stone detection but useful for identifying obstruction. Signs of a renal stone on US include echogenic focus with shadowing and twinkle artifact on color Doppler imaging.
- CT: 99% of stones are visible on unenhanced CT. Overall, best test for stone characterization, assessing size, location, and composition (calcium vs uric acid). Dual-energy CT is now routinely utilized for aiding characterization of stone composition.

REFERENCES

Brisbane, W., Bailey, M. R., & Sorensen, M. D. (2016). An overview of kidney stone imaging techniques. *Nature Reviews. Urology, 13*(11), 654–662.

Cheng, P. M., Moin, P., Dunn, M. D., Boswell, W. D., & Duddalwar, V. A. (2012). What the radiologist needs to know about urolithiasis: Part 1 pathogenesis, types, assessment, and variant anatomy. *AJR. American Journal of Roentgenology, 198*(6), W540–W547.

Kambadakone, A. R., Eisner, B. H., Catalano, O. A., & Sahani, D. V. (2010). New and evolving concepts in the imaging and management of urolithiasis: urologists' perspective. *Radiographics, 30*(3), 603–623.

CASE 29

Bladder Cancer

1. B, D. Magnetic resonance imaging (MRI) shows a large mass arising from the right lateral bladder wall, most compatible with primary bladder cancer. Although much less likely, metastatic involvement from direct extension of prostate, colorectal, and cervical carcinoma is possible as well. Benign bladder processes such as cystitis usually present as diffuse symmetric bladder wall thickening and are unlikely in this case.
2. C. Transitional cell carcinoma (TCC) accounts for >90% of all epithelial tumors, although up to 25% of tumors can contain areas with other histologic features such as clear cell, glandular cell, sarcomatoid, and squamous cell components.
3. D. Magnetic resonance imaging (MRI) has been shown to better depict intramural tumor invasion as well as extravesical extension and allows differentiation between muscle-invasive and nonmuscle-invasive disease.
4. C. The bladder tumor, mucosa, and submucosa enhance early after contrast administration while the muscle layer maintains its hypointensity and enhances late (60 seconds).

Comment

- Introduction: primary bladder neoplasms account for 2% to 6% of tumors, with bladder cancer ranked as the fourth most common malignancy in the United States.
- Bladder neoplasms can arise from any of the bladder wall layers; however, epithelial tumors are the most common with transitional cell carcinoma being the commonest histology.
- Other primary epithelial tumors include squamous carcinoma, adenocarcinoma, small cell/neuroendocrine carcinoma, carcinoid, and melanoma.
- Bladder cancer is more common in men than in women with the male:female ratio of 3–4:1 and is diagnosed at a more advanced stage and with a higher mortality rate in women.
- The pathogenesis for urothelial tumors is direct prolonged contact of the bladder urothelium with urine containing excreted carcinogens predominantly from cigarette smoking.

Case 28 is online only and accessible at www.expertconsult.com.

Smokers have four times the risk of bladder cancer, and cigarette smokers account for one-third to one-half of all cases of bladder cancer.

- Presentation: patient symptoms are all nonspecific and may include gross or microscopic hematuria, voiding symptoms such as frequency, dysuria, pelvic pain, and pressure.
  - More than 80% of patients with bladder cancer have hematuria, which is typically macroscopic and painless.
- Imaging:
  - Ultrasound is not routinely used for staging of bladder cancer but if incidentally found often appears as a polypoid or plaquelike hypoechoic lesion that projects into the bladder.
  - Computed tomography (CT) is the primary imaging modality for bladder cancer.
    - Imaging should be performed in the nephrographic phase before the excreted IV contrast material reaches a bladder so that the enhancing tumor can be visualized against a background of low attenuation urine within the bladder.
    - On delayed scanning, the lesion appears as a filling defect against a background of high attenuation contrast material within the bladder.
    - CT does not typically allow for the diagnosis of flat lesions and lesions at the bladder base adjacent to the prostate gland due to the presence of benign prostatic hypertrophy in some of the patients.
- MRI:
  - Tumor has an intermediate signal on T2 weighted images, slightly higher than that of the bladder wall.
  - On T1 weighted images, the tumor has an intermediate signal with enhancement seen in the tumor after gadolinium injection.
  - Peak enhancement of the tumor is earlier than that of the bladder wall, which is helpful if dynamic imaging is performed.
  - High-resolution fast spin echo T2 weighted images of the bladder obtained in three orthogonal planes with a small field of view and large matrix can be used to evaluate the detrusor muscle for tumor depth and invasion of the surrounding organs.

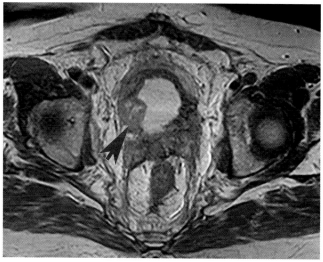

Fig. 29.1 Axial T2 weighted magnetic resonance image (MRI) shows intermediate signal intensity mass along the right lateral wall of the bladder (*red arrow*) consistent with transitional cell carcinoma.

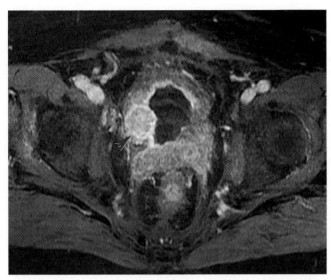

Fig. 29.2 Axial postcontrast T1 weighted magnetic resonance image (MRI) at 60 seconds shows enhancing mass in the right lateral bladder wall *(red arrow)* consistent with transitional cell carcinoma; however, at this late phase the muscular layer shows enhancement as well, compared to the early phase.

- Multifocal nature transitional cell carcinoma: TCCs are commonly multifocal, ~2% of patients with bladder TCC have synchronous upper tract TCC and 6% will have metachronous upper tract disease. Also 40% of patients with upper tract TCC will have bladder cancer.
- Treatment: is strongly influenced by tumor stage.
  - Superficial tumors can be treated with local transurethral resection with or without intravesical therapy.
  - The primary surgical procedure for bladder cancer is cystectomy, which is adequate for early stages.
  - For advanced diseases, chemotherapy, radiation therapy, and surgery are used.

REFERENCES

Kundra, V., & Silverman, P. M. (2003). Imaging in oncology from the University of Texas M. D. Anderson Cancer Center. Imaging in the diagnosis, staging, and follow-up of cancer of the urinary bladder. *AJR. American Journal of Roentgenology, 180*(4), 1045–1054. doi:10.2214/ajr.180.4.1801045.

Raman, S. P., & Fishman, E. K. (2014). Bladder malignancies on CT: The underrated role of CT in diagnosis. *AJR. American Journal of Roentgenology, 203*(2), 347–354. doi:10.2214/AJR.13.12021.

Verma, S., Rajesh, A., Prasad, S. R., Gaitonde, K., Lall, C. G., … Mouraviev, V. (2012). Urinary bladder cancer: Role of MR imaging. *Radiographics, 32*(2), 371–387. doi:10.1148/rg.322115125.

CASE 30

Urethral Diverticulum

1. A, B. Location of the cystic mass inferior to the bladder and in close approximation to the urethra and vagina suggests bladder diverticulum or carcinoma to be unlikely. This location is typical for vaginal cyst or urethral diverticulum.
2. B. Since the Skene gland ducts terminate in the middle to the distal urethra near the 3-o'clock and 9-o'clock positions, most diverticula are located in the posterior lateral wall of the middle third of the urethra.
3. C. Malignancy arising in a urethral diverticulum is seen as enhancing soft tissue mass within the diverticulum. Evaluation of urethral diverticulum should include postcontrast imaging if areas of wall thickening or soft tissue masses are seen within the diverticulum.
4. A, C, D. Recurrent infection in urethral diverticula is seen in 30% to 50% of patients. Calculus formation associated with urethral diverticulum is seen in about 1.5% to 10% of cases. Both benign and malignant tumors can develop in urethral diverticula, with adenocarcinoma being the most common malignancy seen.

Comment

- Introduction: a urethral diverticulum is a focal outpouching of the urethra and occurs more commonly in women than in men.
  - Represents either an infected paraurethral gland that has ruptured in the urethra or a prolapse of the urethral wall through a defect in the periurethral fascia.
  - May be either asymptomatic or manifest nonspecific symptoms of lower genitourinary tract pathology.
  - Classic clinical presentation is a soft, slightly tender badge and a lesion causing dysuria, dyspareunia, and dribbling incontinence.
  - Incidence ranges between 0.6% and 5% but rates as high as 40% have been found.
  - Recurrent infection in the diverticula is seen in 30% to 50% of patients. They are also common in patients with previous gonococcal infection.
  - Calculus formation associated with urethral diverticulum has been found in 1.5% to 10% of cases. Stagnation of infected urine enhances salt deposition nidi of desquamated mucoid slough, which eventually consolidates into calculi. Most calculi consist of calcium oxalate or calcium phosphate.
  - Both benign and malignant tumors can develop in urethral diverticula with malignancy mainly consisting of transitional cell carcinoma, adenocarcinoma, or squamous cell carcinoma. Adenocarcinoma is the most common diverticula malignancy occurring in 60% of cases.
- Pathogenesis: can be a congenital disorder but it is more commonly acquired presenting in adult life.
  - Most commonly infected paraurethral gland is the etiology.
  - Infection leads to duct obstruction with retention cyst or abscess formation, which eventually ruptures in the urethra, creating the diverticulum's neck or ostium.
  - The periurethral glands, known as Skene glands, provide urethral lubrication with mucous production. The ducts of these glands terminate in the middle to the distal urethra near the 3-o'clock and 9-o'clock positions, hence most diverticula are located in the posterior lateral wall of the middle third of the urethra.
  - Urethral diverticula can be single or multiple and can extend around the urethra partially ("saddlebag" or "horseshoe") or completely, varying in size from a few millimeters to ≥5 cm.
- Imaging:
  - MRI: a urethral diverticular cavity can be well seen as single or multiple and as unilocular or multilocular.
    - T2-weighted imaging is preferred for the detection of hyperintense fluid in a diverticulum.
    - A diverticulum with circumferential involvement of the urethra may be seen ("saddlebag" or "horseshoe" diverticulum).
    - Intravenous gadolinium-based contrast material administration aids in the detection of inflammation and of the rare diverticular adenocarcinoma.
    - Malignancy arising from a diverticulum can be visualized as enhancing soft tissue within the diverticulum.
    - Infected diverticula can be unilocular and contain a thick-walled or multiple septa, which enhances on postcontrast imaging.

- MRI may be performed with a torso phased-array coil or an endoluminal (endorectal, endovaginal, or endourethral) coil. Phased-array endoluminal MRI is the most accurate method for identifying and characterizing female urethral diverticula.
- Ultrasound can also be used in the assessment of urethral diverticula. Transperineal ultrasound may be useful for better visualization of the urethra. Transluminal ultrasound can be performed with the transvaginal, transurethral, or transrectal approach.
  - Urethral diverticula are seen as cystic masses adjacent to the urethra with debris within them if the diverticulum is infected.
  - Solid masses can be seen in patients with malignancy arising in the urethral diverticulum.
  - Color Doppler flow ultrasound provides information about the vascularity of the diverticular content and septa. Blood flow can be detected in thickened septa and solid tumors suggesting possible malignancy.

REFERENCES
Chou, C. P., Levenson, R. B., Elsayes, K. M., Kin, Y. H., Fu, T. Y., … Chiu, Y. S. (2008). Imaging of female urethral diverticulum: An update. *Radiographics, 28*, 1917–1930.
Hosseinzadeh, K., Furlan, A., & Torabi, M. (2008). Pre- and postoperative evaluation of urethral diverticulum. *AJR. American Journal of Roentgenology, 190*, 165–172.

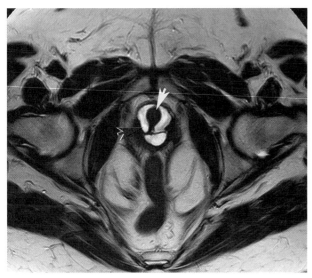

Fig. 30.1 Axial T2 weighted magnetic resonance image (MRI) shows high signal intensity cystic area *(red arrow)* circumferentially engulfing the urethra *(yellow arrow)*. A single thin separation is seen along the posterior aspect; however, no areas of nodularity are seen within this cystic area. This is consistent with a "saddlebag" or "horseshoe" urethral diverticulum.

CASE 31
Acute Emphysematous Cystitis

1. A, B, D. Figures show air in the region of the bladder in a curvilinear appearance, which would suggest presence of air in the bladder wall; however, air in the subcutaneous tissues or pelvic abscess would have a similar appearance as well. Air in the uterus will not have a curvilinear appearance but will be linear and vertical in appearance.
2. B. Patients with diabetes mellitus are at higher risk for development of emphysematous cystitis. Bladder calculus, malignant involvement, or fistulization to bowel are not considered to be risk factors for emphysematous cystitis.
3. B, C, D. Computed tomography (CT) features of emphysematous cystitis include thickening of the bladder wall, intraluminal air, and intramural air.
4. A, B, C. Complications of emphysematous cystitis include rupture, renal pyelitis, and ureteritis.

Comment

- Background: emphysematous cystitis is a relatively rare and complicated urinary tract infection (UTI) primarily observed in diabetic middle-aged women.
  - Presentation is variable and patients can be asymptomatic or present with dysuria, hematuria, abdominal pain, and urinary urgency and frequency and in a few cases with pneumaturia.
  - At-risk factors include patients with diabetes mellitus, obstructive uropathy, immunodeficiency, neurogenic bladder, and recurrent UTIs.
- Imaging:
  - Radiographs: show curvilinear or mottled areas of radiolucency outlining the bladder wall with or without luminal gas. Intraluminal gas will be seen as a gas-filled level that changes with position.
  - US: may show abnormal and thickened bladder wall. It can also show echogenic gas within the bladder wall with dirty shadowing artifact.
  - CT: is a highly sensitive examination and allows for early detection of intraluminal or intramural gas.
- Complications of emphysematous cystitis include ureteric and renal parenchymal extension and bladder rupture with sepsis and peritonitis.
- Treatment for emphysematous cystitis involves broad-spectrum antimicrobial therapy, hyperglycemic control, and adequate urine drainage with correction of possible bladder outlet obstruction when present.

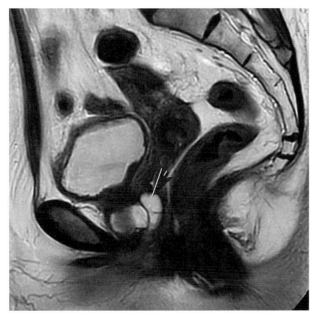

Fig. 30.2 Sagittal T2 weighted magnetic resonance image (MRI) shows high signal intensity cystic area *(red arrow)* inferior to the bladder in the midurethra. This is consistent with a "saddlebag" or "horseshoe" urethral diverticulum.

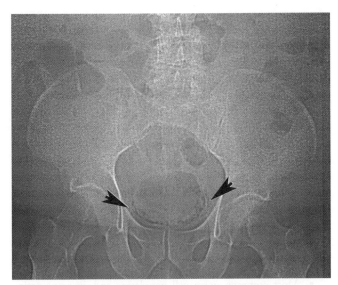

Fig. 31.1 Radiograph showing curvilinear air in the region of the bladder *(arrows)* outlining the bladder.

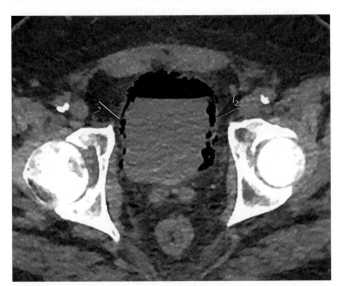

Fig. 31.2 Axial computed tomography (CT) image through the pelvis shows presence of air in the bladder wall *(red arrow)* consistent with emphysematous cystitis.

REFERENCES

Eken, A., & Alma, E. (2013). Emphysematous cystitis: The role of CT imaging and appropriate treatment. *Canadian Urological Association Journal, 7*(11-12), E754–E756. doi:10.5489/cuaj.472.

Grayson, D. E., Abbott, R. M., Levy, A. D., & Sherman, P. M. (2002). Emphysematous infections of the abdomen and pelvis: A pictorial review. *Radiographics, 22*(3), 543–561. doi:10.1148/radiographics.22.3.g02ma06543.

Joseph, R. C., Amendola, M. A., Artze, M. E., Casillas, J., Jafri, S. Z., ... Dickson, P. R. (1996). Genitourinary tract gas: Imaging evaluation. *Radiographics, 16*(2), 295–308. doi:10.1148/radiographics.16.2.8966288.

CASE 32

Extraperitoneal Bladder Rupture

1. A. Figures demonstrate bladdery injury. No pelvic mass, vascular injury, or fracture is shown.

2. C. Figures demonstrate contrast extravasation to the prevesical space (space of Retzius). Neither Morison pouch (hepatorenal fossa) nor the pouch of Douglas (retrouterine space in females), is depicted. No contrast is shown in the rectovesical space, the most gravity-dependent site for fluid accumulation in a male.

3. C. The bladder injury shown is best characterized as extraperitoneal bladder rupture. There is no contrast extravasation surrounding bowel loops to indicate intraperitoneal or combined injury. Bladder contusion has no detectable imaging abnormality.

4. D. Extraperitoneal bladder rupture most commonly results from blunt abdominal trauma, including motor vehicle crashes, falls, and crush injuries.

Comment

Bladder Trauma

- Most frequently result from:
  - Motor vehicle crashes
  - Falls
  - Crush injuries
  - Blunt trauma to the lower abdomen
  - 60% to 90% of patients with bladder injury have associated pelvic fracture

Role of Imaging

- In a trauma patient, gross hematuria with pelvic fracture is an absolute indication for dedicated bladder imaging (passive excretion after IV contrast administration may be insensitive)
- Relative indications:
  - Gross hematuria without pelvic fracture
  - Microhematuria with pelvic fracture
  - Microhematuria
- Fluoroscopic and computed tomography (CT) cystography have similar test performance.

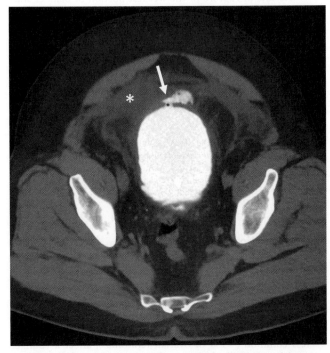

Fig. 32.1 Axial image demonstrates contrast opacification of the bladder, and fluid and stranding in the adjacent prevesical fat *(asterisk)*. There is an anterior bladder wall defect with extravasated contrast beyond the bladder wall *(arrow)*.

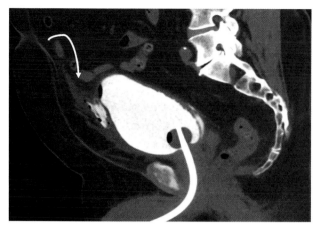

Fig. 32.2 Sagittal image shows no contrast above the level of the peritoneal reflection *(curved arrow),* indicating extraperitoneal bladder rupture.

Classification of Bladder Injury

- Contusion
  - Mucosal injury; no detectable imaging abnormality
- Extraperitoneal
  - Accounts for ~60% of bladder injuries
  - May result from bladder wall tears, or laceration of bladder by associated pelvic fracture
  - Extravasation pattern is confined to extraperitoneal space of the pelvis (molar-tooth appearance), though in complex injuries may extend to abdominal wall, penis, scrotum, and perineum
- Intraperitoneal
  - Accounts for one-third of bladder injuries
  - Sudden impact or compression in the setting of a bladder full of urine results in acutely elevated intraluminal bladder pressure
  - Results in rupture of the weakest portion of bladder wall, the bladder dome
  - As the dome is covered by peritoneum, injury results in intraperitoneal pattern of extravasation, outlining bowel loops and mesenteric fat
- Combined
  - Account for 5% of major bladder injuries
  - Refers to the presence of both intraperitoneal and extraperitoneal injury

REFERENCES

Ramchandani, P., & Buckler, P. M. (2009). Imaging of genitourinary trauma. *American Journal of Roentgenology, 192,* 1514–1523.

Tirkes, T., Sandrasegaran, K., Patel, A. A., Hollar, M. A., Tejada, J. G., … Tann, M. (2012). Peritoneal and retroperitoneal anatomy and its relevance for cross-sectional imaging. *Radiographics, 32,* 437–451.

CASE 34

Mature Cystic Teratoma

1. A, C, D. Those that would be included are hemorrhagic cysts, mature cystic teratoma, and cystadenoma.
2. D. Presence of low signal on fat-suppressed T1 weighted images is specific for teratomas.
3. C. Immature teratomas differ from mature cystic teratomas in that they demonstrate clinically malignant behavior, are much less common (<1% of ovarian teratomas), affect a younger age group (usually during the first two decades of life), and are

Case 33 is online only and accessible at www.expertconsult.com.

histologically distinguished by the presence of immature or embryonic tissues.
4. A. Torsion is the most common complication seen in mature cystic teratomas.

Comment

Background

- Ovarian teratomas are the most common germ cell neoplasms seen in ~0.1% of the general population.
- There are three types of ovarian teratomas: mature cystic, immature, and mono dermal.
- Mature cystic teratomas (MCTs) are cystic tumors composed of well-differentiated derivations from at least two of the three germ cell layers (ectoderm, mesoderm, and endoderm).
  - Account for 99% of ovarian teratomas
  - Affect a younger age group (mean patient age, 30 years) than epithelial ovarian neoplasms
  - Bilateral in ~10% of cases
  - Most common germ cell neoplasms and, in some series, the most common ovarian neoplasms removed at surgery. It is also the most common ovarian mass in children.
  - Most mature cystic teratomas are asymptomatic. Abdominal pain or other nonspecific symptoms occur in the minority of patients. They grow slowly at an average rate of 1.8 mm/year.
  - Mature cystic teratomas requiring removal can be treated with simple cystectomy.
  - Mature cystic teratomas are filled with sebaceous material, which is liquid at body temperature and semisolid at room temperature.
    - The wall of the cyst has squamous epithelium, and hair follicles, skin glands, muscle, and other tissues lie within the wall.
    - A raised protuberance is seen projecting into the cyst cavity known as the Rokitansky nodule with hair, bone, or teeth seen arising from this protruberance.
    - Ectodermal tissue (skin derivatives and neural tissue) is always present, mesodermal tissue (fat, bone, cartilage, muscle) is present in over 90% of cases, and endodermal tissue (e.g., gastrointestinal and bronchial epithelium, thyroid tissue) is seen in the majority of cases.
    - Adipose tissue is present in 67% to 75% of cases, and teeth are seen in 31% of cases.
  - Contain adipose tissue (up to 75%) and are composed of cysts containing fatty sebum (>99%). This microscopic fat can be detected on computed tomography (CT) and magnetic resonance imaging (MRI) with frequency selective fat suppression.
  - Microscopic intracellular fat can be detected an MRI with chemical shift imaging (CSI) on in-phase and out-of-phase gradient echo images. Detection of fat in an ovarian mass is diagnostic of a teratoma.
  - Fat fluid level can often be seen within a teratoma as well as a mural nodule.
- Immature teratomas account for <1% of ovarian teratomas.
  - Contain immature, embryonic tissue types and tend to contain small amounts of adipose tissue
  - More solid and tend to be larger than mature cystic teratomas (MCTs)
  - Display malignant behavior such as capsular invasion and rapid growth as well as infiltration of adjustment tissues and peritoneal implants
- Monodermal teratomas are composed predominantly of a single tissue type such as thyroid tissue in struma ovarii.
  - They do not contain fat.

- Imaging:
  - US: preferred imaging modality. Typically seen as a cystic adenexal mass with some mural components. Spectrum of findings include:
    - Diffusely or partially echogenic mass with posterior sound attenuation owing to sebaceous material and hair within the cyst cavity
    - Dermoid plug or Rokitansky nodule: most common sonographic feature and appears as an echogenic mass within the cyst made up of hair, teeth, or fat
    - Dermoid mesh: appearance on ultrasound is of multiple small hyperechoic lines and dots within the cyst forming a meshlike picture. These echogenic foci are small hairs floating in the cystic fluid.
    - Tip of the iceberg sign: the appearance of a hyperechoic area, the base of which cannot be visualized. This is the result of a mass made up of matted hair and sebum casting an echogenic shadow.
    - Fat-fluid level: also known as a hair-fluid level or fluid-fluid level is believed to be the result of layering of serous fluid and sebum.
  - No internal vascularity on color Doppler.
  - MRI:
    - The sebaceous component of mature cystic teratomas has very high signal intensity on T1 weighted images, similar to retroperitoneal fat; however, hemorrhage appears bright on T1 weighted images as well.
    - The signal intensity of the sebaceous component on T2 weighted images is variable, usually approximating that of fat.
    - Fatty contents of a mature cystic teratoma can be distinguished from hemorrhage in an endometrioma by three methods: (1) chemical shift artifact in the frequency-encoding direction; (2) gradient-echo imaging with an echo time in which fat and water are in opposite phase and can demonstrate fat-water interfaces and mixtures of fat and water; and (3) sequences with frequency-selective fat saturation that suppress the high signal of teratomas and help distinguish them from hemorrhagic lesions

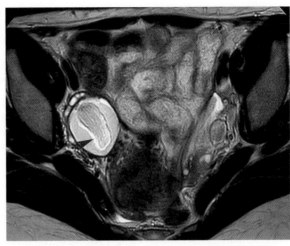

Fig. 34.2 Axial T2 weighted magnetic resonance image (MRI) shows cystic mass in the right ovary with central hyperintense components *(red arrow)*.

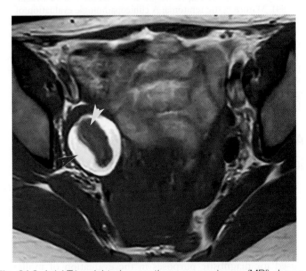

Fig. 34.3 Axial T1 weighted magnetic resonance image (MRI) shows hyperintense areas *(red arrow)* within the mass in the right ovary with central hypointense components *(yellow arrow)*, likely due to fluid.

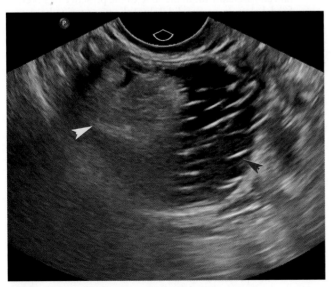

Fig. 34.1 Transvaginal ultrasound image of the ovary shows a cystic mass with hypoechoic lines and dots *(red arrow)* and lobular echogenic solid tissue within the cyst *(yellow arrow)*.

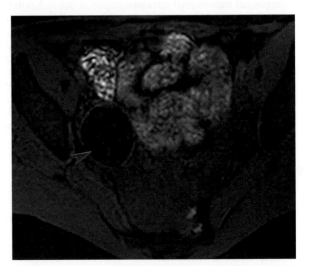

Fig. 34.4 Axial T1 fat suppressed magnetic resonance image (MRI) shows signal drop in the peripheral hyperintense component *(red arrow)* seen on the nonfat suppressed image, which would be consistent with fat and hence a mature cystic teratoma.

- Management: uncomplicated ovarian teratomas tend to be asymptomatic and are often discovered incidentally.
  - They are predisposed to ovarian torsion (up to 16%) and may then present with acute pelvic pain.
  - Other less likely complications include rupture (1–4%), malignant transformation (1–2%), superimpose infection (1%), and autoimmune hemolytic anemia (1%).
  - Initial serial follow-up for lesions <7 cm to monitor growth is considered, beyond which resection is advised.
  - Laproscopic approach is used for masses <8 cm to avoid intraoperative tumor spillage that can lead to postoperative peritonitis and adhesion formation.

REFERENCES

Brown, M. F., Hebra, A., McGeehin, K., & Ross III, A. J. (1993). Ovarian masses in children: A review of 91 cases of malignant and benign masses. *Journal of Pediatric Surgery, 28,* 930–933.

Caruso, P. A., Marsh, M. R., Minkowitz, S., & Karten, G. (1971). An intense clinicopathologic study of 305 teratomas of the ovary. *Cancer, 27,* 343–348.

Comerci Jr., J. T., Licciardi, F., Bergh, P. A., Gregori, C., & Breen, J. L. (1994). Mature cystic teratoma: A clinicopathologic evaluation of 517 cases and review of the literature. *Obstetrics and Gynecology, 84,* 22–28.

Matz, M. H. (1961). Benign cystic teratomas of the ovary. *Obstetrical & Gynecological Survey, 16,* 591–605.

Talerman, A. (1994). Germ cell tumors of the ovary. In: R. J. Kurman (Ed.), *Blaustein's pathology of the female genital tract* (4th ed., pp. 849–914). New York, NY: Springer-Verlag.

Togashi, K., Nishimura, K., Itoh, K., Fujisawa, I., Sago, T., … Minami, S. (1987). Ovarian cystic teratomas: MR imaging. *Radiology, 162,* 669–673.

CASE 35

Bicornuate Uterus

1. A, B, C, D. Müllerian duct anomalies comprise unicornuate uterus, uterus didelphys, bicornuate uterus, and septate uterus.
2. C. Magnetic resonance imaging (MRI) provides clear delineation of the internal and external uterine anatomy in multiple planes and, more importantly, reliable depiction of the external uterine contour. Computed tomography (CT) is not used for diagnostic purposes in the evaluation of müllerian duct anomalies. Hysterosalpingograhy does not allow assessment of the uterine fundus, which is the key to differentiating septate uterus from bicornuate uterus. Traditional two-dimensional transvaginal ultrasonography is not as helpful as three-dimensional ultrasonography with coronal plane reconstruction for visualizing the uterine fundus.
3. B. A fundal cleft >1 cm has been reported to be 100% sensitive and specific in differentiation of fusion anomalies (didelphys and bicornuate) from reabsorption anomalies (septate and arcuate).
4. A, B, D. Women with uterine didelphys can be asymptomatic or may present with dyspareunia especially in the presence of longitudinal uterovaginal septum. Increased preterm birth rates have also been reported in these women. Infertility is not associated with uterine didelphys.

Comment

- Background: uterine didelphys is a type of müllerian duct anomaly (class III) with duplication of the reproductive structures with the duplication limited to the uterus and cervix that is uterine didelphys and bicollis (two cervices).
  - Stems from complete midline nonfusion of the müllerian duct result in functional horns (hemiuteri) and cervices. Because fusion occurs in quarter to cranial direction, the vagina is often fused and presents as a single vagina.
  - Duplication of the vulva, bladder, urethra, vagina, and anus may also occur.
- Accounts for approximately 5% to 11% of müllerian duct anomalies.
- There is an association of this anomaly with concomitant appearance of both hemivagina and ipsilateral renal agenesis.
- In cases where concomitant renal agenesis is noted, there tends to be a prevalence of the anomaly to the right site.
- Clinical manifestation: most patients are asymptomatic but some present with dyspareunia or dysmenorrhea in the presence of a varying degree of longitudinal uterovaginal septum. Spontaneous abortion rates of 32% and preterm birth rates of 28% have been reported in women with uterus didelphys. Fetal growth restriction also appears to be increased.
- Classification of müllerian duct anomalies was developed by the American Fertility Society.
  - Class I anomalies consist of segmental agenesis and variable degrees of uterovaginal hypoplasia.
  - Class II anomalies are unicornuate uteri that represent partial or complete unilateral hypoplasia.
  - Class III anomalies comprise of uterus didelphys in which duplication of the uterus results from complete nonfusion of the müllerian ducts.
  - Class IV anomalies are bicornuate uteri that demonstrate incomplete fusion of the superior segments of the uterovaginal canal.
  - Class V anomalies are septate uteri that represent partial or complete nonresorption of the uterovaginal septum after fusion of the paramesonephric ducts. Septate uterus is the most common müllerian duct anomaly (55%) and is associated with some of the poorest reproductive and obstetric outcomes.
  - Class VI anomalies are adequate uteri that result from near-complete resorption of the septum.
  - Class VII anomalies comprise secondly of in utero diethylstilbesterol exposure.
- Imaging findings:
  - Hysterosalpingogram (HSG) separates oblong endometrial cavities with contrast opacification of fallopian tubes. The presence of an obstructed transverse septum may result in nonpacification of the ipsilateral uterine horn and is a potential pitfall leading to the misdiagnosis of unicornuate uterus.
  - US: true coronal image can help differentiate fusion (didelphys and bicornuate) anomalies from reabsorption (septate and arcuate) anomalies due to the presence of a uterine fundal cleft. In uterus didelphys, the two uterine horns are widely divergent with separate, noncommunicating endometrial cavities. Two cervices and duplicated upper vaginas can also be seen with ultrasound, though duplication of the vagina (hemivaginal septum) may not be apparent.
  - MRI: is much more accurate in differentiating between anomalies of fusion and anomalies of resorption.
    - Two widely divergent uterine horns and two separate cervices are seen with a cleft external fundal contour of the uterus.
    - A fundal cleft >1 cm has been reported to be 100% sensitive and specific in differentiation of fusion anomalies (didelphys and bicornuate) from reabsorption anomalies (septate and arcuate).
    - In uterus didelphys, the endometrial-to-myometrial ratio as well as the zonal anatomy are normal.
    - Duplication of the proximal vagina may be visualized at MRI, and this may be further improved by instillation of viscous liquid, such as ultrasound gel, into the vagina before imaging.
    - The presence of a unilateral hemivaginal septum obstructing one of the uterine horns will cause that horn to be markedly distended from blood products, demonstrating high signal intensity at T1 weighted imaging.

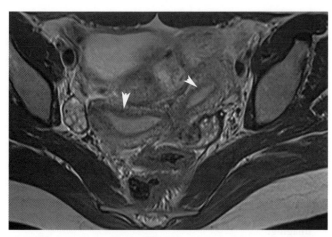

Fig. 35.1 Axial T2 weighted magnetic resonance image (MRI) of the pelvis through the uterine body shows a bicornuate uterus with two horns (*arrows*) seen in the pelvis.

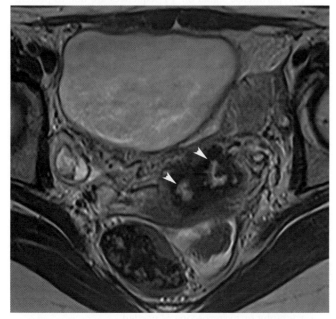

Fig. 35.2 Axial T2 weighted magnetic resonance image (MRI) of the pelvis through the cervix region shows duplicated cervical canal (*arrows*). This is consistent with uterine didelphys and bicollis.

REFERENCE

Behr, S. C., Courtier, J. L., & Qayyum, A. (2012). Imaging of müllerian duct anomalies. *Radiographics*, *32*, E233–E250.

CASE 36

Vaginal Wall Cyst

1. A, B, C. Location of the cyst inferior to the bladder as seen on the sagittal image suggests cystocele to be unlikely in this case. Gartner duct cyst and Bartholin cyst are vaginal wall cysts located at different levels within the vagina, which can help differentiate between the two. A urethral diverticulum is also possible in this case due to its close approximation to the urethra as seen on the axial image.
2. D. Vaginal wall cyst can be seen on any imaging modality; however, magnetic resonance imaging (MRI) best characterizes the anatomic location of the cyst and helps differentiate them from other regional cystic structures.
3. C. Location of the cyst within the vagina can help differentiate between the different types of vaginal wall cysts. All of the uncomplicated vaginal wall cysts appear hyperintense on T2 weighted images. A fluid level can be seen in these cysts in the presence of either hemorrhage or infection. Wall enhancement on postcontrast T1 weighted images is most commonly seen in the presence of infection.
4. A. Sagittal plane is most helpful for evaluation of the vaginal wall cysts, since the anatomic location of the level of the cyst in the vagina can help differentiate between the different types of vaginal wall cysts.

Comment

Introduction

- Vaginal cysts are typically seen as incidental findings on imaging.
- Most cysts are benign and remain small.
- Do not require surgical excision; however, they may be symptomatic when they are large in size or infected.
- Magnetic resonance imaging (MRI) is the best modality for characterization of the anatomic location of the cyst and to differentiate from other regional cystic structures.
- Imaging:
  - Typically well-circumscribed lesions that are isointense relative to fluid at MRI
  - Can be markedly heterogenous at imaging if they have proteinaceous content or are infected
- Different types of cysts seen in the vagina include Gartner duct cyst, Bartholin gland cyst, and Skene gland cyst and can be differentiated from each other and from Nabothian cysts on the basis of location.

Gartner Duct Cyst

- Develop from the vestigial remnants of the mesonephric duct or wolffian ducts.
- Most commonly develop in the anterior lateral wall of the upper vagina, about the level of the inferior border of the pubic symphysis.
- Can be associated with anomalies of the metanephric urinary system.
- Lined with nonmucinous cuboidal or columnar epithelium.
- Usually small and clinically silent but sometimes can be large enough to produce symptoms and cause mass effect on the urethra giving rise to urinary symptoms.
- Bartholin cyst, urethral diverticulum, and cystocele are other common differential diagnoses.

Bartholin Gland Cyst

- Arise in the superficial perineal pouch of the urogenital triangle and the ducts open into the posterior lateral aspect of the vaginal vestibule.
- They develop as a result of an obstruction of the gland duct by a stone or stenosis related to prior infection or trauma.
- Most common vulvar cysts, ranging in size from 1 to 4 cm.
- Patients are often asymptomatic but can present with mild dyspareunia in second or third decade of life or present with pain when the cyst is infected.
- Imaging:
  - CT: appear as hypoattenuating or hyperattenuating cyst near the vaginal introitus
  - MRI: appear as solitary round to oval cysts
    - Low to intermediate in signal intensity on T1 weighted images depending on the mucin content of the cyst fluid
    - Hyperintense on T2 weighted images

- Simple cysts are thin walled and unilocular, but septations can be seen. The cyst wall may be thickened and show enhancement if infected.
- Treatment
  - Symptomatic cysts are treated by means of marsupialization or surgical excision.

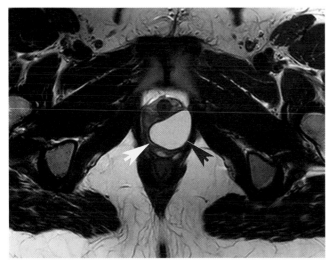

Fig. 36.1 Axial T2 weighted magnetic resonance image (MRI) shows T2 hyperintense mass *(red arrow)* in the region of the vagina, posterior to the urethra and anterior to the rectum. This was seen to arise from the anterior vaginal wall *(yellow arrow)* and hence was consistent with a Gartner duct cyst.

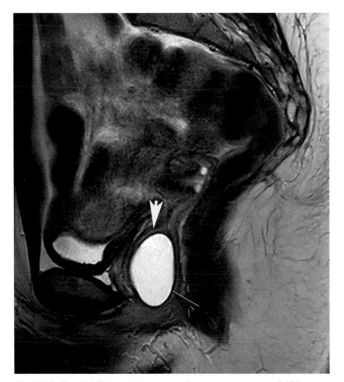

Fig. 36.2 Sagittal T2 weighted magnetic resonance image (MRI) shows T2 hyperintense mass *(red arrow)* in the region of the vagina, posterior to the urethra and anterior to the rectum. This was seen to arise from the anterior vaginal wall *(yellow arrow)* and hence was consistent with a Gartner duct cyst.

- Infected cysts are treated by incision and drainage with a definitive treatment after resolution of infection.
- A rare complication is development of squamous cell carcinoma or adenocarcinoma in a Bartholin gland duct or cyst, respectively.

Skene Gland Cysts

- Skene glands are paired structures located near the external urethral meatus, with ducts draining directly into the urethra lumen.
- Distinguished from urethral diverticula by their location, since urethral diverticula are usually midurethral in location.
- Can cause ureteral obstruction if large in size or cause urinary tract infections.
- Usually asymptomatic but may require drainage or excision due to superimposed infection.
- Imaging:
  - MRI: they are T2 hyperintense if uncomplicated and appear round in shape.
  - May have fluid level if complicated with debris or hemorrhage.
  - Hyperintense signal on T1 sequences are due to proteinaceous material.

REFERENCES
Chou, C. P., Levenson, R. B., Elsayes, K. M., Lin, Y. H., Fu, T. Y., … Chiu, Y. S. (2008). Imaging of female urethral diverticulum: An update. *Radiographics, 28,* 1917–1930.
Walker, D. K., Salibian, R. A., Salibian, A. D., Belen, K. M., & Palmer, S. L. (2011). Overlooked diseases of the vagina: A directed anatomic-pathologic approach for imaging assessment. *Radiographics, 31,* 1583–1598.

CASE 38
Endometrial Carcinoma

1. A, B, C. Hyperplasia, polyps, and endometrial carcinoma have overlapping imaging features and can present as thickening of the endometrium or have a masslike appearance. The masslike lesions shown in the figures are centered in the endometrial cavity and hence unlikely to be cervical carcinoma.
2. B. Endometrial thickness >5 mm in the setting of postmenopausal bleeding seen at transvaginal ultrasound should be investigated further with biopsy and potentially sonohysterography or hysteroscopy as needed.
3. B. Evaluation of the myometrium for disruption or discontinuity of the junctional zone, which is the inner myometrium visualized on magnetic resonance imaging (MRI) as a T2 dark band at the margins of the endometrial canal, is essential for staging of endometrial carcinoma. In postmenopausal women, the junctional zone may be focally indistinct, and when it is not visible but the interface between the endometrial and the myometrium is sharp and smooth, deep endometrial invasion is unlikely.
4. A, B, C, D. All of the conditions mentioned are risk factors for development of endometrial carcinoma.

Comment

- Background: endometrial carcinoma (EC) is the most common malignant neoplasm of the female genital tract in United States and the fourth most common cancer in women.
  - Most are postmenopausal with a mean age of diagnosis of 68 years old; however, up to 15% of cases may occur in premenopausal women.

Case 37 is online only and accessible at www.expertconsult.com.

- Most common genetic syndrome associated with endometrial carcinoma is hereditary nonpolyposis colorectal cancer (HNPCC) or Lynch syndrome.
- Risk factors for EC include conditions promoting increased exposure to unopposed estrogen such as hormonal replacement therapy, obesity, nulliparity, and tamoxifen therapy. Increased rate of obesity and aging population are contributory factors to the increased prevalence of EC.
- Patients with endometrial carcinoma typically present with abnormal uterine bleeding in postmenopausal women, and the diagnosis is confirmed based on the results of evaluation of endometrial biopsy, endometrial curettage, or hysterectomy specimens.
- Endometrial carcinomas have been classified into two types:
  - Type I neoplasms (most common) include endometrial adenocarcinomas, which arise from atypical endometrial hyperplasia and are estrogen dependent.
  - Type II neoplasms include more aggressive histologic variants such as clear cell, serous carcinomas, and uterine carcinoma sarcomas.
- Imaging findings: ultrasound is usually the first examination performed in women with history of vaginal bleeding.
  - US:
    - Premenopausal patients: the endometrium demonstrates a wide spectrum of appearances secondary to physiologic and hormonal changes; 15 to 16 mm is considered the upper limit of normal in premenopausal patients.
    - Postmenopausal endometrium: normal endometrium should appear thin, homogenous, and echogenic.
      - Most authors consider 5 mm as the upper limit of normality for endometrial thickness in postmenopausal women, which has a sensitivity of 96% and specificity of 61% in the diagnosis of EC in postmenopausal women with abnormal uterine bleeding.
      - Other ultrasound imaging features include heterogeneity, focal thickening, irregular endometrial margins, a polypoid mass in the endometrial cavity, intrauterine fluid collection, and frank myometrial invasion.
  - CT: is generally not used for initial diagnosis of endometrial carcinoma, and is useful for evaluation of more advanced disease with extrauterine spread, lymphadenopathy, and metastatic disease beyond the pelvis. EC may appear on CT as a dilated hypoenhancing endometrial cavity with or without enhancing solid nodules.
  - MRI: considered the most accurate imaging technique for preoperative assessment of endometrial cancer due to its excellent soft tissue contrast resolution.
    - Can accurately depict the depth of myometrial invasion, which is the most important morphologic prognostic factor and correlates with tumor grade, presence of lymph node metastasis, and overall patient survival.
    - EC usually appears hyperintense to isointense on T1 weighted images, and hyperintense or heterogenous on T2 weighted images, relative to normal endometrium and shows mild enhancement after IV contrast injection.
    - EC has restricted diffusion demonstrating high signal intensity on DWI images and low signal intensity on the apparent diffusion coefficient (ADC) maps.
    - The presence of myometrial invasion is suggested by an irregular interface and/or loss of the normal endometrium-myometrium interface.
    - Some limitations of MRI include distortion of the uterine anatomy by leiomyomas, presence of adenomyosis, and when the tumor involves the cornu of the uterus.

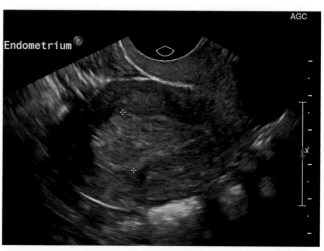

Fig. 38.1 Sagittal image from a B-mode transvaginal ultrasound shows uniform thickening of the endometrium. Differentials for this thickening in this postmenopausal woman would include hyperplasia, polyps, and endometrial carcinoma.

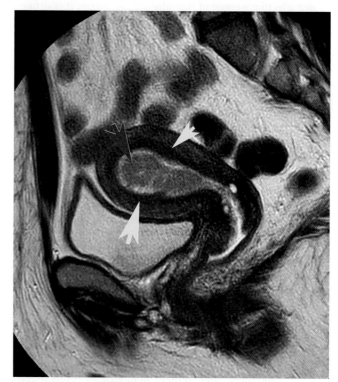

Fig. 38.2 Sagittal T2 weighted magnetic resonance image (MRI) of the pelvis shows expanded endometrial cavity filled with a mass with intermediate T2 signal *(red arrow)*. The underlying junctional zone *(yellow arrow)* is preserved as a thin T2 dark line in a myometrium and hence there is no tumor invasion into the myometrium.

REFERENCES

Beddy, P., Moyle, P., Kataoka, M., Yamamoto, A. K., Joubert, I., … Lomas, D. (2012). Evaluation of depth of myometrial invasion and overall staging in endometrial cancer: Comparison of diffusion-weighted and dynamic contrast-enhanced MR imaging. *Radiology, 262*(2), 530–537.

Faria, S. C., Devine, C. E., Rao, B., Sagebiel, T., & Bhosale, P. (2019). Imaging and staging of endometrial cancer. *Seminars in Ultrasound, CT and MRI, 40*(4), 287–294.

Wright, J. D., Barrena Medel, N. I., Sehouli, J., Fujiwara, K., & Herzog, T. J. (2012). Contemporary management of endometrial cancer. *Lancet, 379*, 1352–1360.

CASE 39

Endometriomas

1. A, C, D. The figures show high signal intensity on T2 and T1 weighted images. This can be seen with fat and blood, and hence hemorrhagic cysts, dermoids, or endometriomas are included in the differential diagnosis.
2. A. Patients with endometriosis are known to have an increased incidence of adenomyosis.
3. A. 1% of endometriomas could potentially undergo malignant transformation typically to endometrioid or clear cell carcinoma.
4. B. Endometriomas can undergo decidualization during pregnancy. In decidualization, there is hypertrophy of the stromal cells of the endometrium located in the endometrioma. The endometrioma increases in size and is more complex in appearance with solid mural nodules or papillary excrescences that may show vascularity on Doppler imaging.

Comment

- Background: endometriosis is a common and important disorder affecting women of reproductive age group. It is defined as the presence of functional endometrial glands and stroma outside the uterine cavity and is considered to be an inflammatory condition.
- Endometriosis is found in 2% to 8% of the general population but is found in 30% to 50% of women diagnosed with infertility.
- Clinical manifestations: endometriosis can be asymptomatic; however, it can also have a wide range of symptoms that can be vague and nonspecific.
  - Common clinical presentation is infertility. Endometriosis is found in approximately 30% to 50% of women diagnosed with infertility.
  - Other common symptoms include pelvic pain, pain with bowel movement, and abnormal uterine bleeding.
  - Rarely patients present with physical signs of endometriosis, which include localized tenderness or nodular masses of the cul-de-sac or uterosacral ligaments.
  - 1% of endometriomas could potentially undergo malignant transformation typically to endometrioid or clear cell carcinoma. These cancers typically occur in women older than age 45 and in endometriomas >9 cm.
- Location: typical location includes ovaries (75%), anterior or posterior cul-de-sac (70%), posterior broad ligament (50%), uterosacral ligament (35%), uterus (10%), and colon (5%).
- Imaging:
  - US: appearance can be highly variable.
    - Typical appearance: unilocular cyst with acoustic enhancement and diffuse homogenous ground-glass echoes as a result of hemorrhagic debris
    - Less typical features include:
      - Multiple locules
      - Hyperechoic wall foci
      - Cystic: solid lesion
      - Anechoic cysts
  - MRI: pathognomonic feature of endometriomas is the shading sign, which can be seen on T2 weighted images
    - T2 shading: reflects the chronic nature of endometriomas and is the result of cyclic bleeding occurring over time. Old blood products contain high iron and protein concentrations, which decrease in T2 relaxation time. Therefore on T2 weighted images endometriomas will show a gradual loss of signal within the lesion with low signal intensity till complete signal void in the dependent portion (shading).
    - T1 weighted images: high signal intensity

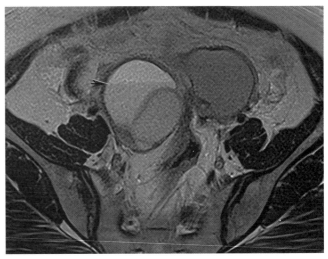

Fig. 39.1 Axial T2 weighted image from magnetic resonance imaging (MRI) showing multiple T2 hyperintense masses in the pelvis with T2 shading within them. Note the fluid level *(arrow)* seen in the right mass, which is consistent with endometriomas.

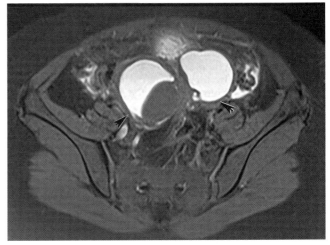

Fig. 39.2 Axial fat suppressed T1 weighted image from magnetic resonance imaging (MRI) showing multiple T1 hyperintense masses *(red arrows)* in the pelvis suggesting presence of hemorrhage within the masses. This is consistent with endometriomas.

- Fluid-fluid levels may also be observed within the lesion
- In some cases, ovaries may be joined together behind the uterus in the pouch of Douglas due to adhesion formation between the adjacent peritoneal surfaces, a sign described at US as "kissing ovaries."

REFERENCES

Bennett, G. L., Slywotzky, C. M., Cantera, M., & Hecht, E. M. (2010). Unusual manifestations and complications of endometriosis—spectrum of imaging findings: Pictorial review. *AJR. American Journal of Roentgenology, 194*(Suppl. 6), WS34–WS46. doi:10.2214/AJR.07.7142.

Foti, P. V., Farina, R., Palmucci, S., Vizzini, I. A. A., Libertini, N., ... Coronella, M. (2018). Endometriosis: Clinical features, MR imaging findings and pathologic correlation. *Insights Into Imaging, 9*(2), 149–172. doi:10.1007/s13244-017-0591-0.

Kawaguchi, R., Tsuji, Y., Haruta, S., Kanayama, S., Sakata, M., ... Yamada, Y. (2008). Clinicopathologic features of ovarian cancer in patients with ovarian endometrioma. *The Journal of Obstetrics and Gynaecology Research, 34*(5), 872–877. doi:10.1111/j.1447-0756.2008.00849.x.

CASE 40

C-Section Defect

1. B. The figure presented shows a hypointense linear area in the anterior lower uterine segment on ultrasound consistent with cesarean section scar.
2. C. Cesarean section scars are best identified on sagittal images on ultrasound, computed tomography (CT), or magnetic resonance imaging (MRI).
3. B. Postmenstrual spotting has been reported in more than twice as many women with a niche compared to those without and patients present with dysfunctional uterine bleeding or spotting 2 to 12 days after the routine menstrual cycle.
4. D. Sonohysterography is the best modality for imaging of the cesarean scar niche, since the fluid or gel instilled into the cavity will distend the niche and make it easily visible.

Comment

- Healed cesarean section scar appears as a narrow transverse line in the anterior lower uterine segment.
- Thinning and retraction of the anterior myometrium creates wedge-shaped defects on both the serosal and endometrial sides. This distortion and prominence of the tissues adjacent to the scar often have an hourglass shape on sagittal views.
- Imaging: Sagittal images are essential to identify cesarean scars on ultrasound (US), computed tomography (CT), or magnetic resonance imaging (MRI).
  - US: chronic cesarean scar site appears as a narrow hyperechoic or hypoechoic line in the thinned anterior lower uterine segment
  - CT: the scar site appears as isoattenuating to mildly hyperattenuating linear area in the anterior lower uterine segment
  - MRI: the scar site appears as a hypointense linear area on T1 and T2 weighted MRI. Focal areas of very low signal intensity can be seen on T1 or gradient echo MRI likely present in susceptibility artifact from surgical material or hemosiderin deposition.
- Cesarean scar niche: in some women there is tethering of the endometrium in the region of the old cesarean scar, creating a potential reservoir or niche that accumulates fluid or blood and may present as postmenstrual spotting or bleeding.
  - A niche is described as indentation of the myometrium of around 1 to 2 mm and is best seen on sonohysterography when it fills up the endometrial cavity distortion with fluid or gel.
  - Scar defects can have different shapes but are most commonly semicircular or triangular.

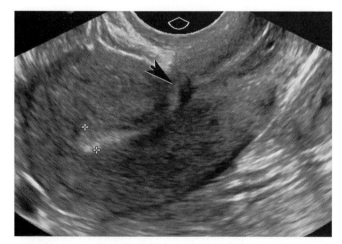

Fig. 40.1 Transvaginal ultrasound image in a sagittal orientation shows small hypoechoic linear area *(red arrow)* in the anterior lower uterine segment consistent with a cesarean section scar.

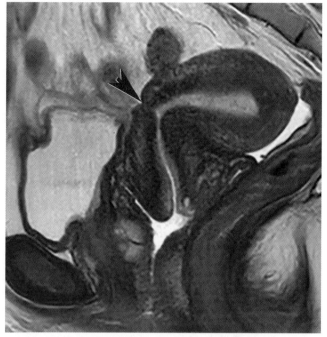

Fig. 40.2 Sagittal T2 weighted magnetic resonance image (MRI) shows a linear hypointense area *(red arrow)* in the lower uterine segment with thinning of the myometrium consistent with cesarean section scar.

REFERENCES

Rodgers, S. K., Kirby, C. L., Smith, R. J., & Horrow, M. M. (2012). Imaging after cesarean delivery: Acute and chronic complications. *Radiographics*, *32*, 1693–1712.

Zimmer, E. Z., Bardin, R., Tamir, A., & Bronshtein, M. (2004). Sonographic imaging of cervical scars after cesarean section. *Ultrasound in Obstetrics and Gynecology*, *23*, 594–598.

CASE 41

Fibroids

1. A. Figures show multiple fibroids in an enlarged uterus.
2. B. Fibroids are influenced by hormones (both estrogen and progesterone) and increase in size during pregnancy.
3. C. Submucosal fibroids are most likely to be symptomatic since they project into the endometrial cavity.
4. B, C. Fibroids with cystic and myxoid degeneration appear to have high signal intensity on T2 weighted images.

Comment

- Background: uterine fibroids, also known as leiomyomas, are the commonest uterine neoplasms.
  - They are benign tumors of smooth muscle origin, with varying amounts of fibrous connective tissue.
  - They are hormone dependent, responding to both estrogen and progesterone; and often increase in size during pregnancy and usually decrease in size after menopause.
  - Majority of women with fibroids are asymptomatic; however, 20% to 50% of them have symptoms such as menorrhagia, pelvic pain and infertility, or complications during pregnancy.
- Classification: uterine fibroids are classified according to their location as submucosal, intramural, or subserosal.
  - Submucosal fibroids are least common but most likely to be symptomatic since they project into the endometrial cavity.
    - Submucosal fibroids can occasionally become pedunculated and prolapse into the cervical canal or vagina.

- Intramural fibroids are the most common type and are usually asymptomatic.
  - They may cause infertility due to compression of the fallopian tubes.
- Subserosal fibroids project exophytically into the abdomen or pelvis and can also become pedunculated.
  - Pedunculated subserosal fibroids can undergo torsion and consequent infarction and thus be a cause of severe abdominal pain.
- Imaging:
  - Plain radiographs: can be identified if calcified or if large and causing compressive symptoms on surrounding bowel
  - US: the preferred initial modality in the imaging fibroids
    - Appear as well-defined, solid masses with a whorled appearance
    - Usually of similar echogenicity to the myometrium, but sometimes may be hypoechoic
    - Can cause the uterus to appear enlarged or may cause an alteration of the normal uterine contour
    - Often show a degree of posterior acoustic shadowing, which is more marked in calcified fibroids
    - Degenerated fibroids may have a complex appearance, with areas of cystic change
    - Doppler US typically shows circumferential vascularity; however, fibroids that are necrotic or have undergone torsion will show absence of flow.
  - CT: scan is not the investigation of choice for the characterization of pelvic masses.
    - Uterine fibroids are often seen incidentally on CT scans performed for other reasons.
    - Typically seen as bulky, irregular uterus or a mass in continuity with the uterus.
    - Degenerated fibroids may appear complex and contain areas of fluid attenuation.
    - Calcification is seen in ~4% of fibroids and is typically dense and amorphous.
  - MRI: is the preferred method for accurately characterizing pelvic masses.
    - On T2 weighted images, fibroids appear as well-defined masses of low signal intensity as compared to the myometrium.
    - On T1 weighted images, they appear isointense to the myometrium.

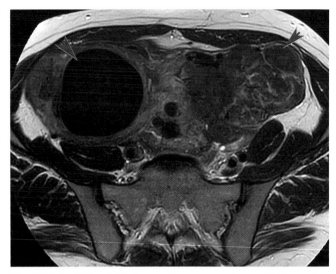

Fig. 41.2 Axial T2 weighted magnetic resonance image (MRI) showing multiple intramural fibroids in the uterus *(red arrows)*.

- Degenerated fibroids have a variable and often heterogeneous appearance, with minimal or irregular enhancement.
- Cystic degeneration results in high signal intensity on T2 weighted images and low signal intensity on T1 weighted images.
- Fibroids that have undergone myxoid degeneration are filled with a gelatinous material and can be difficult to differentiate from fibroids that have undergone cystic degeneration; however, they typically appear as more complex cystic masses.
- Red, or carneous, degenerated fibroids have a peripheral rim of low signal on T2 weighted images and high signal on T1 weighted images

REFERENCES

Murase, E., Siegelman, E. S., Outwater, E. K., Perez-Jaffe, L. A., & Tureck, R. W. (1999). Uterine leiomyomas: histopathologic features, MR imaging findings, differential diagnosis, and treatment. *Radiographics*, 19(5), 1179–1197.

Wilde, S., & Scott-Barrett, S. (2009). Radiological appearances of uterine fibroids. *The Indian Journal of Radiology & Imaging*, 19(3), 222–231. doi:10.4103/0971-3026.54887.

CASE 42

Ovarian Vein Thrombosis

1. B, D. Computed tomography images show filling defect within the left ovarian vein representing left ovarian vein thrombosis. The gonadal vein is not completely opacified. Mixing flow artifact can be seen as a filling defect and may simulate thrombus.
2. A. Predisposing factors for ovarian vein thrombosis include hypercoagulability, stasis of blood flow, and recent cesarean section.
3. D. The most common presenting signs and symptoms of ovarian vein thrombosis include triad of right lower abdominal or flank pain, fever resistant to antibiotic therapy, and palpable cordlike tender abdominal mass.
4. B. Ovarian vein thrombosis is observed almost exclusively in females. The right side is more frequently affected and occurs more commonly in puerperium and postpartum periods than in early pregnancy.

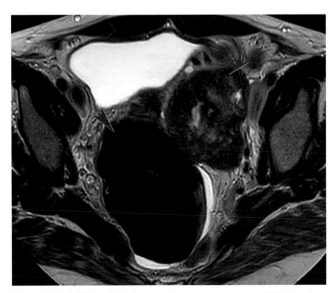

Fig. 41.1 Axial T2 weighted magnetic resonance image (MRI) showing two large subserosal fibroids arising from the uterus *(red arrows)*.

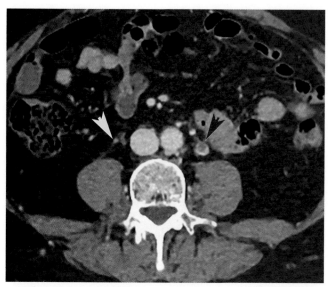

Fig. 42.1 Axial postcontrast computed tomography image through the midabdomen shows dilated left ovarian vein with a filling defect within it *(red arrow)*. This suggest ovarian vein thrombosis. Note normal appearance of the right ovarian vein *(yellow arrow)*.

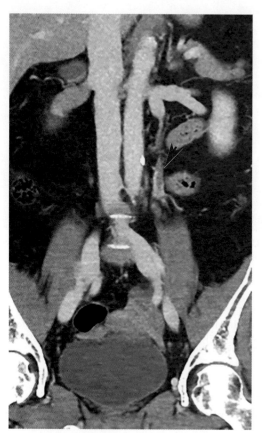

Fig. 42.2 Coronal postcontrast computed tomography image through the midabdomen shows dilated left ovarian vein with a filling defect within it *(red arrow)*. This suggest ovarian vein thrombosis.

Comment

- Ovarian vein thrombosis occurs most commonly in postpartum patients and can result in pulmonary emboli.
- Incidence of postpartum ovarian vein thrombosis is 1 in 600 to 1 in 2000 deliveries.
- Ovarian veins originate from the plexus in the broad ligament near the ovary and fallopian tube and communicate with the uterine plexus and then course upward anterior to the psoas muscle and the ureter.
  - Right ovarian vein drains into the inferior vena cava.
  - Left ovarian vein drains into the left renal vein in most individuals.
- Ovarian vascular pedicle sign: can help in localizing origin of pelvic masses by tracing the ovarian veins retrograde to the adnexa.
- Ovarian vein thrombosis can also occur in patients with pelvic inflammatory disease, oncology patients, and is a complication of pelvic surgery.
- Imaging:
  - US: may be difficult to visualize ovarian vein due to overnight bowel gas. Ovarian veins are seen as tubular subvention in hypoechoic structures in the adnexa adjacent to the ovarian arteries. If the ovarian veins are identified, absence of Doppler flow can be a diagnostic feature of ovarian vein thrombosis.
  - CT: tubular structure with an enhancing wall and low attenuation thrombus in the expected location of the right ovarian vein.
- Treatment: anticoagulation and antibiotics if necessary

REFERENCE

Karaosmanoglu, D., Karcaaltincaba, M., Karcaaltincaba, D., Akata, D., & Ozmen, M. (2009). MDCT of the ovarian vein: Normal anatomy and pathology. *AJR. American Journal of Roentgenology, 192,* 295–299.

CASE 43

Normal Ovaries and Corpus Luteum

1. B, D. The volume and maximal diameter of ovaries and ovarian follicles and the number of ovarian follicles differ significantly with age but not between the two ovarian phases of the menstrual cycle. Corpus luteum is seen in the postovulatory luteal ovarian phase and secretory uterine phase and is occasionally hemorrhagic. Ovarian stroma becomes edematous with a bank torsion and not in response to cyclical changes.
2. A. The zonal anatomy of ovaries is best seen on magnetic resonance imaging (MRI) on T2 weighted images.
3. A. A corpus luteum cyst develops when the corpus luteum fails to regress after ablation and instead enlarges with or without hemorrhage.
4. D. The ring-of-fire sign is the presence of ringlike peripheral hypervascularity on color Doppler imaging with a characteristic low impendance and high diastolic flow. This sign can be seen in highly vascular pelvic lesions such as corpus luteum and in ectopic pregnancy.

Comment

- Menstrual cycle/ovarian cycle: each menstrual cycle can be divided into three phases on the basis of events in the ovary (ovarian cycle) and in the uterus (uterine cycle based on the changes in the endometrium). These cycles are controlled by the endocrine system and physiologic hormonal variations.
  - Ovarian cycle: phases in the ovarian cycle are follicular phase, ovulation, and luteal phase. In each ovarian cycle a few follicles are stimulated by the follicles' terminating

hormone (FSH); however, only one dominant follicle can reach majority and will contain the ovum. During ovulation, the ovum is released from the mature follicle under the influence of the luteinizing hormone (LH). During the luteal phase, the pituitary hormones FSH and LH cause the remaining parts of the dominant follicles to transform into the corpus luteum, which produces progesterone.

- Uterine menstrual cycle includes menstruation, proliferative phase, and secretory phase.

- Imaging findings:
  - The ovaries in women of reproductive age show a distinct zonal anatomy on T2 weighted images: low-intensity cortex containing high-intensity follicles and intermediate-intensity medulla. During the menstrual phase, the ovaries shrink and have smaller follicles and demonstrate lower signal intensity of the medulla due to decreased water content within the stroma. During periovulation, the ovaries reach their maximum size and have an enlarged dominant follicle. The medulla has high signal intensity due to T2 prolongation caused by vascularized edematous changes in the stroma.
  - In postmenopausal women, the ovaries shrink to half the size of those in premenopausal women, and the zonal anatomy on T2 weighted images becomes obscure.

- Corpus luteum: after ablation, the developing corpus luteum contains a heterogenous population of cells that induces steroidogenic luteal cells.
  - Corpus luteum maintains a high degree of vascularization, which is seen as a ring of fire sign: the presence of ringlike peripheral hypervascularity with a characteristic low impedance, high diastolic flow pattern. Other features on imaging include thick-walled or an ovarian lesion with convoluted wall, which may be hemorrhagic.
  - Corpus luteum is essential for establishing and maintaining pregnancy, since it secretes progesterone, which is a steroid hormone responsible for the desidualization of the endometrium.
  - Seen at the end of luteal phase or during pregnancy. When associated with pregnancy, most corpus luteum cysts spontaneously involute at the end of the second trimester.
  - Follicular cyst develops when a dominant follicle does not rupture or release the ovum and instead grows and turns into a cyst. They resolve spontaneously in two or three menstrual cycles.

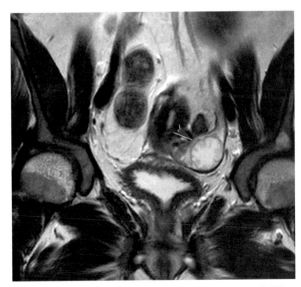

Fig. 43.1 Coronal T2 weighted magnetic resonance image (MRI) showing a cyst *(red arrow)* in the left ovary with crenulated appearance. This was consistent with a corpus luteum cyst.

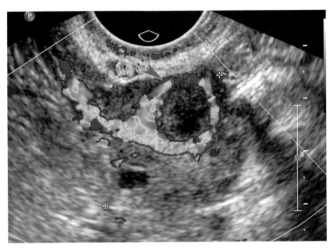

Fig. 43.2 Color Doppler image of the left ovary showing a cyst with a thick irregular wall with a ring of fire sign *(red arrow)* around it. This was consistent with a corpus luteum cyst.

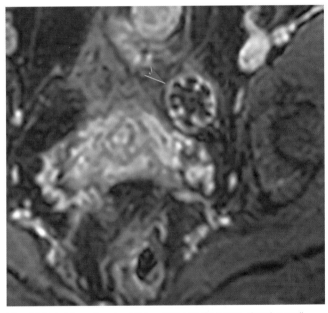

Fig. 43.3 Axial postcontrast T1 weighted MRI image showing wall enhancement in the cyst in the left ovary *(red arrow),* which as an irregular thickened wall consistent with a corpus luteum cyst.

REFERENCE
Takeuchi, M., Matsuzaki, K., & Nishitani, H. (2010). Manifestations of the female reproductive organs on MR images: Changes induced by various physiologic states. *Radiographics, 30,* 1147.

CASE 44

Proximal Fallopian Tube Occlusion/Hydrosalpinx

1. D. Intraperitoneal free spill of contrast is not shown, indicating bilateral proximal fallopian tube occlusion.
2. B. The globular area of filling at the left adnexa represents hydrosalpinx.
3. C. From the ovary, an ovum sequentially traverses the infundibulum, ampulla, and isthmus of the fallopian tube.
4. B. Hysterosalpingography is typically performed during the midproliferative phase, between days 7 and 10.

Comment

Diagnosis and Imaging Findings

A range of imaging examinations is used in the evaluation of subfertility, a condition of reduced fertility despite a prolonged period of unwanted nonconception. (Infertility encompasses a more stringent definition of inability to conceive despite regular unprotected intercourse over 1 year.) Imaging exams include ultrasonography (US), hysterosalpingo-contrast-enhanced US, magnetic resonance imaging (MRI), and hysterosalpingography (HSG).

HSG is typically performed between days 7 and 10 of the menstrual cycle, for fluoroscopic assessment of the uterine cavity and fallopian tubal patency. The cervix is cannulated under direct visualization, and contrast material is injected via catheter for retrograde opacification of the uterus and fallopian tubes, until intraperitoneal spillage of contrast is confirmed bilaterally.

Intraperitoneal free spill of contrast is typically seen as contrast pools with concave margins, the latter imposed by adjacent pelvic organs such as the ovaries and bowel loops. Gentle turning of the patient under fluoroscopic visualization can help accentuate free intraperitoneal contrast. HSG has sensitivity and specificity of 92% and 86%, respectively, for detecting bilateral tubal disease. Stasis of tubal contrast is interpreted as a sign of tubal occlusion. The opacification of tubular or globular contrast pools with convex margins may signify the presence of peritubal adhesions, hydrosalpinx, or hematosalpinx, such as can be seen in endometriosis. In the setting of endometriosis, the presence of hydrosalpinx reduces the probability of conceiving by half, and doubles the rate of spontaneous abortion.

HSG may also demonstrate intrauterine filling defects, or intrauterine abnormalities, including the spectrum of congenital uterine abnormalities that may impact fertility. Intrauterine filling defects may represent endometrial polyps, submucosal fibroids, or intrauterine adhesions (Asherman syndrome).

Treatment

Multiple treatment options are available when tubal occlusion is detected. These include surgical laparoscopic salpingectomy and fluoroscopically guided fallopian tube recanalization.

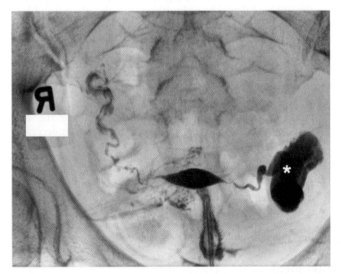

Fig. 44.1 Spot fluoroscopic image during hysterosalpingography demonstrates a globular area of filling at the left adnexa *(asterisk),* representing hydrosalpinx. Intraperitoneal free spill of contrast is not shown, indicating bilateral proximal fallopian tube occlusion.

REFERENCES

Simpson, W. L., Beitia, L. G., & Mester, J. (2006). Hsterosalpinography: A reemerging study. *Radiographics, 26,* 419–431.

Vickramarajah, S., Stewar, V., van Ree, K., Hemingway, A. P., Crofton, M. E., & Bharwani, N. (2017). Subfertibiliy: What the radiologist needs to know. *Radiographics, 37,* 1587–1602.

CASE 45

Adenomyosis

1. A, B, D. T2 weighted image shows hyperintense foci in the myometrium with intervening dark signal as seen in adenomyosis. Most fibroids are well-defined lesions, which are hypointense on T2 weighted images due to the presence of smooth muscle within. Cystic changes can be seen in fibroids in the presence of cystic degeneration; however, this is seen in well-defined lesions. Myometrial contractions resolve with time and do not show cystic areas within them. Endometrial carcinomas arise within the endometrium and may extend into the myometrium; however, they are mildly hyperintense on T2 weighted images.

2. A. T2 hyperintense foci seen in the myometrium adjacent to the endometrium is the most specific feature for adenomyosis and is due to islands of ectopic endometrial tissue and cystic dilatation of glands seen in this region.

3. B. The junctional zone is an area of high signal intensity seen on T2 weighted images between the endometrium and myometrium.

4. D. A junctional zone a thickness of <8 mm generally exclusive diagnosis of adenomyosis. Junctional zone >12 mm is associated with a sensitivity and specificity of 93% and 91%, respectively, and is considered a strong indicator for adenomyosis.

Comment

- Background: adenomyosis is a nonneoplastic condition, pathologically characterized by benign invasion of ectopic endometrium into the myometrium with adjacent smooth muscle hyperplasia.
  - Reported prevalence of adenomyosis in hysterectomy specimens varies from 5% to 70%.
- Clinical manifestation: adenomyosis occurs mainly in premenopausal women, particularly those who are multiparous.
  - Symptoms are nonspecific, and common symptoms include dysmenorrhea, menorrhagia, and abnormal uterine bleeding.
  - Patients frequently have associated disorders, most commonly leiomyoma and endometriosis.
- Imaging findings:
  - US:
    - Asymmetric myometrial thickening
    - Subendometrial linear striations and/or cysts, which may produce the characteristic "Venetian blinds sign"
    - Hypervascular on color Doppler imaging
  - MRI: is an accurate, noninvasive modality for diagnosing adenomyosis with a high sensitivity (78–88%) and specificity (67–93%).
    - Adenomyosis appears as either diffuse or focal thickening of the junctional zone forming an ill-defined area of low signal intensity, occasionally with embedded bright foci on T2 weighted images.
    - Areas of low signal intensity on T2 weighted images correspond to smooth muscle hyperplasia, and bright foci on T2 weighted images correspond to islands of ectopic endometrial tissue and cystic dilatation of glands.
    - When menstrual hemorrhage occurs within these ectopic endometrial tissues, signal intensity on T1 weighted images may become high.
    - The most important MRI criterion for diagnosis of adenomyosis is maximal junctional zone (JZ) thickness (JZ_{max}) ≥12 mm, which is associated with a sensitivity and a specificity of 93% and 91%, respectively.

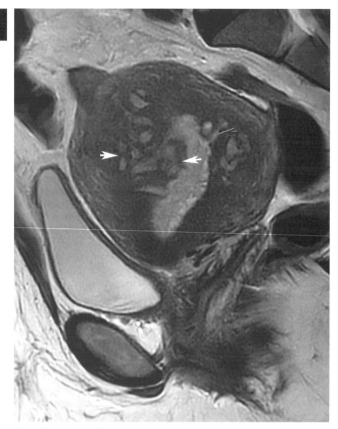

Fig. 45.1 Sagittal T2 weighted image through the uterus, which shows thickening of the junctional zone *(between the two white arrows)* with cystic spaces in the myometrium *(red arrow)*, which are due to extension of the endometrium into the myometrium.

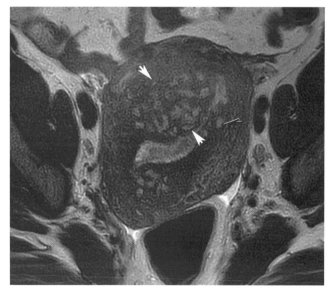

Fig. 45.2 Axial T2 weighted image through the uterus, which shows thickening of the junctional zone *(between the two white arrows)* with cystic spaces in the myometrium *(red arrow)*, which are due to extension of the endometrium into the myometrium.

- Other criteria include:
  - Ratio of JZ_{max} over the full myometrium thickness measured at the same place ($ratio_{max}$) >40% (sensitivity 65%, specificity 93%)
  - Difference in maximal and minimal thicknesses in both anterior and posterior portions of the uterus (JZ differential = JZ_{diff}) of >5 mm (sensitivity and specificity of 70% and 85%, respectively)
  - The presence of a big smooth regular uterus (sensitivity 23%, specificity 98%)
  - Myometrial cysts (<3 mm in size) are pathognomonic of adenomyosis; however, they are seen in only half the cases on T2 weighted images.
- Management: treatment for adenomyosis depends on the patient's symptoms, age, and desire for future fertility. The definitive treatment is hysterectomy, but initially less invasive approaches include nonsteroidal antiinflammatory drugs, menstrual-suppression hormonal therapy with danazol (oral or intrauterine device [IUD]) or gonadotropin-releasing hormone (GnRH) agonist, endometrial resection or ablation, and uterine artery embolization (UAE).

REFERENCES

Ascher, S. M., Arnold, L. L., Patt, R. H., Schruefer, J. J., Bagley, A. S., ... Semelka, R. C. (1994). Adenomyosis: Prospective comparison of MR imaging and transvaginal sonography. *Radiology, 190,* 803–806.

Azziz, R. (1989). Adenomyosis: Current perspectives. *Obstetrics and Gynecology Clinics of North America, 16,* 221–235.

Bazot, M., Cortez, A., Darai, E., Rouger, J., Chopier, J., ... Antoine, J. M. (2001). Ultrasonography compared with magnetic resonance imaging for the diagnosis of adenomyosis: Correlation with histopathology. *Human Reproduction, 16,* 2427–2433.

Reinhold, C., McCarthy, S., Bret, P. M., Mehio, A., Atri, M., ... Zakarian, R. (1996). Diffuse adenomyosis: Comparison of endovaginal US and MR imaging with histopathologic correlation. *Radiology, 199,* 151–158.

CASE 46
Testicular Torsion

1. B. The major diagnostic consideration for acute onset of scrotal pain without prior trauma includes testicular torsion, epididymitis, epididymoorchitis, torsion of the testicular appendage, strangulated inguinal hernia, and testicular neoplasm. Color Doppler ultrasound in the figures shows absence of right testicular blood flow. The right testis is slightly enlarged and heterogenous in appearance. In a patient with acute onset of scrotal pain, the findings are characteristic of testicular torsion.
2. D. Bell clapper deformity is a congenital anomaly in which there is lack of normal attachment of the testes to the posterior scrotal wall and the testes can twist freely within the tunica vaginalis, predisposing it to torsion.
3. B. In patients with acute testicular torsion, testicular salvage rates decrease with prolonged ischemia. During the first 6 hours, testicular salvage rates are nearly 100%. It decreases to 70% between 6 and 12 hours and is only 20% between 12 and 24 hours.
4. A. Torsion of the spermatic cord initially results in testicular venous outflow obstruction, followed by arterial obstruction. The right and left testicular arteries originate from the anterior aspect of the abdominal aorta just distal to the renal arteries. Color and power Doppler ultrasound have higher sensitivity and specificity than grayscale ultrasound in detecting testicular torsion.

Comment

- Testicular torsion occurs when the testis torts on the spermatic cord.
- Most common symptom is acute testicular pain.

- Majority are either spontaneous or in the setting of minor/incidental trauma.
- First venous and later arterial flow is obstructed.
- Extent of testicular ischemia will depend on the degree of twisting (180–270 degrees) and the duration of torsion.
- Testicular salvage is more likely in patients treated within 4 to 6 hours after onset of torsion.
- Two types are recognized:
  - Extravaginal: seen mainly in newborns and occurs prenatally in most cases
  - Intravaginal: can occur at any age but more common in adolescents
    - Predisposing factor is the bell clapper deformity in which the tunica vaginalis joins high on the spermatic cord leaving the testis free to rotate.
- Imaging:
  - US: modality of choice for evaluating the potentially torsed testis
    - Key findings include
      - Twisting of spermatic cord: most sensitive and specific finding in both complete and incomplete torsion
      - Altered blood flow
        - Incomplete torsion: elevated resistive index >0.75 and to and for flow
        - Complete torsion: absence of blood flow in both testis and epididymis
      - Increased size of testis and spididymis
      - Homogenous echotexture early and then heterogenous echotexture after 24 hours, which implies necrosis
      - Reactive hydrocele
      - Reactive thickening of scrotal skin with hyperemia and increased flow on color Doppler
      - Whirlpool sign in the spermatic cord: the intrascrotal portion of the edematous cord appears as a round, ovoid, or curled echogenic extratesticular mass with epididymal head wrapped around it
      - Orientation of the testis, cord, and epididymis may be inverted
- Treatment: key is rapid diagnosis and surgical intervention
  - Likelihood of salvage is directly related to the time of onset and detorsion
    - <6 hours: 100% salvage
    - 6 to 12 hours: 50%
    - 12 to 24 hours: 20%

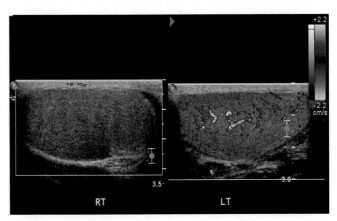

Fig. 46.1 Color Doppler ultrasound image of the right and left testes side-by-side shows normal intratesticular flow in the left testes but absence of flow in the right testes.

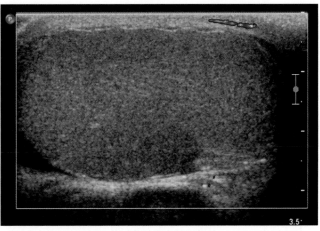

Fig. 46.2 Sagittal color Doppler ultrasound image of the right testes shows complete absence of intratesticular flow.

REFERENCES

Aso, C., Enríquez, G., Fité, M., Torán, N., Piró, C., … Piqueras, J. (2005). Gray-scale and color Doppler sonography of scrotal disorders in children: An update. *Radiographics, 25*, 1197–1214.

Bhatt, S., & Dogra, V. S. (2008). Role of US in testicular and scrotal trauma. *Radiographics, 28*, 1617–1629.

Vijayaraghavan, S. B. (2006). Sonographic differential diagnosis of acute scrotum: Real-time whirlpool sign, a key sign of torsion. *Journal of Ultrasound in Medicine, 25*, 563–574.

CASE 47

Fournier Gangrene

1. A, B, C, D. Multiple foci of soft tissue gas and extensive soft tissue inflammation are highly suspicious for Fournier gangrene in this patient. Soft tissue gas can also be seen postoperatively and secondly to penetrating injury and decubitus ulcer.
2. B. All illicit disorders have unknown predisposing factors of Fournier gangrene, but diabetes mellitus is the most commonly associated predisposing factor and is seen in 20% to 70% of patients with Fournier gangrene.
3. C. Computed tomography (CT) is a modality of choice in patients with Fournier gangrene and may confirm the diagnosis in clinically equivocal cases, depict the source of infection, and determine the extent of the disease before surgery. Plain radiography may show soft tissue gas, and ultrasonography may depict fluid and gas of the subcutaneous tissues, but extent of the disease is incompletely evaluated. Magnetic resonance imaging (MRI) shows the soft tissue involvement better than CT; however, it does not show the presence of gas well.
4. B. Fournier gangrene is usually polymicrobial infection, including both aerobic and anaerobic bacteria. Major and complete surgical deployment with intravenous administration of broad-spectrum antibiotics is the treatment of choice. Infection in Fournier gangrene spreads along the fascial planes and can extend into the abdominal wall, retroperitoneum, and thigh. Men are 10 times more commonly affected than women.

Comment

- Fournier gangrene (FG) is a fulminant form of infective necrotizing fasciitis of the perineal, genital, or perianal regions, which commonly affects men but can also occur in women and children.
- Source of infection in the vast majority of cases is either perineal or genital skin infections. Anorectal or urogenital and

perineal trauma, including pelvic and perineal injury or pelvic interventions, are other causes of FG.

- Comorbid systemic disorders such as diabetes mellitus and alcohol misuse are seen. Diabetes mellitus is reported to be present in 20% to 70% of patients with FG and chronic alcoholism in 25% to 50% of patients.
- Cultures from the wounds commonly show polymicrobial infections by aerobes and anaerobes. On an average, at least three organisms are cultured from each diagnosed patient.
- Infection commonly starts as a cellulitis adjacent to the portal of entry, depending on the source of infection, commonly in the perineum or perianal region. Crepitus of the inflamed tissues is a common feature because of the presence of gas-forming organisms.
- Spread of infection is along the facial planes. The subcutaneous emphysema in Fournier gangrene dissects along fascial planes and can extend from the scrotum and perineum to the inguinal regions, thighs, abdominal wall, and retroperitoneum.
- Imaging: CT plays an important role in the diagnosis as well as the evaluation of disease extent for appropriate surgical treatment. CT has greater specificity for evaluating disease extent than radiography, US, or physical examination.
  - CT: features include soft tissue thickening and inflammation. CT can demonstrate asymmetric fascial thickening, any coexisting fluid collection or abscess, fat stranding around the involved structures, and subcutaneous emphysema secondary to gas-forming bacteria.
  - Radiography: hyperlucencies representing soft tissue gas may be seen in the region overlying the scrotum or perineum.
  - US: thickened, edematous scrotal wall. The thickened scrotal wall contains hyperechoic foci that demonstrate reverberation artifacts, causing "dirty" shadowing that represents gas within the scrotal wall.
  - Up to 90% of patients with Fournier gangrene have been reported to have subcutaneous emphysema, so that at least 10% do not demonstrate this finding.
- Treatment: includes hemodynamic stabilization, intravenous administration of broad-spectrum antibiotics using multiple antimicrobial agents, and immediate and complete surgical debridement of the necrotic tissue.

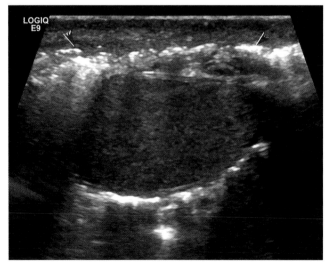

Fig. 47.1 Sagittal ultrasound image of the right scrotum shows normal appearance of the right testes with linear echogenic area seen in the subcutaneous tissues (*red arrow*) consistent with air. Scrotal thickening is also present, which suggests diagnosis of Fournier gangrene.

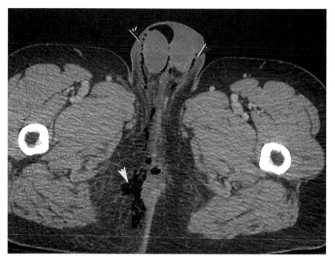

Fig. 47.2 Axial noncontrast computed tomography (CT) image shows extensive soft tissue swelling and inflammation and multiple foci of gas (*red arrows*) in the perineum extending into the scrotum and subcutaneous tissue of the gluteal region on the right side (*yellow arrow*). This confirmed the diagnosis of Fournier gangrene.

REFERENCES

Levenson, R. B., Singh, A. K., & Novelline, R. A. (2008). Fournier gangrene: Role of imaging. *Radiographics, 28,* 519–528.

Thwaini, A., Khan, A., Malik, A., Cherian, J., Barua, J., … Shergill, I. (2006). Fournier's gangrene and its emergency management. *Postgraduate Medical Journal, 82,* 516–519.

CASE 48

Esophageal Adenocarcinoma, With Esophageal Stent Migration

1. C. In a patient with relevant risk factors, circumferential distal esophageal narrowing and irregularity must be viewed with high suspicion for esophageal malignancy.
2. A. In the distal esophagus, adenocarcinoma is more likely than squamous cell carcinoma. Achalasia typically demonstrates pronounced dilatation of the upper to midesophagus. Herpes esophagitis typically demonstrates multiple fine esophageal ulcers.
3. C. While smoking and alcohol use are risk factors common to both esophageal squamous cell carcinoma and adenocarcinoma, Barrett esophagus represents a risk factor for adenocarcinoma.
4. C. The figures demonstrate migration of the esophageal stent, proximal to the distal esophageal malignancy. The patient would benefit from endoscopic intervention to reposition the esophageal stent.

Comment

Diagnosis and Imaging Findings

While the most prevalent of primary esophageal malignancies worldwide is squamous cell carcinoma, esophageal adenocarcinoma has become the predominant type of esophageal cancer in North America and Europe, and is most commonly seen in the distal third of the esophagus. Imaging findings of advanced disease typically include irregular mural thickening and mucosal abnormality, in a circumferential pattern (so-called apple-core lesion).

Risk factors for esophageal adenocarcinoma are gastroesophageal reflux disease (GERD) and obesity. A precursor lesion to adenocarcinoma is Barrett esophagus, whereby the normal squamous epithelium is replaced by intestinal columnal epithelium. While Barrett esophagus can be detected endoscopically, it is not reliably assessed by radiologic examination. In analogous terms, alcohol and tobacco use are the main risk factors of squamous cell carcinoma, and esophageal squamous dysplasia is the precursor lesion.

Treatment

In the United States, the overall 5-year survival rate for patients with esophageal adenocarcinoma is 17%. Most tumors are found when regional or distant metastatic disease is already present; endoscopic ultrasonography and positron emission tomography positively impact staging accuracy.

Disease limited to the esophageal mucosa can be treated endoscopically. Surgical esophagectomy, without or with neoadjuvant chemotherapy, is the preferred approach to locally advanced tumors.

In cases deemed unresectable, patients can undergo endoscopic stenting to relieve obstructive symptoms. Acute complications include esophageal perforation, bleeding, and bronchotracheal compression. Delayed complications include perforation, stent migration, tumor ingrowth, stent occlusion or food impaction, and mucosal erosion/bleeding.

REFERENCES

Gollub, M. J., Gerdes, H., & Bains, M. S. (1997). Radiographic appearance of esophageal stents. *Radiographics, 17,* 1169–1182.

Rustgi, A. K., & El-Serag, H. B. (2014). Esophageal carcinoma. *New England Journal of Medicine, 371,* 2499–2509.

CASE 49

Cricopharyngeal Bar

1. B. Cricopharyngeal bar represents hypertrophic prominence or spasm of the cricopharyngeus muscle.
2. B. The typical location of cricopharyngeal bar is anterior to lower cervical vertebrae, C4–C6.
3. A. Cricopharyngeal bar is a smoothly marginated posterior filling defect, which moves with swallowing.
4. A. Based on the imaging findings, cricopharyngeal bar is the best choice. Ulcer, Barrett esophagus, and squamous cell carcinoma present as irregularly marginated mucosal or mural masses.

Comment

Diagnosis and Imaging Findings

The radiologic finding of focal prominence at the junction of the hypopharynx and cervical esophagus is commonly referred to as a cricopharyngeal bar. Ascribed to hypertrophic prominence or fibrosis of the cricopharyngeus muscle, it is typically seen as a smooth, posterior filling defect of the esophagus at the level of C5–C6. Its prevalence has been reported in 5% to 19% of unselected series, and may be found in an asymptomatic patient, or a patient with dysphagia.

Management

In an asymptomatic patient, no treatment is indicated. In a patient with symptomatic dysphagia, varying treatment pathways include endoscopic dilatation, laser ablation, and surgical myotomy.

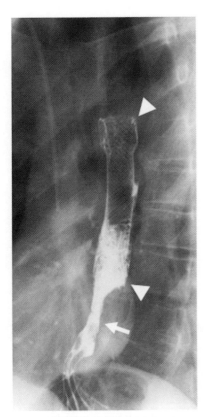

Fig. 48.1 Contrast esophagram. At base magnification, a stent is shown in the midthoracic esophagus *(arrowheads),* proximal to a circumferential segment of irregular distal esophageal narrowing *(white arrow).*

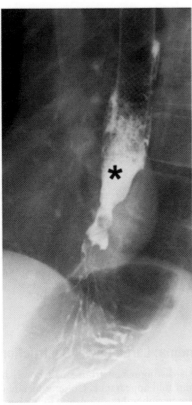

Fig. 48.2 Contrast esophagram. Magnified image confirms luminal narrowing, and retained contrast proximally *(asterisk),* indicating partial obstruction by tumor due to stent migration.

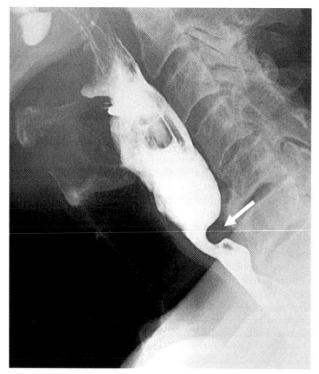

Fig. 49.1 Lateral image from a single contrast esophagram, centered on the cervical esophagus. There is a smoothly marginated posterior filling defect at the C5–C6 level, representing cricopharyngeal bar *(arrow)*.

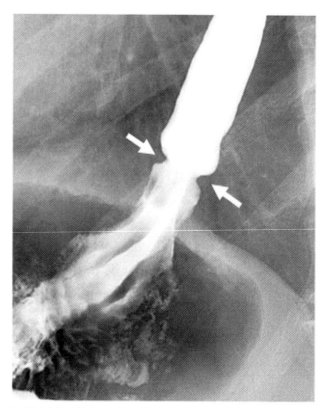

Fig. 50.1 Magnified spot fluoroscopic image from a contrast esophagram demonstrates a smooth marginated filling defect at the anterior and posterior margin of the distal esophagus *(arrows)*.

REFERENCES

Azpeitia Armán, J., Lorente-Ramos, R. M., Gete García, P., & Collazo Lorduy, T. (2019). Videofluoroscopic evaluation of normal and impaired oropharyngeal swallowing. *Radiographics, 39,* 78–79.

Carucci, L. R., & Turner, M. A. (2015). Dysphagia revisited: Common and unusual causes. *Radiographics, 35,* 105–122.

CASE 50

Schatzki Ring

1. A. The figure demonstrates a filling defect at the anterior and posterior aspect of the distal esophagus. Outpouching, contrast extravasation, and air-fluid level are findings of diverticulum, perforation, and enteric stasis/obstruction, respectively; these are not depicted.
2. B. The contour is smooth; the appearance on the anterior and posterior aspect of the image makes this most likely a circumferential finding.
3. A. A smoothly marginated circumferential filling defect of the distal esophagus is a typical appearance of Schatzki ring.
4. D. The etiology of Schatzki ring is idiopathic.

Comment

Diagnosis and Imaging Findings

A Schatzki ring is a thin, smooth circumferential narrowing of the gastroesophageal junction. At pathologic analysis, it represents a mucosal shelf overlying an annular band of connective tissue and smooth muscle, triangle shaped in cross section.

The finding has been reported in 6% to 14% of barium esophagrams. While the majority are incidentally detected, when symptomatic, Schatzki ring represents the most common cause of dysphagia for solids and food impaction in adults. It has been reported that all rings <13 mm in diameter are symptomatic (Schatzki rule).

Schatzki ring can be associated with hiatal hernia and reflux esophagitis; however, the prevalence of these findings in the general population make for inconclusive analysis.

Differential considerations include the esophageal A-ring, though this is typically found 2 to 3 cm proximal to the gastroesophageal junction, and rarely symptomatic. Esophageal web is typically a noncircumferential finding. Reflux-related stricture and esophageal carcinoma are alternative considerations if the contours are irregular and extensive.

Treatment

Symptomatic Schatzki ring is treated with endoscopic dilatation; this is typically accompanied by acid suppression/proton-pump inhibitor therapy.

REFERENCES

Patel, B., Han, E., & Swan, K. (2013). Richard Schatzki: A familiar ring. *AJR. American Journal of Roentgenology, 201,* W678–W682.

Smith, M. S. (2010). Diagnosis and management of esophageal rings and webs. *Gastroenterology & Hepatology, 6,* 701–704.

CASE 52

Contrast Enema; Large Bowel Obstruction

1. D. Colon is distinguished from small bowel by its caliber, position, and fold appearance. Colon typically demonstrates large caliber, peripheral position, and folds that incompletely

Case 51 is online only and accessible at www.expertconsult.com.

traverse the full diameter of the bowel loop (haustra); small bowel demonstrates relatively small caliber, central position, and folds that traverse the full diameter of the bowel loops.

2. B. Small bowel folds are termed plicae circularis or valvulae conniventes, while large bowel folds are termed haustra.

3. B. The figure of the contrast enema demonstrates contrast distending the rectum, and then tapering rapidly at a focal transition point in the rectosigmoid colon. The findings most likely represent large bowel obstruction.

4. D. Each of the choices may represent an underlying etiology of large bowel obstruction: obstructing mass, stricture related to acute or chronic inflammation, and serosal or peritoneal metastatic disease.

Comment

Diagnosis and Imaging Findings

While large bowel obstruction is less common that small bowel obstruction by a fourfold to fivefold margin, it represents an abdominal emergency with high morbidity and mortality if left untreated.

The most common cause of large bowel obstruction is primary colonic malignancy, accounting for >60% of cases in one study. Major sites of obstruction include the cecum, hepatic and splenic flexures, and rectosigmoid colon. Colonic volvulus and complications of diverticulitis represent other common etiologies. Uncommon etiologies include intussusception, hernia, fecal or foreign-body impaction, and extrinsic compression by pelvic or peritoneal disease.

While abdominal radiography can distinguish large from small bowel obstruction, computed tomography (CT) is the gold standard for diagnosis (sensitivity and specificity of 96% and 93%, respectively). Contrast enema can be performed in some instances to help distinguish large bowel obstruction from colonic pseudoobstruction, or confirm suspected volvulus.

Typical CT findings of large bowel obstruction include dilated large bowel proximal to a transition point, with decompressed

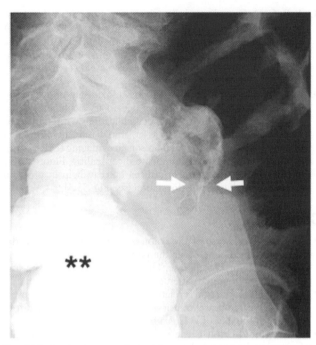

Fig. 52.2 Contrast enema. Lateral fluoroscopic spot image of the pelvis shows contrast distending the rectum *(double asterisk),* with abrupt narrowing at the rectosigmoid colon, at a focal transition point with irregular margins *(arrows).*

bowel distal to the point of obstruction. CT can also help to identify underlying etiologies such as colonic mass, volvulus, sequelae of diverticulitis, or complications such as perforation and pneumatosis intestinalis. An important mimic of large bowel obstruction is adynamic ileus, which typically demonstrates bowel dilatation without transition point, and often includes diffuse small bowel dilatation.

Treatment

Taking into account the wide range of possible underlying etiologies of large bowel obstruction, definitive treatment typically involves surgical decompression of distended colon, resection of the obstructed segment, and either formation of end colostomy or enterostomy with closure of the distal colonic/rectal stump, or primary surgical anastomosis. Among patients with high risk of surgical morbidity, endoscopic placement of a colonic stent to reestablish colonic patency may represent a temporizing or palliative measure.

REFERENCES
Jaffe, T., & Thomspon, W. M. (2015). Large-bowel obstruction in the adult: Classic radiographic and CT findings, etiology, and mimics. *Radiology, 275,* 651–663.
Sawai, R. S. (2012). Management of colonic obstruction: A review. *Clinics in Colon and Rectal Surgery, 25,* 200–203.

CASE 53

Diverticulitis

1. C. The contrast enema demonstrates a colovesical fistula in this patient with acute or chronic sigmoid diverticulitis. There is no drainable collection or stricture on the provided figures. An underlying colon cancer would need to be excluded with colonoscopy.

2. D. The sigmoid colon is the most common site of diverticulosis due to its narrow caliber and higher intraluminal pressure relative to other segments of the colon.

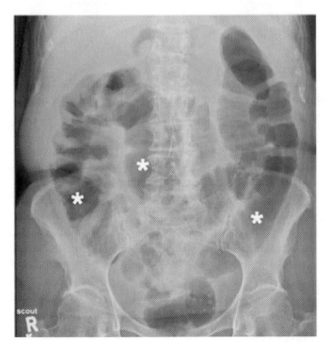

Fig. 52.1 Contrast enema. Frontal scout image demonstrates diffuse air-filled dilatation of ascending, transverse, and descending/sigmoid colon *(asterisks).*

3. A, B, C, D. Complicated diverticulitis may result in abscess or peritonitis due to rupture and spillage of bowel contents. A reactive small or large bowel obstruction can occur due to the inflammation caused by acute diverticulitis. Chronic inflammation related to repeated episodes of acute diverticulitis may result in development of a stricture.

4. B. Computed tomography (CT) is the mainstay of evaluating for suspected acute diverticulitis due to its availability, rapid acquisition, and ability to detect complications with high accuracy. Plain film can be used as an initial modality to detect pneumoperitoneum. Magnetic resonance imaging (MRI) is not routinely used in evaluating acute diverticulitis. Fluoroscopic enema is also not routinely utilized but can help in problem solving for leak or fistula formation (see Fig. 53.3).

Comment

- Diverticular disease of the colon is a common disease of the Western world. The older the patient, the greater the likelihood of having the disease. However, there is an increasing incidence in younger patients in the past 30 to 40 years.
- Diverticular formation is related to increased intraluminal pressures, decreased bowel transit times, and diminishing quantities of fiber in the diet of Western industrialized countries.
- The sigmoid colon is the most common site of diverticular formation because it has the narrowest caliber and highest intraluminal pressure.
- Most patients are asymptomatic or manifest vague abdominal discomfort. Some will present with abdominal pain (typically in the left lower quadrant) and may exhibit fever, leukocytosis, and change in bowel habits. A small group experience rectal bleeding, although a massive rectal bleed secondary to diverticulosis is uncommon (<5%).
- About 15% of patients with diverticulosis develop frank diverticulitis.
- The pathogenesis of diverticulitis is thought to be infection secondary to impacted fecal matter within the diverticula, local peridiverticular inflammation, and frank diverticulitis (if untreated) with pericolonic abscess formation.
- Some of the abscesses drain spontaneously via communication with the colonic lumen. Most do not and will require percutaneous drainage or surgical intervention.
- In addition to abscess formation, additional complications of diverticulitis may include fistula formation (to bladder, vagina, skin, or other bowel segments), small bowel obstruction, or peritonitis related to perforation.

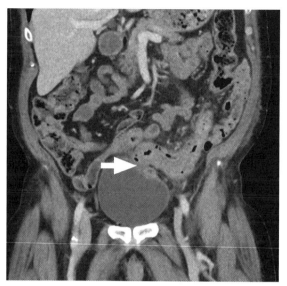

Fig. 53.2 Coronal reformatted CT of the lower abdomen and pelvis demonstrating abutment of the dome of the bladder *(arrow)*, which was thickened in this patient with acute or chronic diverticulitis.

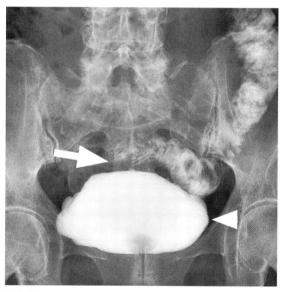

Fig. 53.3 Fluoroscopic contrast enema shows opacification of the sigmoid colon *(arrow)* and urinary bladder *(arrowhead)*, confirming the presence of a colovesical fistula as suspected on computed tomography (CT) in Figs. 53.1 and 53.2.

- Segmental colonic resection may be necessary in cases of complicated or recurrent diverticulitis.
- Computed tomography is the imaging study of choice for detecting acute diverticulitis and its complications.
- Imaging findings of diverticulitis:
  - CT: segmental bowel wall thickening with pericolonic fat stranding adjacent to an inflamed colonic diverticula. Complicated cases may show perforation, abscess formation, or fistula.

REFERENCES

Dickerson, E. C., Chong, S. T., Ellis, J. H., Watcharotone, K., Nan, B., … Davenport, M. S. (2017). Recurrence of colonic diverticulitis: Identifying predictive CT findings-retrospective cohort study. *Radiology, 285*(3), 850–858.

Pereira, J. M., Sirlin, C. B., Pinto, P. S., Jeffrey, R., Stella, D. L., & Casola, G. (2004). Disproportionate fat stranding: A helpful CT sign in patients with acute abdominal pain. *Radiographics, 24*(3), 703–715.

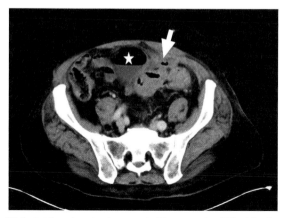

Fig. 53.1 Axial postcontrast computed tomography (CT) of the lower abdomen shows inflammation of the fat adjacent to the sigmoid colon with a small focus of extraluminal air *(arrow)*. There is an adjacent air-fluid level *(star)*, compatible with a fistula or abscess.

CASE 54

Colon Cancer

1. D. Colon cancer is most prevalent in the rectosigmoid colon (~50%).
2. D. Of these choices, the most common site of metastatic colon cancer is the liver.
3. C. Serum CEA (carcinoembryonic antigen) can be used in the follow-up evaluation of treated colon cancer. CA 19-9 is a tumor marker of pancreatic origin. CA 125 is a tumor marker of ovarian pathology. 5-HIAA is a surrogate marker for serotonin and may be elevated among patients with neuroendocrine tumors.
4. B. According to the CT Colonography Reporting and Data System, a small polyp is defined by size of 6 to 9 mm.

Comment

Colorectal Cancer (CRC)

- Third-most common cancer worldwide; 10% of all new cancer diagnoses
- Staging, per American Joint Committee on Cancer (AJCC, 8th ed.) TNM system:
  - T (tumor), depth of involvement of wall of colon or rectum
  - N (node), tumor involvement in locoregional lymph nodes
  - M (metastasis), spread to other organs
- In the United States, screening for colorectal cancer is recommended for adults age 50 to 75 years (earlier for patients at high risk).
  - Colorectal adenocarcinoma is believed to develop from adenomas, or precancerous growths over the course of ~10 years.
  - Screening is directed to the detection and removal of adenomas (polyps).
  - Optical colonoscopy is the gold standard screening test for CRC.

CT Colonography (CTC)

- Alternative to optical colonoscopy (OC)
  - Sensitivity of CTC for CRC, 96%
- Advantages of CTC
  - Minimally invasive compared to OC, no need for sedation
  - Relatively short examination time (15 minutes)
  - Low risk of perforation (0.005–0.03% for CTC, compared to 0.03–0.7% for OC)
- Disadvantages
  - Polyp detection by CTC requires follow-up OC for polyp removal
  - Use of ionizing radiation
- CTC reporting (C-RADS, CT Colonography Reporting and Data System)
  - Polyp: a structure with homogeneous soft tissue attenuation, arising from colonic mucosa by a fixed point of attachment, projecting into lumen
  - Mass: any colonic lesion with soft tissue attenuation, >3 cm
  - Polyp size
    - Diminutive (<6 mm); variably reported
    - Small (6–9 mm)
    - Large (10–30 mm)
  - Polyp morphology
    - Pedunculated: defined by the presence of a stalk
    - Sessile: base width greater than vertical height
    - Flat: plaquelike morphology, protrudes <3 mm from mucosa
  - Segmental location
    - Six segments: rectum, sigmoid, descending, transverse, ascending, cecum

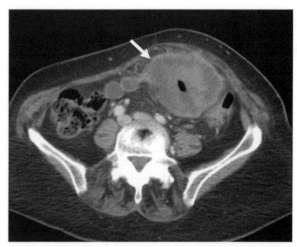

Fig. 54.1 Contrast-enhanced computed tomography (CT) of the abdomen. Axial image demonstrates hypoenhancing mass encasing a loop of bowel in the left midabdomen *(arrow)*.

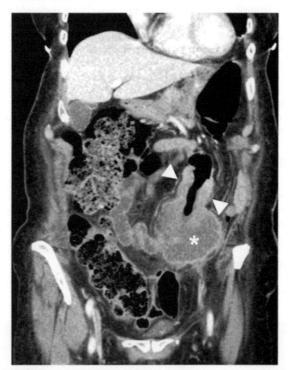

Fig. 54.2 Contrast-enhanced computed tomography (CT) of the abdomen. Coronal image localizes the mass *(asterisk)* to the transverse colon, with an associated segment of concentric colonic wall thickening *(arrowheads)*.

- Based on findings, C-RADS category and management recommendations are assessed for colonic and extracolonic findings

REFERENCES

de Gonzalez, A. B., Kim, K. P., & Yee, J. (2010). CT colonography: Perforation rates and potential radiation risks. *Gastrointestinal Endoscopy Clinics of North America, 20,* 279–291.

Pickhardt, P. J., Hassan, C., Halligan, S., & Marmo, R. (2011). Colorectal cancer: CT colonography and colonoscopy for detection—systematic review and meta-analysis. *Radiology, 259,* 393–405.

Zalis, M. E., Barish, M. A., Choi, J. R., Dachman, A. H., Fenlon, H. M., … Ferrucci, J. T. (2005). CT colonography reporting and data system: A consensus proposal. *Radiology, 236,* 3–9.

CASE 55
Pseudomembranous Colitis

1. B. The appearance of thickened haustral folds on computed tomography (CT) or radiography is referred to as thumb-printing. Comb sign refers to engorgement of the vasa recta in the small bowel mesentery, classically seen in Crohn's disease. The double bubble sign describes adjacent air-filled structures in neonates due to duodenal atresia. Steinstrasse, meaning "stone street" in German, is the descriptor for stacked stones layering in the ureter.
2. C. Pancolitis in an ill patient with marked submucosal colonic edema, as shown in Figs. 55.1, 55.2, and 55.3, most likely represents pseudomembranous colitis. The appearance can be similar to that of ulcerative colitis but is not typical for Crohn's disease. Ischemic colitis and typhlitis (or neutropenic enterocolitis) are not causes of pancolitis. Ischemia classically affects a watershed area such as the splenic flexure, while typhlitis occurs in the right colon and may involve the terminal ileum.
3. A, C. The mainstay of treatment for pseudomembranous colitis is antibiotic therapy with vancomycin or metronidazole. Fecal transplant has recently emerged as a new therapeutic option. Surgical resection and chemotherapy are not treatment options for pseudomembranous colitis.
4. B. Dilation of the transverse colon to >6 cm is concerning for toxic megacolon, which increases the risk for perforation. Accordion sign describes the appearance of the colon due to mucosal hyperenhancement and marked submucosal edema and thickening. Ogilvie syndrome is colonic pseudo-obstruction; pneumatosis refers to air within the bowel wall.

Comment

- Pseudomembranous colitis (also known as *Clostridioides difficile* colitis, formerly *Clostridium difficile* colitis) is an infectious/inflammatory colitis associated with recent antibiotic use. Its incidence continues to increase in hospitalized patients with high mortality if not properly detected and treated.
- Signs and symptoms include abdominal pain, diarrhea, fever, and leukocytosis.
- If untreated, pseudomembranous colitis can lead to sepsis, toxic megacolon, and perforation.

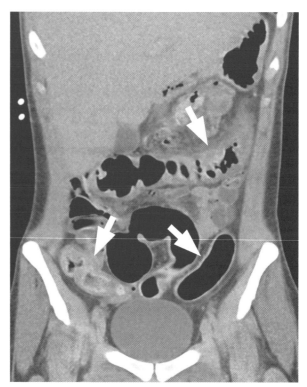

Fig. 55.2 Coronal reformatted computed tomography (CT) of the abdomen demonstrates the pancolonic nature of the inflammatory colitis *(arrows)* in this patient.

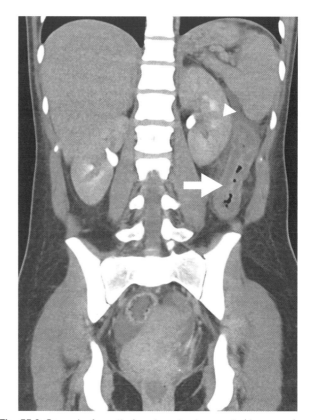

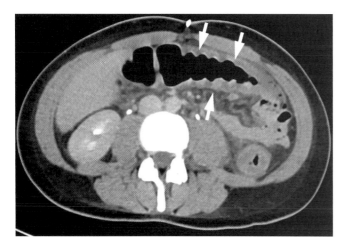

Fig. 55.1 Axial contrast-enhanced computed tomography (CT) of the abdomen shows marked thickening of the haustral folds of the transverse colon *(arrows)*. This pattern gives the appearance of thumbprinting.

Fig. 55.3 Coronal reformatted post-contrast computed tomography (CT) of the abdomen shows the degree of submucosal edema *(arrow)* typically seen in pseudomembranous colitis caused by *C. difficile* infection. Pericolonic stranding is also noted *(arrowhead)*.

- Treatment involves intravenous fluid resuscitation and administration of vancomycin or metronidazole. Recently, fecal transplant has become a viable treatment option as well.
- Pseudomembranous colitis is typically a pancolitis, involving the entirety of the colon. This pattern can be similar to that of ulcerative colitis.
- Imaging findings of pseudomembranous colitis:
  - Plain film: can be negative in the early stages of disease. In the later stages, colonic dilation, wall thickening, and thumbprinting may be identified. Fulminant disease may result in toxic megacolon, characterized by dilation of the transverse colon to >6 cm with loss of haustral marking and pseuopolyps. Free air may be seen when the colon has perforated.
  - CT: findings may include bowel wall thickening, thumbprinting, accordion sign (resembling the appearance of accordion folds due to hyperenhancing colonic mucosa against thickened edematous submucosa), pericolonic fat stranding, and ascites.

REFERENCES
Kirkpatrick, I. D., & Greenberg, H. M. (2001). Evaluating the CT diagnosis of clostridium difficile colitis: Should CT guide therapy? *AJR. American Journal of Roentgenology*, 176(3), 635–639.
Ramachandran, I., Sinha, R., & Rodgers, P. (2006). Pseudomembranous colitis revisited: Spectrum of imaging findings. *Clinical Radiology*, 61(7), 535–544.

CASE 56

Acute Appendicitis CT and US

1. B. A blind-ending tubular structure is seen in the right lower quadrant with inflammation about it and is consistent with acute appendicitis.
2. D. High-density areas seen within the right lower quadrant in the tubular structure best represent appendicoliths.
3. C. Appendicolith is not considered to be a specific sign for appendicitis.
4. C. Ultrasound is specifically preferred in children and young women for the evaluation of acute appendicitis, due to the lack of ionizing radiation.

Comment

- Appendicitis is inflammation of the vermiform appendix.
- Acute appendicitis is typically a disease of children and young adults of the peak incidence in the second and third decades of life.
- Patients typically present with umbilicus pain, which within a day or later localizes to McBurney point with associated fever, nausea, and vomiting.
- Appendicitis is typically caused by obstruction of the appendiceal lumen with the resulting buildup of fluid, secondary infection, venous congestion, ischemia, and necrosis. Obstruction may be caused by lymphoid hyperplasia, appendicolith, foreign bodies, Crohn's disease, or other rare causes (including stricture, tumor, and parasite).
- Imaging findings:
  - Plain radiograph: appendicolith can be visualized in approximately 7% to 15% cases. If an inflammatory process is present, displacement of cecal gas with mural thickening may be evident. Small bowel obstruction with small bowel dilatation and air fluid levels is seen in ~40% of patients with perforation.

- US: graded compression with a linear probe over the site of maximal tenderness by gradually increasing pressure exerted to displace normal overlying bowel gas can help with identifying the appendix. Findings supportive of the diagnosis of appendicitis include:
  - Aperistaltic, noncompressible, dilated appendix >6 mm in outer diameter
  - Hyperechoic appendicolith with posterior acoustic shadowing
  - Echogenic prominent pericecal and periappendiceal fat
  - Periappendiceal fluid collection
  - Wall thickening (≥3 mm)
  - Mural hyperemia with color flow Doppler
  - Periappendiceal reactive nodal prominence/enlargement
- CT: is highly sensitive (94–98%) and specific (up to 97%) for the diagnosis of acute appendicitis and allows for evaluation of alternative causes of abdominal pain. CT findings include:
  - Appendiceal dilatation >6 mm in diameter
  - Wall thickening >3 mm and enhancement
  - Cecal bar sign (arrowhead sign): thickening of the cecal apex
  - Periappendiceal inflammation: fat stranding, thickening of the lateroconal fascia mesoappendix, extraluminal fluid, phlegmon, abscess
  - Focal wall nonenhancement representing necrosis (gangrenous appendicitis)
  - Appendicolith and periappendiceal reactive nodal enlargement are nonspecific findings
- MRI: recommended as a second-line modality for suspected acute appendicitis in pregnant patients when available. Imaging findings are similar to those seen on ultrasound and CT scan.

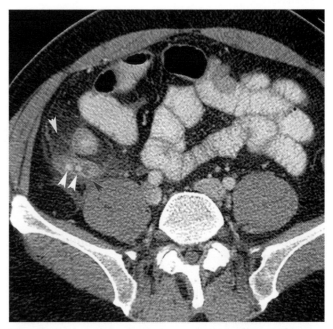

Fig. 56.1 Axial contrast-enhanced computed tomography (CT) image through the lower abdomen shows a tubular, blind-ending structure *(red arrow)* in the right lower quadrant with high-density structures within it, which are consistent with appendicoliths *(white arrows)*. Note fat stranding *(yellow arrow)* around the inflamed appendix in the right lower quadrant due to periappendiceal inflammation.

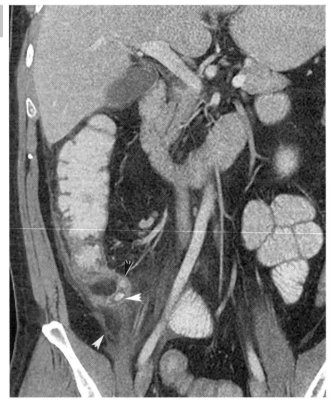

Fig. 56.2 Coronal contrast-enhanced computed tomography (CT) image through the lower abdomen shows a tubular, blind-ending structure *(red arrow)* in the right lower quadrant with high-density structures within it, which are consistent with appendicoliths *(white arrow)*. Note fat stranding *(yellow arrow)* around the inflamed appendix in the right lower quadrant due to periappendiceal inflammation.

REFERENCES

Mostbeck, G., Adam, E. J., Nielsen, M. B., Claudon, M., Clevert, D., … Nyhsen, C. (2016). How to diagnose acute appendicitis: Ultrasound first. *Insights Into Imaging, 7*, 255–263.

Pinto Leite, N., Pereira, J. M., Cunha, R., Pinto, P., & Sirlin, C. (2005). CT evaluation of appendicitis and its complications: Imaging techniques and key diagnostic findings. *AJR. American Journal of Roentgenology, 185*, 406–417.

Puylaert, J. B. (1986). Acute appendicitis: US evaluation using graded compression. *Radiology, 158*, 355–360.

Smith, M. P., Katz, D. S., Lalani, T., Carucci, L. R., Cash, B. D., … Kim, D. H. (2015). ACR appropriateness Criteria® right lower quadrant pain—suspected appendicitis. *Ultrasound Quarterly, 31*, 85–91

CASE 60

Intraperitoneal Free Air on Supine Abdominal Radiograph

1. C. The radiograph demonstrates pneumoperitoneum.
2. A. The radiograph is likely obtained in the supine position, as three signs of intraperitoneal free air on supine radiograph are shown. Pneumoperitoneum on an erect abdominal radiograph typically shows free air under the right hemidiaphragm.
3. E. The continuous diaphragm sign, falciform ligament sign, and Rigler sign are depicted on the abdominal radiograph.

Cases 57–59 are online only and accessible at www.expertconsult.com.

4. A. An erect chest radiograph is the most sensitive radiographic technique for detection of pneumoperitoneum.

Comment

Diagnosis and Imaging Findings

The presence of gas in the peritoneal cavity is referred to as pneumoperitoneum. While this may be a benign or expected finding in immediate postsurgical patients, or in patients with peritoneal indwelling catheters (e.g., peritoneal dialysis catheter), its presence may signify advanced abdominopelvic pathology, including bowel perforation secondary to trauma, ulcer, infection, obstruction, malignancy, and necrosis.

An erect chest radiograph is the most sensitive radiograph for detection of pneumoperitoneum. In the upright or erect position, air is shown as abnormal lucency under the diaphragm (typically on the right). Radiographic sensitivity for detection of pneumoperitoneum decreases with small volume of intraperitoneal free air and with recumbent or supine patient position.

Radiologic signs of intraperitoneal free air are predicated on the observation of abnormal lucency at the interface to bowel, peritoneal ligaments, and the body wall.

Bowel Signs

- Rigler sign: air outlining both sides of a bowel loop, resulting in the bowel wall being shown as a line and not an edge or interface
- (Telltale) triangle sign: a triangular pocket of air at the intersection of three loops of bowel

Peritoneal Ligament Signs

- Continuous diaphragm sign/saddlebag/mustache sign: air underneath the central tendon of the diaphragm in the midline
- Silver/falciform ligament sign: air outlines the falciform ligament
- Inverted V sign: air outlines lateral umbilical ligaments (inferior epigastric vessels)

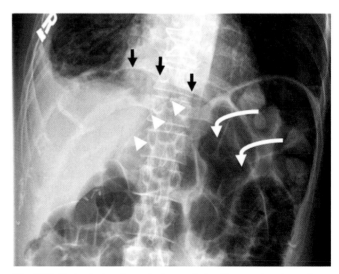

Fig. 60.1 Abdominal radiograph demonstrates three supine signs of intraperitoneal free air: abnormal transverse lucency at the diaphragm, the continuous diaphragm sign *(arrows);* oblique line of the right/paramedian upper abdomen, the falciform ligament sign *(arrowheads);* abnormal lucency outlining both sides of the wall of a loop of bowel, Rigler sign *(curved arrows).*

Organ or Body Wall Signs

- Lucent liver sign: air anterior to the liver results in reduction of normal liver opacity
- Football sign: abdominal cavity outlined by gas, typically in massive pneumoperitoneum
- Doge cap sign: triangular collection of gas in Morison pouch.

Treatment

The finding of intraperitoneal free air should trigger investigation for underlying etiologies; CT of the abdomen/pelvis may be indicated for radiologic evaluation.

REFERENCES

Levine, M. S., Scheiner, J. D., Rubesin, S. E., Laufer, I., & Herlinger, H. (1991). Diagnosis of pneumoperitoneum on supine abdominal radiographs. *American Journal of Roentgenology, 156,* 731–735.

Sureka, B., Bansal, K., & Arora, A. (2015). Pneumoperitoneum: What to look for in a radiograph? *Journal of Family Medcine and Primary Care, 4,* 477–478.

Fair Game

CASE 61

Hepatocellular Carcinoma

1. A. The images demonstrate an infiltrative arterially enhancing mass in the right lobe of the liver with tumor thrombus extending along the right portal vein. Neuroendocrine tumor metastases and hepatic adenoma are both arterially enhancing lesions but should not show tumor thrombus and do not typically show this infiltrative pattern. Cholangiocarcinoma does not demonstrate this pattern of arterial enhancement and only exceedingly rarely presents with tumor thrombus.
2. B. Hepatitis B infection remains the leading cause of HCC worldwide, largely due to the endemic nature of the disease in Asia. Alcohol and hepatitis C are more common etiologies in the Western world. Nonalcoholic fatty liver disease (NAFLD) is a rapidly emerging liver condition leading to a rampant increase in cirrhosis worldwide with subsequent risk for HCC.
3. A, B, C, D. The major diagnostic features of HCC on imaging are nonrim arterial phase hyperenhancement, nonperipheral washout, capsular enhancement, and threshold growth (>50% increase in 6 months).
4. D. Of patients with HCC, 50% to 75% exhibit elevated levels of alpha-fetoprotein (AFP). It is a useful marker in disease surveillance and monitoring for response to therapy. CEA is often elevated in colorectal cancer. CA 19-9 elevation can be associated with pancreatic ductal adenocarcinoma or biliary carcinoma (cholangiocarcinoma). CA-125 is most commonly associated with ovarian cancer.

Comment

- Hepatocellular carcinoma (HCC) is the most common primary malignancy of the liver (followed by cholangiocarcinoma).
- HCC is the fifth most common cancer worldwide and the third most common cause of cancer-related death.
- Worldwide, the leading cause of HCC is chronic hepatitis B infection (particularly endemic in Asia). Alcohol abuse contributes to a much higher prevalence of HCC in the Western world. Other risk factors for development of hepatocellular carcinoma include hepatitis C infection, biliary cirrhosis, aflatoxins, congenital biliary atresia, and inborn errors of metabolism (e.g., alpha-1 antitrypsin deficiency, hemochromatosis, Wilson disease).
- HCC is most commonly a disease of middle-aged to elderly adults and is more common in men.
- Diagnosis may be made on surveillance imaging for high-risk patients or symptoms such as weight loss, abdominal pain, palpable mass, jaundice, or hemorrhage.
- Alpha-fetoprotein (AFP) is elevated in 50% to 75% of HCC cases.
- Treatment options for HCC include resection, liver transplantation, and locoregional therapy with thermal ablation (microwave ablation or radiofrequency ablation), transarterial chemoembolization (TACE), transarterial radioembolization (TARE), or selective internal radiation therapy (SIRT).
- HCC can appear as a focal dominant mass, multifocal process, or infiltrative disease.
- The major diagnostic imaging features of HCC include nonrim arterial phase hyperenhancement, nonperipheral washout, capsular enhancement, and threshold growth (>50% increase in 6 months).

- Many classification systems exist for characterizing and stratifying features of focal lesions in high-risk patients, notably the Liver Imaging Reporting and Data System (LI-RADS).
- Imaging findings of hepatocellular carcinoma:
  - US: Variable appearance, particularly with the typically heterogeneous appearance of the background liver in patients with chronic liver disease. Characteristic appearance on contrast-enhanced ultrasound is arterial-phase enhancement with portal venous washout.
  - CT: Variable depending on pattern (i.e., focal vs infiltrative), but characteristic features include arterial enhancement, portal venous/equilibrium phase enhancement, and

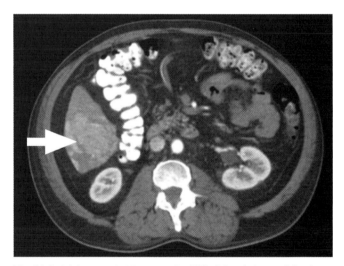

Fig. 61.1 Axial computed tomography (CT) of the abdomen following intravenous (IV) and oral contrast demonstrates heterogeneous enhancement in the inferior right hepatic lobe *(arrow)*.

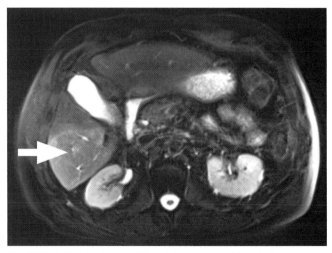

Fig. 61.2 Axial fat-saturated T2 weighted image of the abdomen shows heterogeneously hyperintense geographic T2 signal in the inferior right hepatic lobe *(arrow)*, corresponding to the enhancement seen in Fig. 61.1.

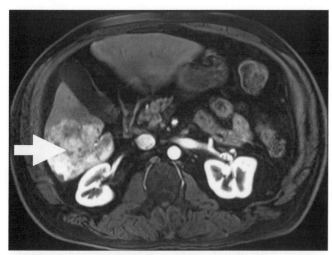

Fig. 61.3 Postcontrast T1 weighted image with fat saturation in the arterial phase shows matching heterogeneous arterial phase hyperenhancement *(arrow)*.

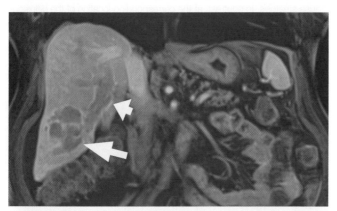

Fig. 61.4 Coronal postcontrast T1 weighted image with fat saturation in the portal venous phase demonstrates infiltrative direct spread of tumor *(arrow)* into the right portal vein *(arrowhead)*. The findings depict hepatocellular carcinoma with tumor thrombus, compatible with LI-RADS TIV categorization.

capsular enhancement. Look for tumor thrombus, which will demonstrate enhancement.
- MRI: Same dynamic contrast-enhanced features as on CT. The tumor is typically intermediate in T2 signal ("evil gray") with restricted diffusion. Diffusion weighted imaging is also helpful in distinguishing tumor thrombus from bland thrombus. It is important to understand contrast physiology if using a hepatocyte-specific contrast agent. For example, lesional hypointensity on the 3-minute phase cannot be characterized as washout with gadoxetic acid.

REFERENCES
Choi, J. Y., Lee, J. M., & Sirlin, C. B. (2014). CT and MR imaging diagnosis and staging of hepatocellular carcinoma: part 1. Development, growth, and spread: Key pathologic and imaging aspects. *Radiology, 272*(3), 635–654.
Nowicki, T. K., Markiet, K., & Szurowska, E. (2017). Diagnostic imaging of hepatocellular carcinoma—a pictoral essay. *Current Medical Imaging Reviews, 13*(2), 140–153.
Reynolds, A. R., Furlan, A., Fetzer, D. T., Sasatomi, E., Borhani, A. A., ... Heller, M. T. (2015). Infiltrative hepatocellular carcinoma: What radiologists need to know. *Radiographics, 35*(2), 371–386.

CASE 62
Fatty Liver; Occult Liver Metastasis

1. D. The CT image shows focal enhancement adjacent to the falciform ligament; at this location, MRI shows focal restricted diffusion, without focal signal loss on opposed phase imaging, most likely representing metastatic melanoma given the provided history.
2. B. The provided images show a background of diffuse fatty liver, confirmed by signal loss on opposed-phase MRI compared to in-phase MRI.
3. C. Contrast-enhanced abdominal CT is typically performed at the following intervals postinjection: early arterial, 15 to 20 seconds; late arterial, 35 to 40 seconds; hepatic or portal venous phase, 70 to 80 seconds; nephrographic phase, 100 to 120 seconds.
4. B. Melanoma, renal cell carcinoma, and neuroendocrine tumors are examples of malignancies that may have hypervascular liver metastases; other examples include choriocarcinoma and thyroid carcinoma. Lung adenocarcinoma metastases are not typically hypervascular.

Comment
Fatty Liver
- High prevalence, 25% to 35% in the United States
- Can result from many different conditions
  - Common: alcoholic liver disease, nonalcoholic fatty liver disease (NALFD, related to obesity and metabolic syndrome), viral hepatitis
  - Uncommon: nutritional or dietary disorder, posttreatment (e.g., radiation), metabolic and storage disorders
- Imaging modalities and features
  - US: liver echogenicity in excess of renal cortex, and loss of definition of diaphragm and intrahepatic architecture
    - Reported sensitivity 60% to 100%, specificity 77% to 95%
  - CT:
    - Unenhanced CT:
      - Intrahepatic vessels are normally hypodense to liver
      - Liver attenuation <40 HU (sensitivity 52.5%, specificity 100%)
      - Or 10 HU less than spleen (sensitivity 60.5%, specificity 100%)
    - Contrast-enhanced (portal venous phase) CT:
      - Liver attenuation 20 HU less than spleen (sensitivity 86%, specificity 87%)
  - MRI:
    - Chemical shift gradient echo (GRE) imaging—comparison of in-phase and opposed-phase images
      - Normal liver: signal intensity is similar between in-phase and opposed-phase images
      - Fatty liver: loss of signal intensity on opposed-phase images compared to in-phase images
      - Sensitivity 81%, specificity 100%
    - Proton density fat fraction (PDFF)
    - MRI spectroscopy (MRS)

Pitfalls of Interpretation

Heterogeneous imaging appearance of fatty liver has varying implications on interpretation:
- Diffuse fatty liver
  - Resultant hypoattenuation of liver may reduce sensitivity of liver lesion detection, including of metastases, on CT

- Patients may benefit from MRI, which offers higher soft tissue contrast, multiphasic postcontrast enhancement, diffusion weighted imaging, and imaging with hepatobiliary contrast agents
- Diffuse fatty liver with areas of focal sparing
  - Focal sparing typically has geographic shape, or found in periportal distribution or surrounding gallbladder
  - Appearance may mimic focal lesion
- Focal fatty change against the background of normal liver
  - Typically around falciform ligament or gallbladder, or periportal distribution
  - Appearance may mimic hypoenhancing mass on contrast enhanced CT
  - More heterogeneous distributions may mimic neoplastic or inflammatory conditions
    - Vessels typically course uninterrupted through fatty change

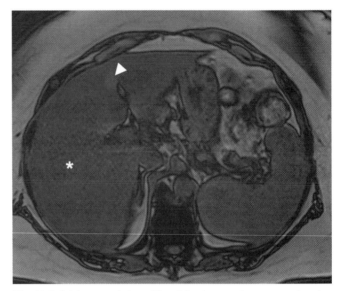

Fig. 62.3 Axial opposed-phase T1 weighted magnetic resonance imaging (MRI) of the liver shows diffuse signal hypointensity (*asterisk*), indicating diffuse steatosis. In contrast, at the corresponding location of the diffusion-restricting focus in Fig. 62.2, there is no focal signal hypointensity.

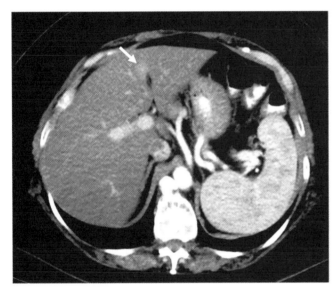

Fig. 62.1 Axial late-arterial contrast-enhanced CT of the upper abdomen demonstrates focal enhancement adjacent to the falciform ligament *(arrow)*.

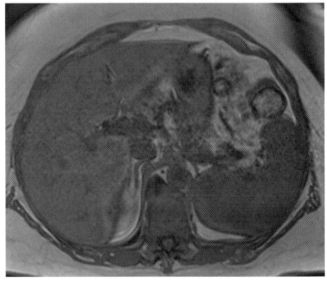

Fig. 62.4 Axial in-phase T1 weighted MR image, for reference.

REFERENCES

Elsayes, K. M., Menias, C. O., Morshid, A. I., Shaaban, A. M., Fowler, K. J., ... Tang, A. (2018). Spectrum of pitfalls, pseudolesions, and misdiagnoses in noncirrhotic liver. *American Journal of Roentgenology, 211,* 97–108.

Hamer, O. W., Aguirre, D. A., Casola, G., Lavine, J. E., Woenckhaus, M., & Sirlin, C. B. (2006). Fatty liver: Imaging patterns and pitfalls. *Radiographics, 26,* 1637–1653.

Jacobs, J. E., Birnbaum, B. A., Shapiro, M. A., Langlotz, C. P., Slosman, F., ... Horii, S. C. (1998). Diagnostic criteria for fatty infiltration of the liver on contrast-enhanced helical CT. *American Journal of Roentgenology, 171,* 659–664.

Lawrence, D. A., Oliva, I. B., & Israel, G. M. (2012). Detection of hepatic steatosis on contrast-enhanced CT images: Diagnostic accuracy of identification of areas of presumed focal fatty sparing. *American Journal of Roentgenology, 199,* 44–47.

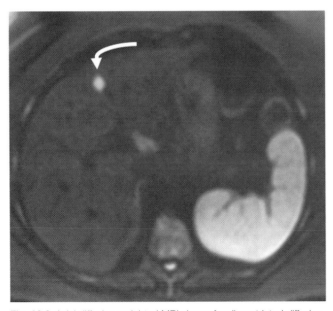

Fig. 62.2 Axial diffusion weighted MRI shows focally restricted diffusion at the corresponding area *(curved arrow)*.

CASE 63

Intrahepatic Cholangiocarcinoma

1. C. The liver lesion demonstrates peripheral rim enhancement with centripetal filling, T2 hypointensity, and restricted diffusion. These findings are most compatible with a fibrotic malignancy, specifically intrahepatic cholangiocarcinoma. Hemangioma is T2 bright and shows peripheral nodular discontinuous enhancement with delayed filling. Hepatocellular carcinoma more typically shows nonrim-like arterial enhancement with washout and intermediate T2 signal. Metastases can have rim enhancement and restricted diffusion, but usually show intermediate T2 signal intensity ("evil gray").
2. D. Patients from Southeast Asia (and the Middle East) exhibit higher rates of developing cholangiocarcinoma relative to the rest of the world, including North America, South America, and Africa.
3. A, B, C, D. There are several known risk factors for development of cholangiocarcinoma, including choledochal cysts, exposure to the contrast agent thorotrast, primary sclerosing cholangitis, and infection with the liver fluke *Clonorchis sinensis*.
4. A, B, D. Intrahepatic cholangiocarcinoma classically shows early peripheral enhancement with gradual centripetal fill-in, retraction of the overlying liver capsule, and upstream segmental biliary ductal dilation. It is not classically T2 hyperintense but rather T2 dark (due to fibrosis) or intermediate in signal.

Comment

- Cholangiocarcinoma is a malignant primary liver tumor arising from the biliary tree. It is the second most common primary liver neoplasm (behind hepatocellular carcinoma).
- Cholangiocarcinoma is a rare malignancy, although more common in Southeast Asia and the Middle East. It portends a poor prognosis with high morbidity.
- Risk factors for cholangiocarcinoma include primary sclerosing cholangitis (PSC), recurrent pyogenic cholangitis, choledocholithiasis, parasitic infection with liver flukes (i.e., *Clonorchis sinensis*), choledochal cysts (including Caroli disease), toxins (e.g., polyvinyl chloride, thorotrast, alcohol), and viral infections (HIV, hepatitis B/C).
- The majority of cholangiocarcinoma occur in an extrahepatic location, while 20% occur as mass-forming intrahepatic tumors.
- Patients may present with painless jaundice. Most cases are unresectable at the time of clinical presentation. Even resectable cases have high mortality.
- Imaging findings of intrahepatic cholangiocarcinoma:
  - US: Irregular homogeneous mass with hypoechoic rim. May demonstrate capsular retraction, which helps narrow the differential diagnosis. With contrast-enhanced ultrasound, the mass shows irregular rim enhancement with heterogeneous central hypoenhancement in the arterial phase and washout on the portal venous/delayed phases.
  - CT: Intrahepatic cholangiocarcinoma is often described as a "cauliflower lesion" due to its morphology. It shows irregular heterogeneous early peripheral enhancement with centripetal filling on more delayed phases. Classic findings include capsular retraction with upstream intrahepatic biliary dilation. Intrahepatic cholangiocarcinoma rarely results in tumor thrombus but often encases the portal venous, hepatic venous, and hepatic arterial system, leading to unresectability.
  - MRI: Similar findings to CT but with increased soft tissue resolution, which helps delineate relationship to vessels and thus resectability. MRI better evaluates extent of disease

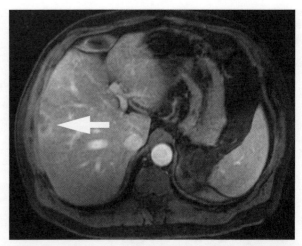

Fig. 63.1 T1 weighted magnetic resonance imaging (MRI) with fat saturation in the portal venous phase showing peripheral enhancement of a solid mass in the right hepatic lobe *(arrow)*.

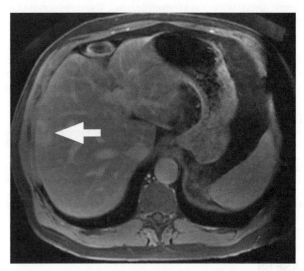

Fig. 63.2 T1 weighted magnetic resonance imaging (MRI) with fat saturation in the equilibrium phase demonstrates progressive centripetal enhancement within the tumor *(arrow)*.

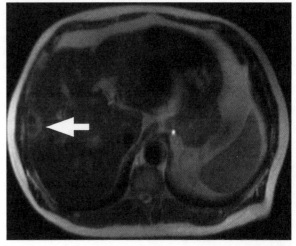

Fig. 63.3 T2 weighted magnetic resonance imaging (MRI) without fat saturation showing central T2 hypointensity with peripheral hyperintensity *(arrow)*. This suggests an underlying central fibrous component.

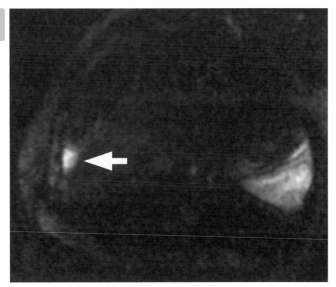

Fig. 63.4 Diffusion weighted image demonstrating intense restricted diffusion *(arrow)* within this intrahepatic mass. The constellation of findings supports a diagnosis of intrahepatic cholangiocarcinoma.

and better outlines the biliary tree. A target appearance with peripheral restriction on diffusion weighted imaging favors cholangiocarcinoma over hepatocellular carcinoma.

REFERENCES
Chung, Y. E., Kim, M. J., Park, Y. N., et al. (2009). Varying appearances of cholangiocarcinoma: Radiologic-pathologic correlation. *Radiographics, 29*(3), 683–700.
Han, J. K., Choi, B. I., Kim, A. Y., et al. (2002). Cholangiocarcinoma: Pictorial essay of CT and cholangiographic findings. *Radiographics, 22*(1), 173–187.
Sainani, N. I., Catalano, O. A., Holalkere, N. S., et al. (2008). Cholangiocarcinoma: Current and novel imaging techniques. *Radiographics, 28*(5), 1263–1287.

CASE 65

Gallbladder Cancer

1. A, D. Gallbladder carcinoma commonly shows invasion into the adjacent liver parenchyma, as seen in this case, due to the fact that venous drainage from the gallbladder drains into segment IV of the liver by short, direct communicating veins that directly enter into the middle hepatic vein radicals or by veins accompanying the extrahepatic ducts into the liver. Gallbladder polyps can be large in size and mimic gallbladder carcinoma.
2. A. More than 80% of gallbladder carcinomas are adenocarcinomas.
3. A, B, C, D. Porcelain gallbladder is associated with gallbladder cancer in 12.5% to 62% of patients. Polyps >10 mm have also been associated with gallbladder carcinoma, and hence in most guidelines cholecystectomy is recommended. Patients with primary sclerosing cholangitis (PSC) and females with Indian ethnicity have a higher incidence of gallbladder carcinoma. In patients with PSC, a substantial number (60%) of gallbladder polyps are malignant.
4. D. Early in the course of the disease patients with gallbladder carcinoma are invariably asymptomatic, and it is commonly detected at an advanced stage due to lack of symptoms.

Case 64 is online only and accessible at www.expertconsult.com.

Comment

- Background: Gallbladder carcinoma is the fifth most common malignancy of the gastrointestinal tract. Highest incidence of gallbladder cancer is seen in South America and Asia while lower incidences are seen in developed regions such as North America and the United Kingdom.
  - It predominantly affects older persons with long-standing cholecystolithiasis and is most common in elderly women (>60 years of age, female to male ratio = 4:1).
  - Chronic inflammation related to gallstones promotes epithelial dysplasia and adenocarcinoma formation; however, only 0.3% to 3% of patients with cholelithiasis develop gallbladder carcinoma and approximately 20% of gallbladder cancer patients show no evidence of previous cholelithiasis.
  - Other risk factors include larger gallstones >3 cm in diameter (10 times greater risk than in patients with stones <1 cm in diameter), porcelain gallbladder (associated with gallbladder cancer in 12.5% to 62% of patients), polyps >10 mm in diameter, anomalous pancreatic of biliary duct junction, obesity, endogenous and exogenous estrogens, segmental adenomyomatosis of the gallbladder, primary sclerosing cholangitis (PSC), and familial tendency.
  - Early patients are asymptomatic; however, it is often detected at an advanced stage due to lack of symptoms.
  - Staging of gallbladder cancer as per the American Joint Committee on Cancer, Eight Edition, ranges from stage 0 to IVb.
    - Stage 0 describes carcinoma in situ when the cancer involves the mucosa only while stage IVb indicates lymph nodal involvement of four or more lymph nodes (N2 disease) on the presence of metastatic disease.
    - Survival in gallbladder cancer patients varies from 80% 5-year survival in those with in situ disease declining to only 8% when lymph nodes are involved and 2% for patients with stage IVb disease.
- Pathology: More than 80% of gallbladder cancers are adenocarcinomas; they can be categorized into papillary, tubular, mucinous, and signet cell types.
- Mode of spread: Invasion of the tumor into the liver and initial location of liver metastasis to the portion adjacent to the gallbladder is due to the fact that venous drainage from the gallbladder drains into segment IV of the liver by short, direct communicating veins that directly enter into the middle hepatic vein radicals or by veins accompanying the extrahepatic ducts into the liver.
  - Vascular invasion is reported in 15% of cases.
  - Lymphatic metastasis is seen to the paraaortic lymph nodes through the pancreaticoduodenal lymph nodes and lymph nodes in the hepaticoduodenal ligament.
  - Transperitoneal spread is common and involves liver, common bile duct, colon, duodenum, pancreas, omentum, and stomach and may manifest as peritoneal carcinomatosis in advanced stages.
  - Neural spread reported in 25% to 35% of cases is a poor prognostic sign.
  - Intraductal spread along the lumen and wall of the ducts is rare and is usually seen in the papillary type of gallbladder carcinoma.
- Diagnosis:
  - US: the most widely used technique in the preoperative study of gallbladder carcinoma and the standard initial study in patients with upper quadrant pain.
    - Early cancer can be seen as a hypoechoic or isoechoic irregularly shaped lesion, appearing as a subhepatic mass that usually masks the gallbladder.

- Ultrasound clues to a polypoid gallbladder carcinoma include a solitary polyp >10 mm, a wide polyp base, focal wall thickening of >3 mm, and coexisting gallstones.
  - At color and spectral Doppler ultrasound, linear color signal at the polyp base and an increased resistive index may indicate a cancerous polyp.
  - At contrast enhanced ultrasound, diffuse or branched enhancement and then abruptly rising, persistent time intensity enhancement curve has been shown to be associated with malignant gallbladder lesions.
- CT: typically gallbladder adenocarcinomas appear as large heterogenous masses, which may have engulfed gallstones or areas of necrosis.
  - Patchy moderate enhancement is usually seen.
  - Features of advanced disease include intrahepatic biliary dilatation, invasion of adjacent structures, lymphadenopathy, peritoneal carcinomatosis, and hepatic or other distant metastasis.
- MRI: the most common pattern of gallbladder carcinoma seen is a masslike or diffuse wall thickening.
  - Focal wall thickening with an eccentric mass is reported in 75% of cases.
  - It is typically hypointense on T1 weighted and hyperintense on T2 weighted images.
  - Concurrent gallstones are seen as filling defects.
  - Following administration of gadolinium contrast, gallbladder carcinoma shows heterogenous arterial enhancement that persists in the venous phase.
  - Adjacent liver invasion, bile duct invasion, lymph node metastasis, and vascular invasion can be easily seen on MRI.
  - Diffusion weighted imaging (DWI) is shown as hyperintensity on DWI images and hypointensity on ADC maps. DWI may increase sensitivity for detection of liver and lymph node metastases.
- FDG-PET: has a high sensitivity and specificity in differentiating between benign and malignant diseases compared to conventional US, CT, and MRI.

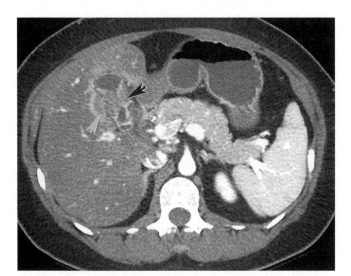

Fig. 65.1 Axial postcontrast computed tomography image at 60 seconds shows a large mass arising from the gallbladder *(red arrow)* and infiltrating into the adjacent liver parenchyma *(blue arrow)*. This was consistent with gallbladder adenocarcinoma.

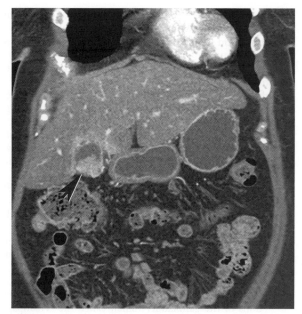

Fig. 65.2 Coronal postcontrast image shows a large enhancing mass in the gallbladder *(red arrow)*. This was consistent with gallbladder adenocarcinoma.

REFERENCES

Gourgiotis, S., Kocher, H. M., Solaini, L., Yarollahi, A., Tsiambas, E., & Salemis, N. S. (2008). Gallbladder cancer. *American Journal of Surgery, 196*(2), 252–264. doi:10.1016/j.amjsurg.2007.11.011.

Kalra, N., Gupta, P., Singhal, M., Gupta, R., Gupta, V., … Srinivasan, R. (2019). Cross-sectional imaging of gallbladder carcinoma: An update. *Journal of Clinical and Experimental Hepatology, 9*(3), 334–344. doi:10.1016/j.jceh.2018.04.005.

McCain, R. S., Diamond, A., Jones, C., & Coleman, H. G. (2018). Current practices and future prospects for the management of gallbladder polyps: A topical review. *World Journal of Gastroenterology, 24*(26), 2844–2852. doi:10.3748/wjg.v24.i26.2844.

CASE 66

Emphysematous Cholecystitis

1. A, B, C, D. Figures show air in the right upper quadrant overlying the liver. This could be within the liver or gallbladder and could also be in an overlying small bowel or large bowel loop.
2. D. Emphysematous cholecystitis is typically associated with *Clostridium* infection.
3. C, D. Atherosclerosis and diabetes mellitus are risk factors for emphysematous cholecystitis.
4. A. Gallbladder perforation is a major complication of emphysematous cholecystitis.

Comment

- Background: Emphysematous cholecystitis (EC) is a rare form of acute cholecystitis where gallbladder wall necrosis causes gas formation in the lumen or wall.
  - Men are affected twice as commonly as women, and the majority of patients are between 50 and 70 years of age.
  - Patients with atherosclerosis and diabetes mellitus are at increased risk for developing EC. The underlying etiology is felt to be due to vascular compromise of the cystic artery leading to gallbladder wall ischemia.
  - Patients with EC have a higher likelihood of having acalculous cholecystitis and gallbladder perforation.
  - Commonly isolated organisms include *Clostridium welchii/perfringens*, *Escherichia coli*, and *Bacteroides fragilis*.

- Clinical manifestation is often insidious and may then progress rapidly. Up to one-third of the patients may be afebrile, and localized tenderness is often not a dominant clinical feature.
- Imaging: EC can be graded radiologically according to the distribution of gas with the gallbladder. Stage I is when the air is confined to the gallbladder lumen; stage II is when there is gas present within the gallbladder wall; stage III is when gas extends to the pericholecystic tissues.
  - On imaging, the condition is diagnosed when there is a radiographic demonstration of air in the gallbladder wall +/= biliary ducts in the absence of an abnormal communication with the gastrointestinal tract.
  - Radiography used to be the mainstay in diagnosis of EC; however, due to its low sensitivity, some cases may be missed.
  - Ultrasound is less sensitive than CT; however, it is highly specific for identifying air in the gallbladder.
    - US may show high echogenic reflectors with low-level posterior shadowing and reverberation artifact ("dirty" shadowing and "ring down" artifact).
    - Another specific sign is presence of small, nonshadowing echogenic foci rising up from the dependent portions of the gallbladder lumen called the "champagne sign."
  - CT is the most sensitive and specific modality for imaging gas within the gallbladder lumen or wall.
    - The general CT features of EC include air in the gallbladder wall or lumen, intraluminal membranes, irregular or absent gallbladder wall, irregular enhancement, and pericholecystic abscess.
    - The presence of pneumoperitoneum is a surgical emergency, as this indicates gallbladder perforation.
    - Due to the presence of concomitant cystic duct obstruction in EC, air is seen in the bile ducts in only 20% of cases.
  - Nuclear medicine hepatobiliary scan cannot differentiate between the different types of acute cholecystitis and shows persistent nonvisualization of the gallbladder with a curvilinear area of increased activity in the region of the gallbladder fossa known as the tissue rim sign. The presence of air, however, cannot be confirmed or excluded with hepatobiliary imaging.
- Treatment is emergent surgical intervention with an overall mortality of 15% to 25%. Percutaneous cholecystostomy tube may be placed as an option in patients who are too unwell for surgery.

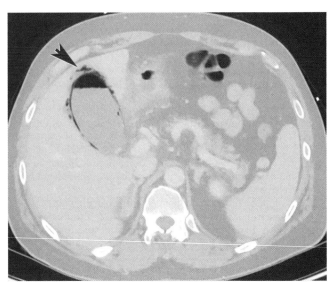

Fig. 66.2 Axial postcontrast computed tomography image in the lung window setting shows air in the gallbladder wall extending into the adjacent liver parenchyma *(red arrow)*. This was consistent with emphysematous cholecystitis.

REFERENCES

Grayson, D. E., Abbott, R. M., Levy, A. D., & Sherman, P. M. (2002). Emphysematous infections of the abdomen and pelvis: A pictorial review. *Radiographics*, *22*(3), 543–561. doi:10.1148/radiographics.22.3.g02ma06543.

Konno, K., Ishida, H., Naganuma, H., Sato, M., Komatsuda, T., … Sato, A. (2002). Emphysematous cholecystitis: Sonographic findings. *Abdominal Imaging*, *27*(2), 191–195. doi:10.1007/s00261-001-0054-3.

Oyedeji, F. O., & Voci, S. (2014). Emphysematous cholecystitis. *Ultrasound Quarterly*, *30*(3), 246–248. doi:10.1097/RUQ.0000000000000101.

CASE 67

Mirizzi Syndrome

1. A, B D, E. The imaging appearance in the figures shows external compression on the common hepatic duct, which appears to have a stricture within it on the ERCP images. This appearance can be seen with all the diseases mentioned except for Bouveret syndrome, which is a rare form of gallstone ileus where the impacted stone leads to a gastric outlet obstruction. The stone enters the stomach through a cholecystogastric or cholecystoduodenal fistula before it gets impacted in the duodenum.
2. C. The most common mechanism of Mirizzi syndrome is believed to be due to a gallstone that is impacted in the infundibulum or cystic duct causing chronic inflammation of the gallbladder and pressure on the common bile duct.
3. A. Surgical treatment of this condition is complicated due to the presence of dense adhesions due to chronic inflammation, and inadvertent ligation of the common hepatic is the most common iatrogenic complication seen.
4. B. Obstructive jaundice is most commonly caused by choledocholithiasis and less commonly due to the other diseases mentioned.

Comment

- Mirizzi syndrome is a rare entity that occurs when a stone becomes impacted in the cystic duct or neck of the gallbladder.
  - Physiologically this condition involves extrinsic compression of the bile duct by pressure applied upon it indirectly by an impacted stone in the cystic duct or neck of the gallbladder.

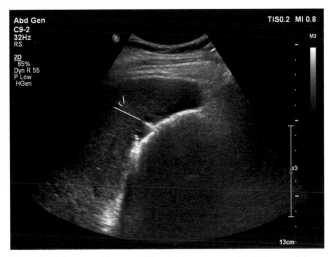

Fig. 66.1 Ultrasound image of the right upper quadrant shows air in the gallbladder wall extending into the liver parenchyma *(arrow)*. This is suspicious for emphysematous cholecystitis.

This type of impaction is very common, but in Mirizzi syndrome a severe local inflammatory response occurs. The inflammatory reaction impinges on the common hepatic and bile ducts, producing varying degrees of narrowing or obstruction. The intrahepatic ducts may become dilated proximal to the obstruction.

- Secondary involvement of major vessels in this region can also occur. In turn, the resulting chronic inflammation and ulceration cause varying degrees of cholecystobiliary fistula, and possibly cholecystoenteric fistula may occur.
- Mirizzi syndrome can be classified into different types, including:
  - Type I, "classic" Mirizzi syndrome
  - Type II cholecystocholedochal fistula with two subtypes: diameter <50% of the CBD and diameter >50% of the CBD
  - Type III, with cholecystoenteric fistula without (a) or with (b) gallstone ileus.
- The major concern is difficulty in making an appropriate diagnosis and performing corrective surgery.
- With the inflammatory mass effect and the bile duct dilation, the condition may mimic a neoplasm of either the gallbladder or the bile ducts.
- Imaging: changes are most confusing on endoscopy retrograde cholangiopancreatography (ERCP).
  - Ultrasound is routinely used as an investigation for biliary disease and can reveal gallstones, biliary ductal dilatation of the common hepatic duct with normal distal CBD, and/or inflammation of the gallbladder due to acute cholecystitis.
  - Although no specific radiologic features of this syndrome can be recognized on CT imaging, this technique can be very effective in detecting the cause and location of biliary obstruction.
  - MRCP is the preferred diagnostic tool and is a noninvasive imaging technique with a 50% diagnostic accuracy rate.

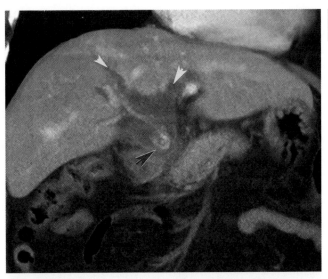

Fig. 67.2 Coronal postcontrast computed tomography (CT) image showing intrahepatic biliary dilatation *(yellow arrow)* with compression of the common bile duct due to a large calculus *(red arrow)* seen at the neck of the gallbladder. This is consistent with Mirizzi syndrome.

MRCP can delineate the typical characteristics of Mirizzi syndrome such as a stone in the common hepatic duct, extrinsic compression of the common hepatic duct, and dilation of the common hepatic duct with normal-size CBD. Presence of inflammation can be seen on MRCP and can also distinguish biliary conditions, including cancer; however, MRCP is not efficient at localizing a cholecystocholedochal fistula.

- Management: surgical management is a mainstay treatment for Mirrizi syndrome.

REFERENCE

Clemente, G., Tringali, A., De Rose, A. M., Panettieri, E., Murazio, M., … Nuzzo, G. (2018). Mirizzi syndrome: Diagnosis and management of a challenging biliary disease. *Canadian Journal of Gastroenterology & Hepatology, 2018*, 6962090. doi:10.1155/2018/6962090.

CASE 68

Primary Sclerosing Cholangitis

1. A, B, C, D. All the responses can have similar imaging features, which include intrahepatic biliary dilatation with multiple short segmental strictures.
2. B. "Beaded appearance" seen in the liver in PSC is described as multifocal annular short segmental strictures in the intrahepatic and/or extrahepatic biliary system alternating with normal ducts.
3. A, B, C, D. All the complications mentioned can be seen in PSC.
4. C. Liver transplantation is the definitive treatment for liver complications in PSC. The other treatments are palliative treatments for complications seen in PSC.

Comment

- Introduction: Primary sclerosing cholangitis (PSC) is a chronic progressive immune-mediated inflammatory disease of the intrahepatic and/or extrahepatic bile ducts.
  - Leads to bile duct fibrosis, multifocal strictures, cholestasis, and biliary cirrhosis.
  - Relatively rare (50 per 100,000 patients), and twice as common in men compared to women

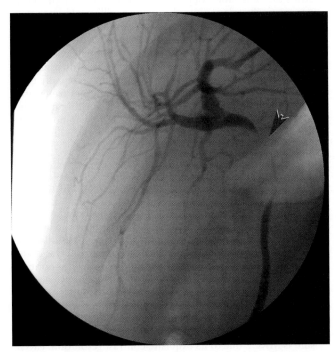

Fig. 67.1 Spot image from endoscopy retrograde cholangiopancreatography (ERCP) showing hepatic biliary dilatation with compression of the common bile duct *(arrow)* at the border from an extrinsic structure. This was shown to be a large calculus at the neck of the gallbladder with surrounding edema compressing on the common bile duct suggesting Mirizzi syndrome.

- Associated with ulcerative colitis and Crohn's disease in 70% of patients.
- Present with cholestatic symptoms: jaundice, pruritis, fatigue, right upper quadrant pain, steatorrhea, and episodes of acute bacterial cholangitis.
- Imaging features of liver disease in PSC:
  - US: dilatation and diffuse echogenic thickening of the extrahepatic ducts.
  - CT: focal, discontinuous, and often peripheral segmental ductal dilatation without associated mass lesion, thickening, and enhancement of the bile ducts due to inflammation. Other features of cirrhosis include atrophy of the left lobe and hypertrophy of the caudate lobe.
  - MRI and MRCP: intrahepatic bile duct dilatation, stenosis, beading, extrahepatic bile duct stenosis, wall enhancement and thickening.
    - Early stage: multifocal annular short segmental strictures in the intrahepatic and/or extrahepatic biliary system alternating with normal ducts or focal mildly dilated ducts (beaded appearance), located at biliary bifurcations.
    - Advanced stages: biliary ducts at the periphery of the liver parenchyma may not be well visualized and may have a "pruned-tree" appearance.
    - Other features: diverticula, webs, and stones.
- Complications of PSC include development of cirrhosis and liver failure, development of associated malignancies such as cholangiocarcinoma, gallbladder cancer, and colorectal cancer.
- Treatment: Oral ursodiol (ursodeoxycholic acid), palliative therapy with endoscopic or percutaneous interventional cholangiographic techniques such as dilation of dominant strictures, placement of stents, or lithotripsy to break intraductal stones. Definitive treatment of liver disease is liver transplantation.

REFERENCES

Gossard, A. A., & Gores, G. J. (2017). Primary sclerosing cholangitis: What the gastroenterologist and hepatologist needs to know. *Clinical Liver Disease, 21*(4), 725–737. doi:10.1016/j.cld.2017.06.004.

Khoshpouri, P., Habibabadi, R. R., Hazhirkarzar, B., Ameli, S., Ghadimi, M., … Ghasabeh, M. (2019). Imaging features of primary sclerosing cholangitis: From diagnosis to liver transplant follow-up. *Radiographics, 39*(7), 1938–1964. doi:10.1148/rg.2019180213.

Vitellas, K. M., Keogan, M. T., Freed, K. S., Enns, R. A., Spritzer, C. E., … Baillie, J. M. (2000). Radiologic manifestations of sclerosing cholangitis with emphasis on MR cholangiopancreatography. *Radiographics, 20*(4), 959–975; quiz 1108–1109, 1112. doi:10.1148/radiographics.20.4.g00jl04959.

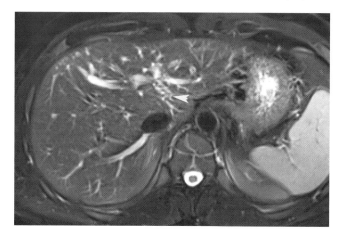

Fig. 68.1 Axial fat-suppressed T2 weighted image from magnetic resonance imaging (MRI) shows multifocal areas of biliary dilatation in the liver (*yellow arrows*).

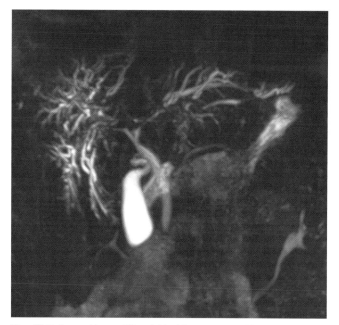

Fig. 68.2 Coronal heavy T2 weighted fat-suppressed image from magnetic resonance cholangiopancreatography (MRCP) shows multiple areas of biliary dilatation and strictures in the liver in both lobes with normal appearance of the extrahepatic bile ducts. This was consistent with primary sclerosing cholangitis (PSC).

CASE 69

Pancreas Divisum

1. B. The axial T2 weighted image and MRCP image demonstrate the classic form of pancreas divisum, in which the dorsal pancreatic duct drains into the minor papilla while a noncommunicating ventral duct empties alongside the common bile duct into the minor papilla. Although controversial, this variant anatomy is considered to be a cause of pancreatitis. Annular pancreas is an anomaly in which a ring of pancreatic tissue surrounds the descending duodenum, potentially compressing and/or obstructing the duodenum. Ansa pancreatica is a variant of ductal anatomy featuring a small branch duct that arises from the dorsal duct to drain into the minor papilla. The duct initially descends caudally before ascending into a loop toward the minor papilla (*ansa* = "handle" in Latin; named for its appearance). Autoimmune pancreatitis is characterized by a "sausage pancreas" appearance in its early stages and later by a soft tissue rind surrounding the gland and "cutoff" of the pancreatic tail.

2. A. Of pancreas divisum cases, 70% are of the Type 1, or "classic," variety. This describes the absence of connection between the dorsal and ventral pancreatic ducts. Type 2 describes absence of the ventral duct, in which the entire pancreas drains into the minor papilla. Type 3 occurs in a small minority; a remnant communication exists between the dorsal and pancreatic ducts. Reverse pancreas divisum describes a small remnant dorsal duct that does not communicate with the main pancreatic duct but drains into the minor papilla.

3. C. The current gold standard for detection of pancreas divisum is MRCP due to its exquisite contrast resolution. ERCP was the traditional method for detection but is invasive and carries a small risk of pancreatitis. Pancreas divisum can be detected on CT but is usually only done so incidentally. Ultrasound is not an option for this diagnosis due to its technical limitations in visualizing this area of the abdomen in most patients.

4. A. Most cases of pancreas divisum are asymptomatic and detected incidentally. Intervention is not necessary in the majority of cases. In patients with recurrent pancreatitis, pancreatic enzyme supplementation, minor papillectomy, and minor papilla stenting are all potential therapeutic options.

Comment

- Pancreas divisum is the most common congenital abnormality of pancreatic duct development. Its incidence ranges from 4% to 10% of the general population with a prevalence of approximately 9% at MRCP, up to 8% at ERCP, and up to 14% in autopsy series.
- Pancreas divisum is most commonly incidental and asymptomatic in affected patients; however, it may be associated with abdominal pain and idiopathic pancreatitis.
- Normal pancreatic development results in the fusion of two separate buds from the midgut at 5 weeks of gestation with associated fusion of the ventral and dorsal pancreatic ducts. Failure of this fusion results in the dorsal duct draining most of the pancreatic gland via the minor papilla (with no communication with the ventral duct and therefore the major papilla in the majority of cases). Despite some controversy, this anatomy is considered a cause of pancreatitis.
- There are three known subtypes of pancreas divisum:
  - Type 1: classic pancreas divisum. Occurs in 70% of cases. No connection between the dorsal and ventral ducts.
  - Type 2: absent ventral duct. Occurs in 20% to 25% of cases. The minor papilla drains the entire pancreatic gland while the major papilla drains the common bile duct.
  - Type 3: functional. Occurs in approximately 5% of cases. An inadequate connection exists between the dorsal and ventral pancreatic ducts.
- "Reverse pancreas divisum" has also been described, in which fusion does occur but a small separate residual dorsal duct drains into the minor papilla.
- A santorinicele can occur in the presence of pancreas divisum. This describes a cystic dilation of the distal dorsal duct immediately upstream from the minor papilla.
- When detected incidentally, pancreas divisum generally does not warrant intervention. However, in a patient with recurrent pancreatitis who is diagnosed with pancreas divisum, management options include surveillance +/− pancreatic enzyme

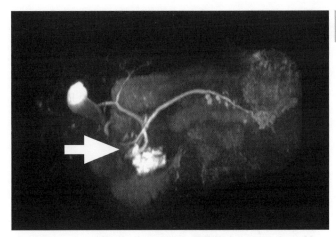

Fig. 69.2 Coronal heavily T2 weighted MRCP image of the pancreaticobiliary system demonstrating a "crossing duct sign" *(arrow)* as seen in pancreas divisum. The main pancreatic duct drains into the smaller minor papilla while the bile duct empties into the major papilla.

supplementation, minor papilla stenting, minor papillectomy, and endoscopic dilatation of potential pancreatic duct stricture.
- Imaging findings of pancreas divisum:
  - ERCP: traditional method of diagnosis. Suspected when injection of the main pancreatic duct at the major papilla fails to demonstrate opacification of the duct at the pancreatic body and tail.
  - CT: may be detected incidentally by a "crossing duct sign" on axial slices, in which the dorsal pancreatic duct crosses over the common bile duct to drain into the minor papilla.
  - MRI: current gold standard for diagnosis. Characterized by drainage of the dorsal duct into the minor papilla with drainage of the noncommunicating ventral duct with the common bile duct into the major papilla (in the classic form). Secretin administration may result in increased sensitivity of detection of classic pancreas divisum and its variants.

REFERENCES

Soto, J. A., Lucey, B. C., & Stuhlfaut, J. W. (2005). Pancreas divisum: Depiction with multi-detector row CT. *Radiology, 235*(2), 503–508.

Turkvatan, A., Erden, A., Turkoglu, M. A., & Yener, O. (2013). Congenital variants and anomalies of the pancreas and pancreatic duct: Imaging by magnetic resonance cholangiopancreatography and multidetector computed tomography. *Korean Journal of Radiology, 14*(6), 905–913.

Yu, J., Turner, M. A., Fulcher, A. S., & Halvorsen, R. L. (2006). Congenital anomalies and normal variants of the pancreaticobiliary tract and the pancreas in adults: Part 2, pancreatic duct and pancreas. *American Journal of Roentgenology, 187*(6), 1544–1553.

CASE 70

Pancreatic Neuroendocrine Tumor

1. A, B, C, D. Pancreatic neuroendocrine tumors are more common in patients with MEN type 1, von Hippel-Lindau disease, tuberous sclerosis, and neurofibromatosis type 1, although they most often occur sporadically.
2. A. Insulinoma is the most common type, accounting for ~40% of functional pancreatic NETs. Gastrinomas are the second most common pancreatic NET, and the most common subtype associated with MEN type 1. Glucagonoma and VIPoma are both rare.
3. C. Glucagonoma is associated with the "4 Ds" of dermatitis, diabetes mellitus, deep vein thrombosis, and depression. Insulinoma may present with Whipple triad (fasting hypoglycemia, symptoms of hypoglycemia, and immediate relief of symptoms after IV glucose administration). Gastrinoma is associated with

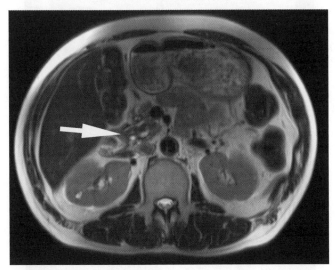

Fig. 69.1 Axial T2 weighted image without fat saturation shows the main pancreatic duct emptying in the minor papilla while the common bile duct drains into the major papilla *(arrows)*.

Zollinger-Ellison syndrome (peptic ulcer disease). VIPoma may demonstrate the clinical triad of watery diarrhea, hypokalemia, and achlorhydria

4. D. The overall sensitivity for detection of pancreatic NET is 90% to 100% with a Ga-68 dotatate scan. In-111 octreotide scans are useful for well-differentiated NETs, with an overall sensitivity of around 80%. F-18 PET CT has poor overall sensitivity unless the tumor is poorly differentiated. MRI demonstrates similar sensitivity to CT.

Comment

- Pancreatic neuroendocrine tumors (NETs)—previously termed *islet cell tumors* due to their derivation from the islets of Langerhans—comprise 1% to 3% of all pancreatic neoplasms, typically occurring in young to middle-age adults with no gender predilection.
- Most pancreatic NETs occur sporadically. The most common associations include multiple endocrine neoplasia (MEN) type 1 (1%–2% of NETs) and von Hippel-Lindau disease. They also occur more commonly in patients with neurofibromatosis type 1 and tuberous sclerosis.
- The majority of pancreatic NETs (~50%–70%) are nonfunctioning and thus do not produce or secrete endocrine products. As such, they can grow to large sizes over a long period of time because they are usually asymptomatic.
- Functional tumors typically present earlier due to clinical manifestations related to their underlying cell line and activity.
  - Insulinoma: Whipple triad—fasting hypoglycemia, symptoms of hypoglycemia, and immediate relief of symptoms after IV glucose administration
  - Gastrinoma: Zollinger-Ellison syndrome
  - Glucagonoma: "4 Ds"—dermatitis (necrolytic migratory erythema, oral rashes), diabetes mellitus, deep vein thrombosis, depression
- Pancreatic NETs are histologically graded by the 2017 World Health Organization classification as well differentiated or poorly differentiated.
  - Well differentiated: divided into grades 1, 2, and 3 according to number of mitoses and Ki-67 index
  - Poorly differentiated: small cell type or large cell type
- Pancreatic NETs are categorized by their markers of neuroendocrine differentiation (chromogranin A and synaptophysin) and their hormone production.
  - Insulinoma: most common sporadic NET; ~40% of functional NETs. Ga-68 dotatate scans show high sensitivity for detection, particularly low-grade and well-differentiated insulinomas. F-18 PET CT is often helpful for higher-grade, poorly differentiated tumors.
  - Gastrinoma: second most common pancreatic NET; most common type in the setting of MEN type 1. Initially present with peptic ulcer disease (PUD). Diarrhea is also common. Hepatic metastases portend a poor prognosis. In-111 octreotide exhibits high sensitivity for detection of gastrinomas.
  - Glucagonoma: most are malignant and large at presentation; ~50% 5-year survival rate.
  - VIPoma: very rare. Classic clinical triad of watery diarrhea, hypokalemia, and achlorhydria (WDHA syndrome).
  - Somatostatinoma: rare; variable presentation. Patients may display "inhibitory syndrome": triad of mild diabetes, cholelithiasis, and diarrhea/steatorrhea.
- Treatment of NETs is surgical if detected early (potentially curable). Long-term survival in patients with metastatic disease is variable, depending on tumor biology and subtype.
- Imaging findings of pancreatic neuroendocrine tumor:
  - US: well-circumscribed, round/oval hypoechoic pancreatic mass. Liver metastases may be targetoid or hyperechoic.
  - CT: smaller tumors are usually hypervascular and well circumscribed. Larger tumors may be heterogeneous and

can demonstrate necrosis, cystic change, and calcifications. About 10% of pancreatic NETs are cystic lesions with a hypervascular rim. Most have a distinct capsule and thus displace rather than invade adjacent structures. However, aggressive tumors can be angioinvasive.

- MRI: similar sensitivity as CT. Typically T1 hypointense and T2 hyperintense relative to normal pancreatic parenchyma; hypervascular on dynamic contrast enhanced sequences.

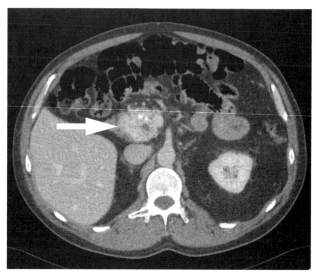

Fig. 70.1 Axial computed tomography (CT) image of the abdomen with intravenous (IV) contrast in the portal venous phase demonstrating a heterogeneous mass in the head of the pancreas *(arrow)* with necrosis and calcifications.

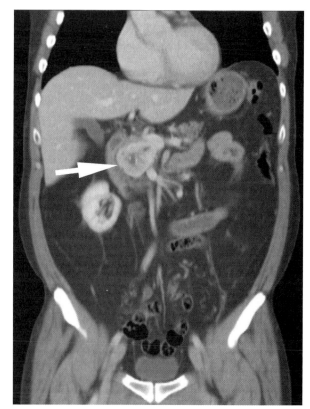

Fig. 70.2 Coronal reformatted computed tomography (CT) image with intravenous (IV) contrast in the portal venous phase better depicts the degree of central necrosis *(arrow)* in the pancreatic tumor.

- Nuclear medicine:
  - In-111 octreotide: overall sensitivity of ~80% (highest in gastrinomas, lowest in insulinomas)
  - F-18 PET CT: limited sensitivity unless poorly differentiated
  - Ga-68 dotatate: up to 90% to 100% overall sensitivity for pancreatic NET detection

REFERENCES

Raman, S. P., Hruban, R. H., Cameron, J. L., Wolfgang, C. L., & Fishman, E. K. (2012). Pancreatic imaging mimics: Part 2, pancreatic neuroendocrine tumors and their mimics. *American Journal of Roentgenology*, *199*(2), 309–318.

Tamm, E. P., Bhosale, P., Lee, J. H., & Rohren, E. M. (2016). State-of-the-art imaging of pancreatic neuroendocrine tumors. *Surgical Oncology Clinics of North America*, *25*(2), 375–400.

CASE 72

Splenic Angiosarcoma With Liver Metastases

1. C. Angiosarcoma is a rare primary malignancy of the spleen. However, it is the most common nonhematolymphatic splenic malignancy. It is an aggressive tumor with a very poor prognosis.
2. B. Splenic angiosarcoma metastasizes to the liver in up to 70% of cases. Spread to the brain, bones, and lungs is also common, but not as frequent as the liver.
3. A. Splenectomy may decrease the risk of splenic hemorrhage from angiosarcoma. Locoregional intervention for angiosarcoma is not typically performed.
4. D. Thorium dioxide (Thorotrast), vinyl chloride, and arsenic are all associated with increased risk of hepatic angiosarcoma but not splenic angiosarcoma.

Comment

- Angiosarcoma is a rare tumor of the spleen but the most common nonhematolymphoid splenic malignancy.
- It is an extremely aggressive neoplasm with a very poor prognosis (usually fatal).
- Metastasis occurs via hematologic dissemination, most often spreading to the liver (70% of cases). Other sites of metastatic spread include the lung, brain, and bone.
- Spontaneous splenic rupture is a complication that can occur in up to 30% of cases.
- Splenectomy prior to rupture may improve patient survival.
- Splenic angiosarcoma occurs in an older patient population with no gender predilection. Presentation is variable and nonspecific.
- There are no known associated risk factors, unlike with hepatic angiosarcoma, which can be associated with occupational exposure to arsenic or vinyl chloride or prior exposure to the intravenous contrast agent thorium dioxide.
- Imaging findings of splenic angiosarcoma:
  - US: heterogeneous echotexture with an enlarged, hypervascular spleen. Single or multiple masses may be present with cystic and/or solid components.
  - CT: single or multiple irregular poorly defined heterogeneous masses within an enlarged spleen. Usually low in attenuation but can vary depending on degree of necrosis and/or hemorrhage. Avid peripheral enhancement on postcontrast imaging. May present with intrasplenic subcapsular hemorrhage or extracapsular hemorrhage (hemoperitoneum).
  - MRI: Intrasplenic masses that are typically hypointense to the spleen on both T1 and T2 weighted images. However, angiosarcoma can also be both T1 and T2 hyperintense due to hemorrhage and/or necrosis. Tumor demonstrates intense heterogeneous enhancement as on CT.

Case 71 is online only and accessible at www.expertconsult.com.

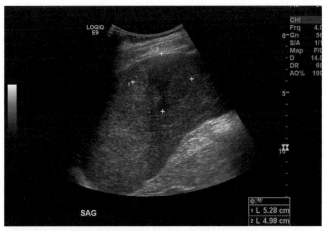

Fig. 72.1 Sagittal ultrasound demonstrating a focal heterogeneous mass in the spleen, measuring approximately 5 cm *(arrow)*.

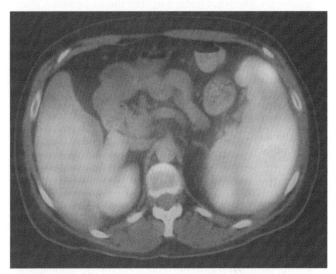

Fig. 72.2 Axial fused positron emission tomography (PET)/computed tomography (CT) image shows intense FDG uptake within the mass *(arrow)* in addition to several other smaller hypermetabolic splenic masses.

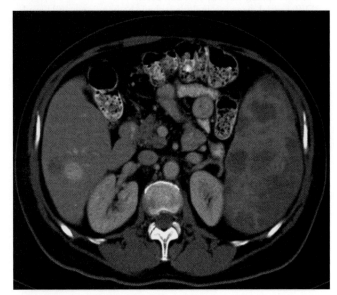

Fig. 72.3 Axial contrast-enhanced computed tomography (CT) demonstrates multiple low attenuation masses in the spleen *(arrow)* along with a hypervascular liver metastasis *(arrowhead)*.

REFERENCES

Ha, H. K., Kim, H. H., Kim, B. K., Han, J. K., & Choi, B. I. (1994). Primary angiosarcoma of the spleen: CT and MR imaging. *Acta Radiologica*, 35(5), 455–458.

Thompson, W. M., Levy, A. D., Aguilera, N. S., Gorospe, L., & Abbott, R. M. (2005). Angiosarcoma of the spleen: Imaging characteristics in 12 patients. *Radiology*, 235(1), 106–115.

CASE 73

Splenic Hamartoma

1. B, C. Multiple splenic hamartomas can be seen in association with both tuberous sclerosis and Wiskott-Aldrich syndrome. They are not associated with von Hippel-Lindau syndrome or Birt-Hogg-Dube syndrome.
2. D. Recent literature suggests that sclerosing adenomatoid nodular transformation (SANT) may represent a fibrosing variation of splenic hamartoma. Littoral cell angioma and hemangioma are distinct entities. Lymphoma can primarily or secondarily involve the spleen but is also a separate disease process.
3. A. Splenic hamartoma can most easily be distinguished on dynamic contrast-enhanced imaging in the arterial phase, where it demonstrates immediate intense heterogeneous enhancement. Hamartomas are more uniform and similar to normal spleen on other phases of contrast.
4. B. Splenic hamartomas are typically heterogeneous and hyperintense on T2 weighted imaging. This can be helpful in identifying it as a distinct lesion from normal spleen. Hamartomas have similar characteristics to background spleen on T1 weighted imaging, diffusion-weighted imaging, and chemical shift imaging.

Comment

- Splenic hamartomas are uncommon lesions that are usually encountered as an incidental finding on imaging.
- Hamartomas in the spleen are usually solitary but can be multiple in patients with tuberous sclerosis or Wiskott-Aldrich syndrome.
- Can occur in any age group with no gender predilection.
- Usually asymptomatic but can result in pain or discomfort if large.
- As with hamartomas of other organs, these lesions represent a disorganized overgrowth of normal parenchyma. As such, they exhibit a similar radiologic appearance to background normal spleen on US, CT, and MRI.
- Differential diagnosis includes splenic hemangioma and lymphangioma. Sclerosing adenomatoid nodular transformation (SANT) may represent a fibrosing form of splenic hamartoma.

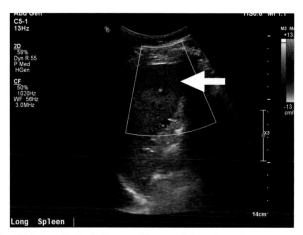

Fig. 73.1 Longitudinal ultrasound image of the spleen demonstrate a focal slightly hyperechoic mass with internal Doppler flow *(arrow)*.

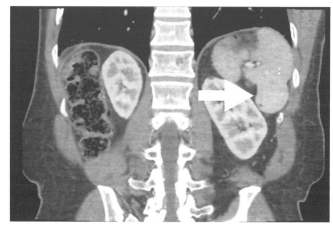

Fig. 73.2 Coronal reformatted contrast-enhanced computed tomography (CT) of the spleen in the late arterial phase demonstrating a focal enhancing mass at the inferior tip of the spleen *(arrow)*.

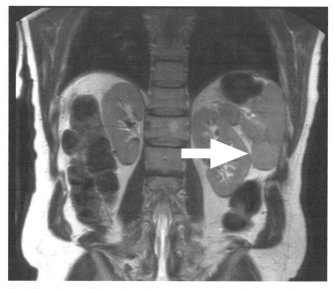

Fig. 73.3 Coronal T2 weighted magnetic resonance imaging (MRI) shows a mildly T2 hyperintense mass *(arrow)* in the inferior spleen.

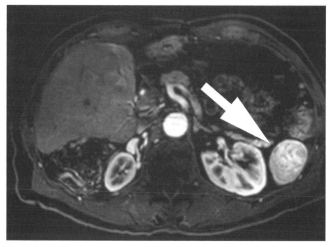

Fig. 73.4 Arterial-phase postcontrast T1 weighted fat-saturated image demonstrating the heterogeneous hypervascular enhancement of the splenic hamartoma *(arrow)*.

- Imaging findings of splenic hamartomas:
  - US: hypoechoic solid masses that can be homogeneous or heterogeneous (due to cystic change or internal hemorrhage); usually hypovascular on Doppler imaging.
  - CT: isodense or slightly hypodense to normal splenic parenchyma. Demonstrates heterogeneous postcontrast enhancement, particularly on the arterial phase.
  - MRI: isointense on T1 weighted images; hyperintense on T2 weighted images. Characteristically demonstrates avid heterogeneous hyperenhancement on immediate postcontrast imaging, which can be a distinguishing feature from splenic hemangioma. Becomes more homogeneous and uniform on more delayed imaging.

REFERENCES

Abbott, R. M., Levy, A. D., Aguilera, N. S., Gorospe, L., & Thompson W. M. (2004). From the archives of the AFIP: Primary vascular neoplasms of the spleen: Radiologic-pathologic correlation. *Radiographics, 24*(4), 1137–1163.

Falk, G. A., Nooli, N. P., Morris-Stiff, G., Plesec, T. P., & Rosenblatt, S. (2012). Sclerosing angiomatoid nodular transformation (SANT) of the spleen: Case report and review of the literature. *International Journal of Surgery Case Reports, 3*(10), 492–500.

Sim, H., In Ahn, H., Han, H., Jun, Y. J., Rehman, A., … Jang, S. M. (2013). Splenic hamartoma: A case report and review of the literature. *World Journal of Clinical Cases, 1*(7), 217–219.

CASE 74

Bilateral Adrenal Hemorrhage

1. A, D. Bilateral adrenal masses developing over a week most likely present hemorrhage especially given clinical history of anticoagulation therapy in a young patient. Adrenal lymphoma can potentially develop over several weeks but is less likely considering the short interval. Adrenal metastasis is unlikely considering patient's young age and lack of prior known malignancy.
2. C. MRI is the most accurate imaging modality for detecting and characterizing adrenal hemorrhage because of its signal characteristics related to the presence of blood products and its ability to evaluate for underlying preexisting neoplasm.
3. A. Trauma typically produces unilateral adrenal hemorrhage.
4. A. Acute adrenal insufficiency is a rare but potentially life-threatening complication when bilateral adrenal gland hemorrhages are present.

Comment

- Introduction and etiology: Hemorrhage of the adrenal gland occurs due to both traumatic and nontraumatic conditions.
  - Nontraumatic adrenal hemorrhage is uncommon and is associated with multiple other conditions.
    - Patients can present with varied symptoms depending on the amount of hemorrhage, sudden or gradual onset of hemorrhage, the ability of the surrounding structures to contain the bleeding, the presence or absence of hemorrhage into the perinephric space, and the functational status of the patient's hemostatic system.
    - Patients may present with gradual-onset upper abdominal or flank pain, or, in the acute presentation, signs of massive blood loss.
    - Approximately 16% to 50% of patients with bilateral adrenal hemorrhages have life-threatening adrenal insufficiency.
  - Traumatic adrenal hemorrhage typically produces unilateral hemorrhage and involves the right adrenal gland more commonly than the left. This may be due to the direct insertion of the right adrenal vein into the inferior vena cava or compression of the right adrenal gland between the liver and spine.

- Nontraumatic adrenal hemorrhage may be due to stress, bleeding diathesis including anticoagulant use, disseminated intravascular coagulopathy and antiphospholipid syndrome, procedures, and intratumoral bleeding. Stress could be in the form of recent surgery, organ failure, sepsis, and pregnancy. Multiple causes can be present at a single time as well.
- Imaging findings: Imaging appearance of adrenal hemorrhage depends on chronicity.
  - Acute hemorrhage is characterized by evolution over time of the attenuation of a nonenhancing mass in one or both adrenal glands. Focal preservation of normal adrenal enhancement may be seen and often has a peripheral distribution. Imaging will show adrenal enlargement of greater than simple fluid attenuation and periadrenal infiltration.
  - On US, acute adrenal hemorrhage may appear as complex hypoechoic solid masses, and the echogenicity gradually decreases as the hematoma resolves, and it may become cystic.
  - On noncontrast CT, acute hemorrhage appears as a high-attenuation mass of the adrenal gland. This may resolve completely or may organize into a chronic cystic collection with or without calcification, which is termed *adrenal pseudocyst*.
  - MRI is the most accurate imaging modality for detecting and characterizing adrenal hemorrhage.
    - In the acute stage (<7 days after onset), the hematoma typically appears isointense and slightly hypointense on T1 weighted images and markedly hypointense on T2 weighted images due to high concentration of intracellular D oxyhemoglobin. In the subacute stage (7 days to 7 weeks after onset), the hematoma appears hyperintense on T1 and T2 weighted images due to the paramagnetic effects of free methemoglobin. In the chronic stage (which typically begins 7 weeks after onset), a hypointense rim is present on T1 and T2 weighted images due to preferential T2 proton relaxation enhancement, which is due to the hemosiderin deposit and presence of a fibrous capsule. Gradient echo imaging is helpful in demonstrating the "blooming effect" (magnetic susceptibility effect) that results from hemosiderin deposition.
- Management: Prompt recognition of adrenal hemorrhage is essential, since, if the patient has acute adrenal insufficiency, adrenal hormone replacement therapy is necessary. Unilateral adrenal hemorrhages can usually be managed conservatively. In nontraumatic adrenal hemorrhage, underlying neoplasm should be ruled out by follow-up imaging.

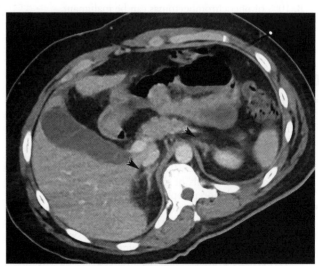

Fig. 74.1 Axial noncontrast computed tomography (CT) obtained 1 week before Fig. 74.2 shows normal bilateral adrenal glands *(arrows)*.

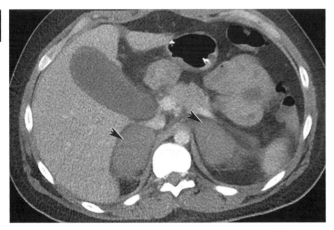

Fig. 74.2 Contrast enhanced axial computed tomography (CT) in late venous phase shows hyperintense bilateral adrenal masses *(arrows)* new from the prior CT (see Fig. 74.1).

REFERENCES

Jordan, E., Poder, L., Courtier, J., Sai, V., Jung, A., & Coakley, F. V. (2012). Imaging of nontraumatic adrenal hemorrhage. *American Journal of Roentgenolgy*, *199*(1), W91–W98. doi:10.2214/AJR.11.7973.

Kawashima, A., Sandler, C. M., Ernst, R. D., Takahashi, N., Roubidoux, M. A., … Goldman, S. (1999). Imaging of nontraumatic hemorrhage of the adrenal gland. *Radiographics*, *19*(4), 949–963. doi:10.1148/radiographics.19.4.g99jl13949.

CASE 75

Pheochromocytoma

1. A. B, C, D. Fat-poor adrenal adenomas are homogenous lesions that show washout of contrast on the delayed images. Appearances of pheochromocytomas can be highly variable. Smaller lesions are typically homogenous; large lesions are more heterogenous, complex, and cystic. Pheochromocytomas can show similar washout characteristics as adrenal adenomas. Adrenocortical carcinoma tends to be large invasive tumors, typically solid, but necrosis and hemorrhage common. Adrenal metastasis can be unilateral or bilateral.
2. D. MIBG scintigraphy is highly specific for pheochromocytomas and paragangliomas and can be used to localize multiple ectopic tumors.
3. B. 10% of pheochromocytomas can be malignant.
4. B. With a history of hypertension symptoms, chemical screening to exclude a pheochromocytoma should precede fine needle aspiration or biopsy of an adrenal mass.

Comment

- Introduction: Pheochromocytoma is a rare lesion most commonly found in the adrenal medulla but may arise in the retroperitoneum ganglia, organ of Zuckerkandl, or urinary bladder.
  - More than 90% of pheochromocytomas are located within the adrenal glands; ~10% are malignant. They arise from the chromaffin cells of the adrenal medulla and typically produce both norepinephrine and epinephrine.
- Clinical manifestations and diagnosis: Hypertension is the most common feature occurring in >90% of patients. Other symptoms include headache, palpitations, and sweating. These are symptoms associated with catecholamine excess.
  - Hypertensive attacks may be induced during anesthesia induction, manipulation of the gland during surgery, percutaneous biopsy, or selective adrenal angiography.

- Approximately 10% of cases are clinically silent with an increasing number of cases seen as incidentalomas on imaging.
- Diagnosis of pheochromocytoma imaging is often challenging due to its complex and variable appearance related to necrosis, fibrosis, cystic and fatty degeneration, and calcification; hence it is described as an "imaging chameleon" mimicking other lesions.
- The plasma catecholamine levels and 24-hour urine free catecholamine and catecholamine metabolite levels are elevated in these patients.
- Imaging findings:
  - US: pheochromocytomas are heterogenous, well encapsulated with hypervascularization and color Doppler, and an early arterial pattern of enhancement at contrast enhanced US
  - CT: pheochromocytomas may present solid, cystic, calcific, and/or necrotic components.
    - Smaller tumors tend to display a more uniform attenuation, with a density of 40 to 50 HU.
    - After contrast administration, pheochromocytomas enhance avidly with some of them showing higher enhancement on the portal venous phase and others on the arterial phase.
    - Pheochromocytomas may show washout characteristics similar to those of adenomas and therefore cannot be reliably differentiated from adenomas using CT washout protocols.
  - MRI: highly sensitive for the diagnosis of pheochromocytomas with a sensitivity of about 98%
    - Pheochromocytoma is slightly hypointense on T1 weighted and hyperintense on T2 weighted images. It does not present loss of signal intensity on opposed-phase images, unlike the typical adenoma.
  - Nuclear medicine test using ^{131}I-MIGB and indium-111 (^{111}In) pentetreotide is often helpful in localizing multiple or ectopic tumors.
- Management: If an adrenal mass is detected in the patient with back chemical evidence of a pheochromocytoma, surgical excision with adequate adrenal blockade is the appropriate treatment.

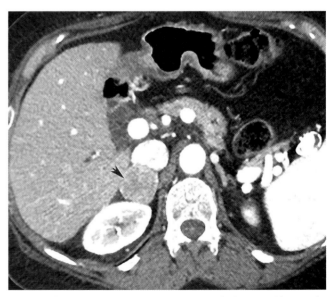

Fig. 75.1 Axial postcontrast computed tomography image at 60 seconds shows a homogenous hypervascular mass in the right adrenal gland *(arrow)*. Left adrenal gland is normal.

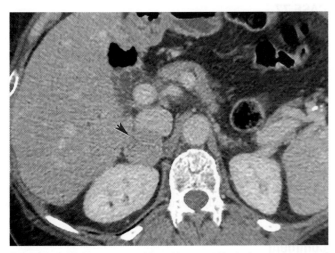

Fig. 75.2 Axial postcontrast delayed image at 5 minutes shows loss of contrast from the right adrenal mass *(arrow)*.

REFERENCES

Albano, D., Agnello, F., Midiri, F., Pecoraro, G., Bruno, A., ... Alongi, P. (2019). Imaging features of adrenal masses. *Insights into Imaging, 10*(1), 1. doi:10.1186/s13244-019-0688-8.

Lockhart, M. E., Smith, J. K., & Kenney, P. J. (2002). Imaging of adrenal masses. *European Journal of Radiology, 41*(2), 95–112. doi:10.1016/s0720-048x(01)00444-2.

CASE 76

Renal Arteriovenous Shunt

1. B, C. Arteriovenous malformation in the kidney will be seen as focal aneurysms and/or focal enhancing mass with only arterial enhancement and direct medication with the renal vein with early enhancement of the renal vein. These features are seen in this particular case. Renal cell carcinomas are also known to enhance avidly; however, the location of these masses in the collecting system associated with the renal arteries does not suggest this diagnosis. Hemorrhagic renal cysts do not have significant arterial enhancement as seen in this particular case. Renal calculi can present as hyperdense lesions seen within the collecting system.
2. B. Percutaneous embolization is favored as a treatment of choice in this entity due to its efficacy and relative lack of invasiveness.
3. C. Hypertension is seen in this entity due to the diversion of blood flow from the renal parenchyma distal to the shunt, resulting in parenchymal ischemia with subsequent renin release, which causes hypertension.
4. D. Renal vein is seen to enhance early in arteriovenous specialists due to the director medication between the artery and vein seen.

Comment

- Background: Renal arteriovenous malformation is a rare condition with the prevalence of ~0.04% of the general population.
- Two etiologies of renal AVMs have been described: congenital and acquired. They can also be classified as traumatic and nontraumatic.
  - Traumatic renal AV shunts are caused by penetrating blunt trauma, percutaneous or open biopsy, or surgery. The most common cause of traumatic renal AV shunts is iatrogenic injury especially percutaneous renal biopsy seen in about 7.4% to 11% of cases after renal biopsy.

- Nontraumatic renal AV shunts are either congenital or acquired with the term *renal AV malformation* representing a congenital AV shunt consisting of clusters of multiple coiled and tortuous vessels and the term *renal AV fistula* representing an acquired nontraumatic shunt that may be caused by a neoplasm, inflammation, or preexisting renal arterial diseases such as renal artery aneurysm, fibromuscular dysplasia, and arterial dissection.
- Clinical manifestation: Renal AV shunts can present with massive hematuria, retroperitoneal hemorrhage, flank pain, hypertension, and high output failure. Some of these cases can be asymptomatic as well, depending on the size of the renal AV shunt.
- Imaging findings:
  - Ultrasound is useful for screening for renal AV shunts especially following a renal biopsy.
    - Appear as a mosaic patterned tissue speckling of perivascular soft tissue caused by tissue vibration, reflecting a rapid flow rate.
    - Small AVFs are not as well seen on grayscale ultrasound; however, large AV fistula may be seen as cystic or tubal anechoic mass, which may be pulsatile with increased velocity flow seen on color Doppler within it.
    - Decrease in the arterial resistance in the arterial waveforms and arterial waveforms in the renal vein are seen on spectral Doppler imaging.
  - CT:
    - Seen as round or oval masses on precontrast CT, which enhance avidly on postcontrast images.
    - Renal vein typically shows an early enhancement due to the direct communication between the artery and the vein within the shunt.
    - Multiple tortuous and dilated vessels within the renal sinus and surrounding pelvicalyceal system.
  - MRI:
    - Tortuous flow void representing the dilated vessels with a high flow within them seen on the precontrast images would suggest an underlying vascular malformation.
    - Time resolved three-dimensional contrast enhanced MR angiography will show similar features as CT.

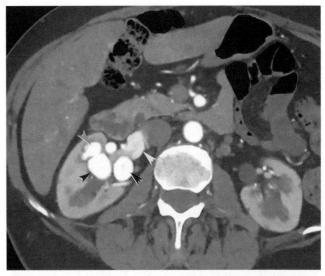

Fig. 76.1 Axial postcontrast computed tomography image shows multiple enhancing masses *(red arrows)* within the right renal collecting system, which are likely due to aneurysms with the arteriovenous malformation *(green arrow)* seen in the renal cortex. Note enlargement of the right renal vein *(yellow arrow)*.

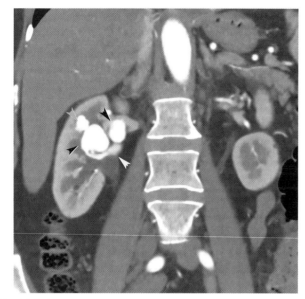

Fig. 76.2 Coronal postcontrast computed tomography image shows multiple enhancing masses *(red arrow)* within the right renal collecting system consistent with aneurysms and arteriovenous malformation seen in the renal cortex *(green arrow)*. Note early enhancement of the right renal vein *(yellow arrow)* due to the arteriovenous shunting.

- Management:
  - Endovascular treatment is the gold standard for treatment of renal AVMs due to its efficacy and relative lack of invasiveness.
    - Associated with the potential risk of complications, including renal infarction and pulmonary embolism, which are secondary to migration of embolic materials. There could also be risk of revascularization and/or incomplete occlusion due to inadequate or incomplete embolization.
  - Surgical treatment is only performed in limited cases in which endovascular embolization has failed or would have been technically difficult.

REFERENCES

Chimpiri, A. R., & Natarajan, B. (2009). Renal vascular lesions: Diagnosis and endovascular management. *Seminars in Interventional Radiology, 26*(3), 253–261.

Cho, K. J., & Stanley, J. C. (1978). Non-neoplastic congenital and acquired renal arteriovenous malformations and fistulas. *Radiology, 129*(2), 333–343.

Gülcü, A., Göktay, Y., Soylu, A., Türkmen, M., Kavukçu, S., … Seçil, M. (2013). Doppler US evaluation of renal biopsy complications in children. *Diagnostic and Interventional Radiology, 19*(1), 15–19.

Kramer, U., Ernemann, U., Fenchel, M., Seeger, A., Laub, G., … Claussen, C. D. (2011). Pretreatment evaluation of peripheral vascular malformations using low-dose contrast-enhanced time-resolved 3D MR angiography: Initial results in 22 patients. *American Journal of Roentgenology, 196*(3), 702–711.

Maruno, M., Kiyosue, H., Tanoue, S., Hongo, N., Matsumoto, S., … Mori, H. (2016). Renal arteriovenous shunts: Clinical features, imaging appearance, and transcatheter embolization based on angioarchitecture. *Radiographics, 36,* 580–595.

Meng, C. H., & Elkin, M. (1971). Immediate angiographic manifestations of iatrogenic renal injury due to percutaneous needle biopsy. *Radiology, 100*(2), 335–341.

Naganuma, H., Ishida, H., Konno, K., Sato, M., Ishida, J., … Komatsuda, T. (2001). Renal arteriovenous malformation: Sonographic findings. *Abdominal Imaging, 26*(6), 661–663.

Stiles, K. P., Yuan, C. M., Chung, E. M., Lyon, R. D., Lane, J. D., & Abbott, K. C. (2000). Renal biopsy in high-risk patients with medical diseases of the kidney. *American Journal of Kidney Diseases, 36*(2), 419–433.

CASE 77
Fibromuscular Dysplasia

1. A, B, C, D. All of these entities should be considered in the differential diagnosis of FMD; however, the classic "string of beads" appearance is seen in the renal arteries in FMD.
2. A. FMD is most commonly described as affecting the renal arteries and, to a lesser extent, internal carotid arteries.
3. B. Angiography is the most appropriate next step in diagnostic examination. Catheter-based angiography remains the gold-standard imaging modality for diagnosis because of its better special resolution.
4. B, C. FMD is most commonly seen in young females. The medial layer of the artery is the most commonly affected layer. The lesion is typically seen in the middle to the distal portion of the renal artery. It has a slowly progressive course.

Comment

- Fibromuscular dysplasia (FMD) is a heterogenous group of vascular lesions characterized by an idiopathic, noninflammatory, and nonatherosclerotic angiopathy of small and midsize arteries.
- Most common in young women with the female-to-male ratio of 3:1 and typically diagnosed between the ages of 30 and 50 years.
- Frequently asymptomatic. Symptomatic patients commonly present with:
  - Hypertension or, less commonly, renal impairment due to renal artery stenosis.
  - CNS symptoms, including headache, neck pain, pulsatile tinnitus, Horner syndrome from transient ischemic attack, stroke, dissection due to carotid and vertebral artery involvement
  - Angina, myocardial infarction, or sudden cardiac death due to coronary artery involvement
  - Symptoms of mesenteric ischemia
- FMD is classified into five categories according to the vessel wall layer affected:
  - Intima: 5%
    - Intimal fiberoplasia
  - Media: 90% to 95%
    - Medial dysplasia (70% commonest type)
    - Perimedial (subadventitial) fibroplasia (15%–20%)
    - Medial hyperplasia (8%–10%)
  - Adventitia: rare
    - Adventitial fibroplasia (1%)
- More commonly classified by Kincaid into the following:
  - Multifocal: multiple stenosis or string of beads aspect
  - Unifocal: short stenosis <1 cm long
  - Tubular: stenosis >1 cm long
  - Mixed types
- May affect any midsize artery in the body and is commonly multifocal and bilateral.
  - Common sites include renal arteries, cervicoencephalic arteries (including internal carotid arteries and vertebral arteries), iliac arteries, celiac trunk and mesenteric arteries, subclavian and axillary arteries.
- Imaging findings:
  - The string-of-beads aspect found in the renal or cervicoencephalic locations on arteriography, CT angiography, or MR angiography is highly suggestive of FMD. Focal or tubular lesions on angiography can also be seen. Another frequent finding suggestive of FMD diagnosis is the presence of a weblike defect at the origin of the internal carotid artery.
  - Arterial dissection can also be seen in a smaller number of cases.
  - Single or multiple aneurysms are frequently seen in FMD patients.

- Treatment/management:
  - Includes medical therapy and surveillance
  - Endovascular therapy for stenosis, dissection, or aneurysms
  - Surgery

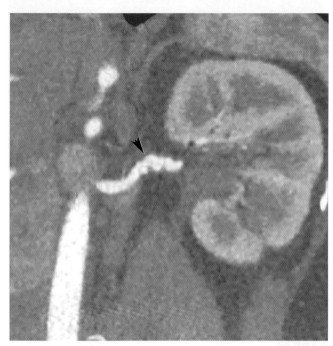

Fig. 77.1 Coronal reformat from a postcontrast computed tomography angiography (CTA) image shows single left renal artery. Alternating areas of focus strictures and aneurysmal dilatation create the typical "string of beads" appearance *(red arrow)* characteristic of fibromuscular dysplasia (FMD).

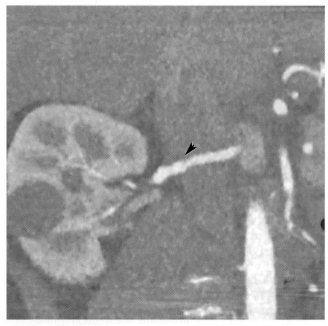

Fig. 77.2 Coronal reformat from a postcontrast computed tomography angiography (CTA) image shows single right renal artery. Alternating areas of focus strictures and aneurysmal dilatation create the typical "string of beads" appearance *(red arrow)* characteristic of fibromuscular dysplasia (FMD).

REFERENCE

Varennes, L., Tahon, F., Kastler, A., Grand, S., Thony, F., … Baguet, J. P. (2015). Fibromuscular dysplasia: What the radiologist should know: A pictorial review. *Insights into Imaging, 6*(3), 295–307. doi:10.1007/s13244-015-0382-4.

CASE 79

Renal Cell Carcinoma With IVC Thrombus

1. A, B, D. Images show a large mass arising in the right kidney with a tumor thrombus seen in the IVC. This appearance can be seen with leiomyosarcoma, renal cell carcinoma, or angiomyolipoma. Hepatocellular carcinoma can present with a tumor thrombus; however, there would not be renal involvement in this instance.
2. D. Tumor invades into the IVC and extends above the diaphragm, hence is at least a T3 lesion.
3. D. Invasion of the Gerota fascia suggests T4 tumor stage.
4. A, B, C. Invasion of Gerota fascia is indicated by an indistinct tumor margin, blurring of the renal outline, and focal thickening of Gerota fascia contiguous with the tumor.

Comment

- Background: Renal cell carcinoma is the eighth most common malignancy affecting adults.
  - Classical presentation: flank pain, hematuria, and palpable flank mass
    - Other presentations:
      - Varicocele formation from tumor thrombus in left renal vein or IVC
      - Paraneoplastic syndromes
        - Polycythemia secondary to excessive secretion of erythropoietin
        - Hypercalcemia from factors regulating calcium
        - Hepatic dysfunction—Stauffer syndrome
- TNM staging

Stage	Description
TX	Primary tumor cannot be assessed
T0	No evidence of primary tumor
T1	Tumor <7 cm in greatest dimension, limited to kidney
	T1a – Tumor <4 cm in greatest dimension, limited to kidney
	T1b – Tumor >4 cm but <7 cm in greatest dimension, limited to kidney
T2	Tumor ≥7 cm in greatest dimension, limited to kidney
T3	Tumor extends into major veins or invades adrenal gland or perinephric tissues, but not beyond Gerota fascia
	T3a – Tumor invades adrenal gland or perinephric tissues but not beyond Gerota fascia
	T3b – Tumor grossly extends into renal vein(s) or vena cava below diaphragm
	T3c – Tumor extends into vena cava above diaphragm
T4	Tumor invades beyond Gerota fascia
NX	Regional lymph nodes cannot be assessed
N0	No regional lymph node metastasis
N1	Metastasis in a single regional lymph node
N2	Metastasis in more than one regional lymph node
MX	Distant metastasis cannot be assessed
M0	No distant metastasis
M1	Distant metastasis

Case 78 is online only and accessible at www.expertconsult.com.

- Imaging: goal of radiologic imaging is to detect and stage the primary tumor
  - Interpretation should include:
    - Tumor size
    - Tumor interface with the renal parenchyma
    - Perinephric tumor extension
    - Local and regional lymph node enlargement
    - The presence and extent of venous invasion
    - Spread into contiguous organs
    - Involvement of the adrenal glands
    - Local or distant metastatic spread
- CT: most widely used
  - Overall accuracy 72% and 90%
  - Clear cell carcinoma is most common subtype
  - Hypervascular lesion
    - Strong enhancement in the corticomedullary phase
  - Frequently heterogeneous due to necrosis, hemorrhage, cystic components, or calcifications
- MRI:
  - Clear cell RCC is usually isointense to hypointense on T1 and hyperintense on T2 weighted images.
  - Do not have extracellular fat
  - 80% of clear cell RCC have intracellular fat, which leads to a drop in signal intensity on T1 opposed-phase images compared to in-phase images
- Perinephric spread: most specific sign of spread is the presence of a discrete mass measuring at least 1 cm in diameter within the perinephric space
  - Imaging:
    - Indistinct tumor margin
    - Blurring of the renal outline
    - Thickening of the perirenal fascia
      - Focal thickening of Gerota fascia contiguous with the tumor tends to be a more reliable indicator of invasion than generalized uniform thickening.
    - Strands of soft tissue spreading into the perinephric fat resulting in webs or wispy densities
- Venous invasion: most important sign is a persistent filling defect within the renal vein or IVC following intravenous contrast medium administration
  - MRI:
    - T1 weighted spin-echo pulse sequences: signal void of flowing blood is replaced by a relatively high signal produced by tumor thrombus
    - Time-of-flight GRE images: tumor thrombus has medium signal intensity and appears as a filling defect

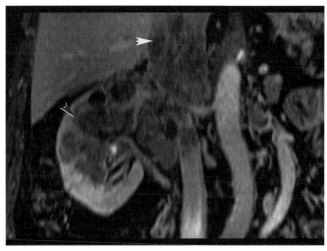

Fig. 79.2 Axial postcontrast T1 weighted image showing a large infiltrative tumor *(red arrow)* occupying almost all of the right kidney with tumor thrombus seen extending into the IVC *(yellow arrow)*.

REFERENCES

Ng, C. S., Wood, C. G., Silverman, P. M., Tannir, N. M., Tamboli, P., & Sandler, C. M. (2008). Renal cell carcinoma: Diagnosis, staging, and surveillance. *American Journal of Roentgenology, 191*(4), 1220–1232.

Reznek, R. H. (2004). CT/MRI in staging renal cell carcinoma. *Cancer Imaging, 4*(Spec No A), S25–S32. doi:10.1102/1470-7330.2004.0012.

CASE 80

Deep Renal Laceration (IV)

1. B. CT images show deep laceration in the left kidney with perirenal hemorrhage and extravasation of contrast on the delayed phase suggestive of Grade IV injury.
2. D. Ideal protocol for imaging kidneys with presence of trauma is a dual phase contrast enhanced CT with arterial and nephrographic phases. Early imaging allows for accurate evaluation of the vasculature. Five-minute delayed CT is useful for evaluation of renal collecting system injuries. Intravenous urography is not routinely used for imaging patients with renal trauma but could be obtained when the patient is rushed straight to the operating room or when CT is unavailable.
3. C. Deep laceration with urinoma formation is consistent with Grade IV AAST injury.
4. C. Grade 4 injuries with laceration involving the collecting system with urinary extravasation need surgical repair.

Comment

- Injury to the kidney seen in approximately 8% to 10% of patients with blunt penetrating abdominal injuries.
- The American Association for the Surgery of Trauma (AAST) renal injury scale is the most widely used grading system for renal trauma. Severity is assessed according to the depth of renal parenchymal damage and involvement of the urinary collecting system and renal vessels.

Grade	Description
I	Subcapsular hematoma or contusion without laceration
II	Superficial laceration <1 cm in depth not involving the collecting system (no evidence of urine extravasation)
	Perirenal hematoma confined within the perirenal fascia

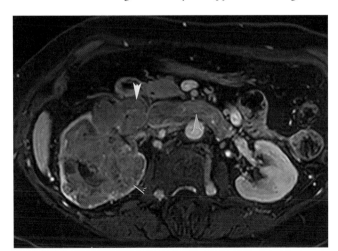

Fig. 79.1 Axial postcontrast T1 weighted image showing a large infiltrative tumor *(red arrow)* occupying almost all of the right kidney with tumor thrombus seen extending into the IVC *(yellow arrow)*. Tumor thrombus is also seen to extend into the left renal vein *(green arrow)*.

Grade	Description
III	Laceration >1 cm not involving the collecting system (no evidence of urine extravasation)
	Vascular injury or active bleeding confined within the perirenal fascia
IV	Laceration involving the collecting system with urinary extravasation
	Laceration of the renal pelvis and/or complete ureteropelvic disruption
	Vascular injury to segmental renal artery or vein
	Segmental infarction without associated active bleeding
	Active bleeding extending beyond the perirenal fascia
V	Shattered kidney
	Avulsion of the renal hilum or laceration of the main renal artery or vein: devascularization of the kidney due to hilar injury; devascularized kidney with active bleeding

- Management:
  - Grade 1: conservative management
  - Grade II: conservative management under close observation
  - Grade III: conservative management under close observation; may be managed surgically if undergoing laparotomy for other abdominal injuries
  - Grade IV: surgical management, especially if undergoing laparotomy for other abdominal injuries
  - Grade V: surgical management
- Category IV injury:
  - Caused by sudden deceleration, which creates tension on the renal pedicle
  - Intravenous urography (IVU) and CT show excretion of contrast material with an intact intrarenal collecting system but with medial perinephric urinary extravasation
  - Ureteropelvic junction injuries are classified into two groups:
    - Avulsion (complete transection)
    - Laceration (incomplete tear)
  - The presence of contrast material in the ureter distal to the ureteropelvic junction helps differentiate laceration from avulsion.

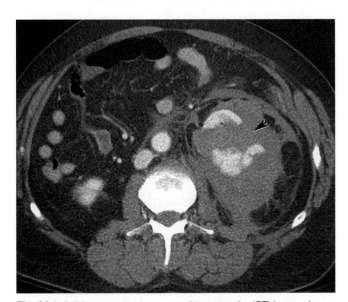

Fig. 80.1 Axial postcontrast computed tomography (CT) image shows deep laceration in the left kidney *(red arrow)* with large perinephric hematoma *(yellow arrow)*.

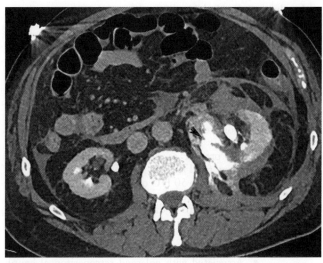

Fig. 80.2 Axial delayed postcontrast computed tomography (CT) image shows extravasation of contrast *(arrow)* medially from the left renal collecting system. This is consistent with Grade IV injury.

REFERENCES

Harris, A. C., Zwirewich, C. V., Lyburn, I. D., Torreggiani, W. C., & Marchinkow, L. O. (2001). CT findings in blunt renal trauma. *Radiographics*, *21*, S201–S214. doi:10.1148/radiographics.21.suppl_1.g01oc07s201.

Kawashima, A., Sandler, C. M., Corl, F. M., West, O. C., Tamm, E. P., ... Fishman, E. K. (2001). Imaging of renal trauma: A comprehensive review. *Radiographics*, *21*(3), 557–574. doi:10.1148/radiographics.21.3.g01ma11557.

Kozar, R. A., Crandall, M., Shanmuganathan, K., Zarzaur, B. L., Coburn, M., ... Cribari, C. (2018). Organ injury scaling 2018 update: Spleen, liver, and kidney. *Journal of Trauma and Acute Care Surgery*, *85*(6), 1119–1122. doi:10.1097/TA.0000000000002058.

Moore, E. E., Shackford, S. R., Pachter, H. L., McAninch, J. W., Browner, B. D., ... Champion, H. R. (1989). Organ injury scaling: Spleen, liver, and kidney. *Journal of Trauma*, *29*(12), 1664–1666.

CASE 81

Renal Lymphoma With Diffuse Infiltration

1. A, B, C, D. Images show an infiltrative mass in the right kidney with multiple hypovascular masses in the left kidney. This is more likely seen in lymphoma or metastasis; however, multifocal renal cell carcinoma or transitional cell carcinoma would have a similar appearance as well.
2. B. Renal lymphoma most commonly presents as multifocal renal masses.
3. A, B, C, D. All of these can be present features of renal lymphoma on CT scan; however, multifocal renal mass is the most common presentation.
4. B, C. PET/CT is helpful for initial staging and follow-up staging of lymphoma.

Comment

- Background: Renal involvement in lymphoma commonly occurs in the presence of widespread nodal or extranodal lymphoma and is classified as secondary renal lymphoma. It is termed *primary renal lymphoma* when only the kidneys are involved without evidence of disease elsewhere. Primary renal lymphoma is exceedingly rare accounting for <1% of extranodal lymphomas.
- Renal lymphoma usually occurs in the setting of widespread non-Hodgkin lymphoma, typically B-cell type intermediate-grade and high-grade tumors or American Burkitt lymphoma.

Involvement by Hodgkin disease is much less common, being seen in <1% of patients at presentation.

- Imaging:
  - US: less sensitive than contrast enhanced CT for detecting renal lymphoma. On ultrasound, renal lymphoma is usually hypoechoic or anechoic. Diffuse nephromegaly may also be seen.
  - CT: secondary renal lymphoma may be unilateral or bilateral, can occur as solitary or multiple focal masses, and may originate from renal parenchyma or from the perinephric space.
    - Can also present as diffuse bilateral nephromegaly without any focal lesions
    - Measures ~30 to 50 HU on unenhanced images
    - Appears hypovascular on contrast enhanced CT
    - Following patterns of disease may be seen on CT:
      - Multiple masses: most common pattern seen in the posterior 60%
        - Typically 1 to 3 cm in size
        - Associated with enlarged retroperitoneal lymph nodes in >50% of cases
      - Single mass: in 20% of cases
        - Up to 15 cm
        - Homogenous, hypodense without cystic change
        - Can have calcifications, hemorrhage, or necrosis within it.
      - Invasion from retroperitoneal nodal mass: in ~30% of cases
        - Usually >10 cm
        - Encasement of vessels without thrombosis is seen; hydronephrosis may be present
      - Diffuse infiltration: in ~20% of cases
        - No discrete masses seen
        - Usually bilateral
        - Usually seen with Burkitt lymphoma
      - Perirenal mass: seen in <10% of cases
        - Appears as perirenal fat stranding, thickening of Gerota fascia and perirenal nodules
    - Atypical patterns include spontaneous hemorrhage, necrosis, heterogenous lesion, cystic changes, and calcifications.
  - MRI: may be useful in patients with renal insufficiency or a history of contrast medium allergy or when there is

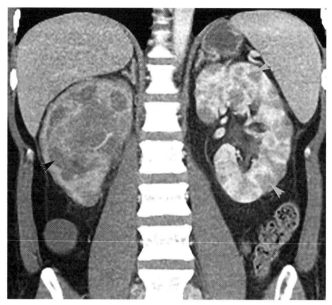

Fig. 81.2 Coronal reformat from a postcontrast computed tomography (CT) image through the abdomen shows diffuse infiltrative mass in the right kidney *(red arrow)*. Multiple hypovascular masses also seen in the left kidney *(green arrow)*. Patient had a history of lymphoma in the mediastinum and hence this was considered to be secondary lymphoma within bilateral kidneys.

increased concern for radiation exposure such as children and young adults
- T1 weighted images appear as hypointense to renal parenchyma
- T2 weighted images appear as isointense or hyperintense to renal parenchyma
- Postcontrast images: poor enhancement compared to the renal parenchyma and delayed enhancement is seen in some lesions
- PET/CT: plays an important role in the evaluation of extranodal lymphoma. Renal lymphoma is intensely FDG-avid whereas RCC, including the papillary and chromophobe subtypes, may not show intense FDG uptake. Also useful in assessing response to therapy.

REFERENCES

Ganeshan, D., Iyer, R., Devine, C., Bhosale, P., & Paulson, E. (2013). Imaging of primary and secondary renal lymphoma. *American Journal of Roentgenology*, *201*(5), W712–W719. doi:10.2214/AJR.13.10669.

Sheth, S., Ali, S., & Fishman, E. (2006). Imaging of renal lymphoma: Patterns of disease with pathologic correlation. *Radiographics*, *26*(4), 1151–1168. doi:10.1148/rg.264055125.

Urban, B. A., & Fishman, E. K. (2000). Renal lymphoma: CT patterns with emphasis on helical CT. *Radiographics*, *20*(1), 197–212.

CASE 82

Angiomyolipoma With Hemorrhage

1. A, B, C. Images show a heterogeneously enhancing mass in the right kidney with a large perinephric hematoma. Hemorrhage can be seen with large renal cell carcinomas, AMLs, or renal cysts. Abscesses are not known to cause perinephric hemorrhage.

2. A. On noncontrast CT, the presence of ROIs containing attenuations of –10 HU or less is a reliable sign of an area of adipose tissue and hence AML.

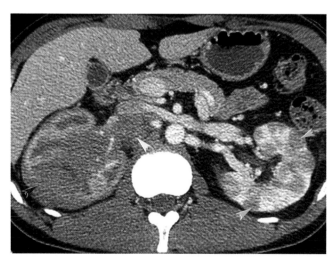

Fig. 81.1 Axial postcontrast computed tomography (CT) image through the abdomen shows diffuse infiltrative mass in the right kidney *(red arrow)* with extension seen into the retroperitoneum *(yellow arrow)*. Multiple hypovascular masses also seen in the left kidney *(green arrow)*.

3. A, B, C. 20% of AMLs are seen in association with tuberous sclerosis complex, neurofibromatosis, and pulmonary lymphangioleiomyomatosis.
4. C, D. T1 hypointense with and T1 hyperintense without fat suppression and India ink artifact at the interface between fat and nonfat components on out of phase images are specific features on MRI for AML.

Comment

- Renal AMLs are the most common benign renal tumors with evidence of varying between 0.2% and 0.6%, with a strong female predilection.
  - They occur as isolated sporadic entities in 80% of cases with the remaining 20% of AMLs seen in association with tuberous sclerosis complex or pulmonary lymphangioleiomyomatosis.
  - They are often found incidentally within the kidneys when imaged for other reasons or as part of screening in patients with tuberous sclerosis.
  - Risk of bleeding in angiomyolipomas is proportional to the size of the lesion, with lesions >4 cm in diameter more prone to spontaneous hemorrhage. Shock due to severe hemorrhage from rupture is described as Wunderlich syndrome.
- Pathology: AMLs are typically composed of small muscle, blood vessels, and adipose tissue. Two histologic types have been described: typical (triphasic) and atypical (monophasic or epithelioid). Approximately 5% of AMLs are fat poor.
- Imaging: The cornerstone of diagnosis on all modalities is redemonstration of macroscopic fat; however, in the setting of hemorrhage or when lesions happen to contain little fat, it may be difficult to distinguish an AML from a renal cell carcinoma.
  - US:
    - Appear as hyperechoic lesions located in the cortex and with posterior acoustic shadowing
    - The echogenicity of the mass is the same as or greater than that of the renal sinus
    - Fat-poor AML has a mixed echotexture, being hyperechoic and isoechoic compared with renal parenchyma

- Fat-invisible AML is homogenously isoechoic with respect to renal parenchyma
- Contrast-enhanced US: enhance peripherally, decreased central enhancement compared with the normal cortex
- CT: acquisition of thin slice sections (1.5–3.0 mm) and obtaining attenuation measurements using small ROIs or even pixel values is helpful for detection of AML.
  - On noncontrast CT, the presence of ROIs containing attenuations of −10 HU or less is a reliable sign of an area of adipose tissue and hence AML.
  - Fat-poor AMLs are heterogeneously isoattenuating or hyperattenuating, since the attenuation value varies according to the size and location of ROI. If an ROI is placed in the region of muscle and vessels, the lesion at attenuation is higher than when an ROI is placed in an area that consists mostly of fat cells.
- MRI: is important to locate fat within a mass by comparing T1 weighted images with and without frequency selective fat suppression
  - A classic fat-rich AML appears T1 hypointense with and T1 hyperintense without fat suppression. This T1 hyperintensity is not a specific characteristics of AML and can also be present in the RCC and hemorrhagic cysts.
  - Another method to evaluate AML is to use in-phase and out-of-phase imaging, which generates India ink artifact at the interface between fat and nonfat components. This can occur either at the interface between the AML and surrounding kidney or between fat and nonfat components of the mass. This can help in evaluation of fat poor AMLs as well.
- Digital subtraction angiography (DSA): angiomyolipomas and hypervascular lesions demonstrating often characteristic features:
  - Arterial phase: a sharply marginated hypervascular mass with intense early arterial network and tortuous vessels giving the sunburst appearance
  - Venous phase: whorled onion peel appearance of peripheral vessels
  - Micro or macro aneurysms
  - Absent arteriovenous shunting
- Radiologic classification of AML:

		Frequency	CT	MRI	US	Amount of fat cells
Sporadic		80%				
	Classic AML	Common	Fat attenuation	Signal loss on FS MRI	Markedly hyperechoic	Abundant
	Fat poor AML	Uncommon	No evidence of fat at noncontrast CT			
	Hyperattenuating AML	Approximately 4.5% of all AMLs	Hyperattenuating (>45 HU), homogenously enhancing or variable enhancement pattern	T2 hypointense No signal loss on CS MRI and no signal loss on FS MRI	Isoechoic	Few or none
	Isoattenuating AML	Rare	Isoattenuating (−10 to −45 HU) and variable enhancement pattern	T2 hypointense Signal loss on CS MRI	Slightly hyperechoic	Scattered
	AML with epithelial cysts	Rare	Hyperattenuating with cysts or multilocular cystic	+/−Signal loss on FS MRI and T2 hypointense in solid component	Unknown	Few or none

		Frequency	CT	MRI	US	Amount of fat cells
	Epithelioid AML	Rare	Hyperattenuating, (>45 HU) heterogeneously enhancing or multicystic Variable enhancement pattern	T2 hypointense in solid component	Unknown	Few or none
Syndromic		20%				
	AML in tuberous sclerosis complex		Variable	Variable	Variable	Any amount
	AML in lymphangi-oleiomyomatosis		Variable	Variable	Variable	Any amount

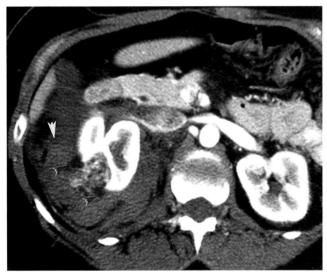

Fig. 82.1 Axial postcontrast computed tomography (CT) image shows a heterogenous mass with fat attenuation within it *(red arrows)* with enhancement within it suggestive of an angiomyolipoma (AML). Large perinephric hematoma *(yellow arrow)* is present, which suggests hemorrhage from the AML.

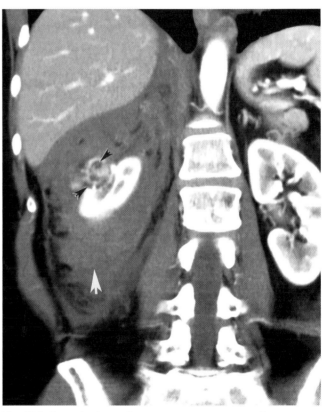

Fig. 82.2 Coronal reformat from a postcontrast computed tomography (CT) image shows a heterogenous mass with fat attenuation within it *(red arrows)* with enhancement within it suggestive of an angiomyolipoma (AML). Large perinephric hematoma *(yellow arrow)* is present, which suggests hemorrhage from the AML.

REFERENCES
Jinzaki, M., Silverman, S. G., Akita, H., Nagashima, Y., Mikami, S., & Oya, M. (2014). Renal angiomyolipoma: A radiological classification and update on recent developments in diagnosis and management. *Abdominal Imaging, 39*(3), 588–604. doi:10.1007/s00261-014-0083-3.
Park, B. K. (2017). Renal angiomyolipoma: Radiologic classification and imaging features according to the amount of fat. *American Journal of Roentgenology, 209*(4), 826–835. doi:10.2214/AJR.17.17973.

Case 83 is online only and accessible at www.expertconsult.com.

CASE 84

Forniceal Rupture

1. A, B, C. Delayed nephrogram, forniceal rupture, and perinephric edema are seen in the images. Renal infarction would be seen as absent enhancement in the affected kidney.
2. B. The renal fornix is the most susceptible part of the renal collecting system to rupture from increased pressure.
3. A, B, C, D. All the conditions listed can result in a delayed nephrogram.
4. D. Wedge-shaped area of decreased renal cortical enhancement is seen in renal infarction and not in forniceal rupture.

Comment

- Renal forniceal or calyceal rupture is a radiographic finding of a perirenal urine leak as a result of ureteric obstruction. A small number of cases have been described from other etiologies, including malignant extrinsic ureteric compression, pregnancy, posterior urethral valves, pelvic-ureteric junction (PUJ) obstruction, vascular extrinsic compression, iatrogenic, and IV fluid administration.
- The renal fornix is the most susceptible part of the renal collecting system to rupture from increased pressure.
- Imaging findings:
  - On noncontrast CT, perinephric low fluid density and fat standing are seen.
  - On contrast administration, delayed nephrogram will be seen on the side of acute obstruction.

- On delayed-phase imaging, contrast will accumulate outside of the collecting system forming a urinoma.
- Delayed nephrogram: absence or reduction of the normal renal parenchyma and enhancement on nephrographic phase imaging
  - Etiology: failure of the normal temporal progression of nephrographic contrast can result from a number of conditions:
    - Obstructive uropathy (most common)
    - Renal vein thrombosis
    - Renal artery stenosis
    - Extrinsic compression (e.g., page kidney)
- Imaging: decreased enhancement seen in the affected kidney compared to the normal kidney with nephrographic enhancement seen in the delayed or urographic phase, which persists for a prolonged period of time

REFERENCE

Gershman, B., Kulkarni, N., Sahani, D. V., & Eisner, B. H. (2011). Causes of renal forniceal rupture. *BJU International, 108*(11), 1909–1911; discussion 1912. doi:10.1111/j.1464-410X.2011.10164.x.

CASE 85

Renal Devascularization (Grade V)

1. D. CT images show complete lack of enhancement of the left kidney with a large perinephric hematoma suggesting devascularization.
2. D. Ideal protocol for imaging kidneys with presence of trauma is a dual-phase contrast-enhanced CT with arterial and nephrographic phases. Early imaging allows for accurate evaluation of the vasculature. Five-minute delayed CT is useful for evaluation of renal collecting system injuries. Intravenous urography is not routinely used for imaging patients with renal trauma but could be obtained when the patient is rushed straight to the operating room or when CT is unavailable.
3. D. Devascularized kidney is consistent with a Grade V AAST renal injury.
4. C. Grade V injuries with complete ureteropelvic disruption and renal pedicle avulsion need surgical repair.

Comment

- Injury to the kidney is seen in approximately 8% to 10% of patients with blunt penetrating abdominal injuries.
- Computed tomography is a modality of choice in evaluation of blunt renal trauma. Multidetector CT is considered the gold-standard method for radiographic assessment of patients with renal trauma. CT scan should be performed after intravenous contrast administration in the following phases: corticomedullary phase 60 to 70 seconds after injection of contrast medium followed by excretory phase at 3 to 5 minutes after injection of contrast.
- The American Association for the Surgery of Trauma (AAST) renal injury scale is the most widely used grading system for renal trauma. Severity is assessed according to the depth of renal parenchymal damage and involvement of the urinary collecting system and renal vessels.

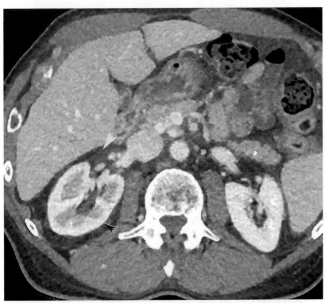

Fig. 84.1 Axial postcontrast computed tomography (CT) image shows decreased enhancement in the right kidney *(red arrow)* compared to the left. Note the perinephric edema *(yellow arrow)* seen around the right kidney.

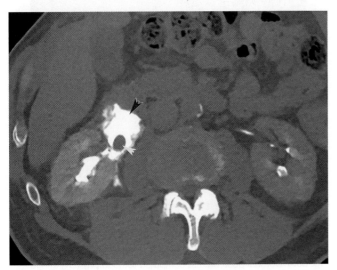

Fig. 84.2 Axial delayed postcontrast computed tomography (CT) image shows accumulation of contrast *(red arrow)* outside the kidney along the right ureter *(yellow arrow)* consistent with forniceal rupture.

Grade	Description
I	Subcapsular hematoma or contusion without laceration
II	Superficial laceration <1 cm in depth not involving the collecting system (no evidence of urine extravasation)
	Perirenal hematoma confined within the perirenal fascia

Grade	Description
III	Laceration >1 cm not involving the collecting system (no evidence of urine extravasation)
	Vascular injury or active bleeding confined within the perirenal fascia
IV	Laceration involving the collecting system with urinary extravasation
	Laceration of the renal pelvis and/or complete ureteropelvic disruption
	Vascular injury to segmental renal artery or vein
	Segmental infarction without associated active bleeding
	Active bleeding extending beyond the perirenal fascia
V	Shattered kidney
	Avulsion of the renal hilum or laceration of the main renal artery or vein: devascularization of the kidney due to hilar injury or devascularized kidney with active bleeding

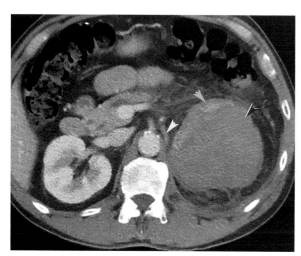

Fig. 85.1 Axial postcontrast computed tomography (CT) image shows complete absence of enhancement in the left kidney *(red arrow)* with no enhancement seen in the left renal artery, which is reduced in caliber *(yellow arrow)*. This is consistent with Grade V devascularization injury. Note the cortical rim sign *(green arrow)* seen due to enhancement of the periphery of the cortex due to capsular blood vessels.

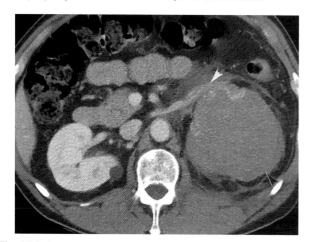

Fig. 85.2 Axial postcontrast computed tomography (CT) image shows complete absence of enhancement in the left kidney *(red arrow)* with partially patent left renal vein *(yellow arrow)*, which is compressed from a large perinephric hematoma. This is consistent with Grade V devascularization injury.

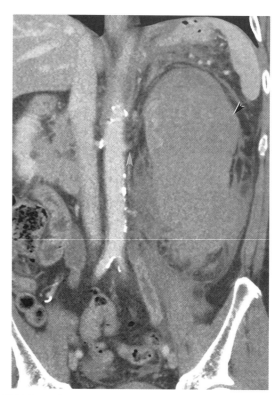

Fig. 85.3 Coronal postcontrast computed tomography (CT) image shows complete absence of enhancement in the left kidney *(red arrow)* with the stump of the left renal artery seen medially *(green arrow)*. This is consistent with Grade V devascularization injury.

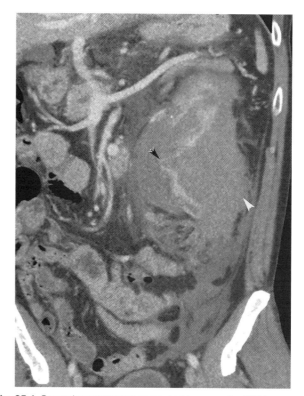

Fig. 85.4 Coronal postcontrast computed tomography (CT) image shows cortical rim sign in the left kidney *(red arrow)* with a large perinephric hematoma *(yellow arrow)*. This is consistent with Grade V devascularization injury.

- Management:
  - Grade 1: conservative management
  - Grade II: conservative management under close observation
  - Grade III: conservative management under close observation; may be managed surgically if undergoing laparotomy for other abdominal injuries
  - Grade IV: surgical management, especially if undergoing laparotomy for other abdominal injuries
  - Grade V: surgical management

REFERENCES

Harris, A. C., Zwirewich, C. V., Lyburn, I. D., Torreggiani, W. C., & Marchinkow, L. O. (2001). CT findings in blunt renal trauma. *Radiographics*, *21*, S201–S214. doi:10.1148/radiographics.21. suppl_1.g01oc07s201.

Kawashima, A., Sandler, C. M., Corl, F. M., West, O. C., Tamm, E. P., … Fishman, E. K. (2001). Imaging of renal trauma: A comprehensive review. *Radiographics*, *21*(3), 557–574. doi:10.1148/radiographics.21.3. g01ma11557.

Kozar, R. A., Crandall, M., Shanmuganathan, K., Zarzaur, B. L., Coburn, M., … Cribari, C. (2018). Organ injury scaling 2018 update: Spleen, liver, and kidney. *Journal of Trauma and Acute Care Surgery*, *85*(6), 1119–1122. doi:10.1097/TA.0000000000002058.

Moore, E. E., Shackford, S. R., Pachter, H. L., McAninch, J. W., Browner, B. D., … Champion, H. R. (1989). Organ injury scaling: Spleen, liver, and kidney. *Journal of Trauma*, *29*(12), 1664–1666.

CASE 86

Urachal Remnant Adenocarcinoma

1. B, C. Presence of a supravesicular mass with calcification is pathognomonic for urachal remnant adenocarcinoma. Bladder diverticulum is in the differential, but uncomplicated diverticulum would not have calcification or soft tissue within. Hematoma is unlikely due to the soft tissue. Bladder carcinoma does not show extensive extravesicular component as seen in this case.
2. B. Since there may not be a patent complication with the umbilicus in this mass due to the different types of connections seen, presentation in urachal remnant carcinoma is typically late with local invasion or metastatic disease seen commonly. This could lead to poor prognosis in this disease.
3. C. Calcifications are present in 70% of cases of urachal adenocarcinoma seen mostly at the periphery, and calcification seen in the midline soft tissue mass along the course of the urachal tract is considered pathognomonic for the diagnosis of urachal adenocarcinoma.
4. A. Sagittal plane is most helpful for evaluation of the urachal abnormalities, since the communication between the bladder and the umbilicus is seen on the sagittal plane.

Comment

- Introduction: The urachus or median umbilical ligament is a midline elongated tubular structure that extends from the anterior dome of the bladder toward the umbilicus.
  - It is a remnant of two embryonic structures: the cloaca, which is a cephalic extension of the urogenital sinus, a precursor of the bladder; and the allantois, which is a derivative of the yolk sac.
  - The structure regresses after birth with a residual fibrous band seen in this region with no known function.
  - In some cases it can persist giving rise to various clinical problems, including abdominal pain and discharging sinus.

- Congenital urachal abnormalities: these are seen twice more commonly in men compared to women. Four types of urachal anomalies are seen:
  - Patent urachus: complication between the bladder and umbilicus through a urachus that has not involuted. This is the commonest type seen in ~50% of cases.
  - Urachal cyst: a fluid-filled dilatation of the urachus seen in ~30% of cases.
  - Umbilical-urachal sinus: blind focal dilation of the umbilical end of the urachus, seen in ~15% of cases.
  - Vesicourachal diverticulum: blind focal dilation of the bladder and of the urachus, seen in ~5% of cases.
- Acquired urachal remnant diseases: urachal remnant can be subject to infection and in some cases the formation of benign or malignant tumors
  - Infection can be lymphatic, hematogenous, or through the bladder and depending on the variation in patency of the urachal lumen may present with drainage of infected fluid along the urachus through the umbilicus or bladder or both directions.
    - Total removal of the cyst wall is essential due to the 30% reinfection rate and possibility of development of malignancy in resected or incompletely resected urachal remnant.
  - Urachal masses are rare, present in <0.5% of all bladder masses, most commonly seen in patients 40 to 70 years of age with two-thirds seen in males
    - Urachal carcinoma predominantly manifest as adenocarcinoma in 90% of cases due to metaplasia of the urachal mucosa into columnar epithelium followed by malignant transformation.
    - Mucin production is found in almost 75% of these cases.
    - Due to their extraperitoneal location, urachal tumors are typically silent with majority of patients showing local invasion or metastatic disease at presentation.
    - Urachal carcinomas may be confused with primary tumors of the bladder dome; however, urachal tumors grow in the perivesical space toward the umbilicus while primary bladder carcinoma arising in the apex will usually have less of an extravesical component.
- Imaging:
  - US: a midline intraabdominal mass superior to the bladder with calcifications and solid components within it.
    - Due to the presence of mucin, increased echogenicity can be seen within this mass instead of an anechoic patent.
  - CT: urachal carcinoma may be solid, cystic, or a combination of the two with the low attenuation components reflecting mucin.
    - Calcification is seen in approximately 50% to 70% of urachal carcinomas, since they are typically mucinous adenocarcinomas, which produce psammomatous calcifications.
      - Calcifications may be punctate, stippled, or curvilinear and peripheral.
      - Calcifications in a midline supravesical mass are considered diagnostic for urachal carcinoma.
  - MRI: sagittal images are most helpful for evaluation of urachal neoplasms.
    - A midline mass with focal areas of heterogenous high signal intensity is seen on T2 weighted images due to the mucin content or due to fluid collection or necrosis.
    - Solid components in the tumor are isointense to soft tissue on T1 weighted images and enhance following intravenous gadolinium contrast administration.

- Prognosis is related to the stage and degree of differentiation but is generally poor due to the presence of local invasion and/or metastatic disease at presentation. Five-year survival rate for urachal adenocarcinoma is variable and has been reported to be ~49% after treatment. Local recurrences are often seen within 2 years of surgery.

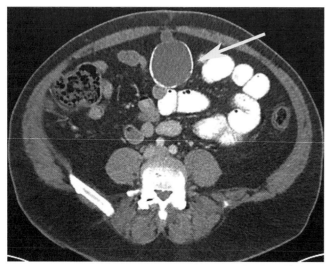

Fig. 86.1 Axial postcontrast computed tomography image at 60 seconds shows an intraabdominal heterogenous low-density mass with peripheral calcifications seen in the midline *(yellow arrow)*. This was consistent with urachal remnant adenocarcinoma.

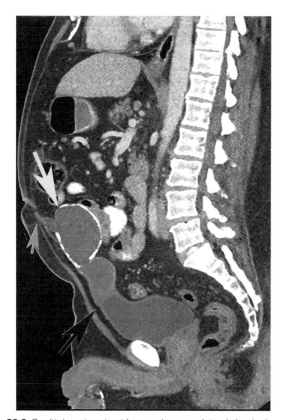

Fig. 86.2 Sagittal postcontrast image shows an intraabdominal heterogenous low-density mass with peripheral calcifications seen in the midline *(yellow arrow)*. This was consistent with urachal remnant adenocarcinoma. Note the relationship to the bladder with close approximation seen on this sagittal image *(red arrow)* and extension to the umbilicus *(green arrow)*.

REFERENCES

Villavicencio, C. P., Adam, S. Z., Nikolaidis, P., Yaghmai, V., & Miller, F. H. (2016). Imaging of the urachus: Anomalies, complications, and mimics. *Radiographics, 36*(7), 2049–2063. doi:10.1148/rg.2016160062.

Yu, J. S., Kim, K. W., Lee, H. J., Lee, Y. J., Yoon, C. S., & Kim, M. J. (2001). Urachal remnant diseases: Spectrum of CT and US findings. *Radiographics, 21*(2), 451–461. doi:10.1148/radiographics.21.2.g01mr02451.

CASE 87
Urethral Diverticulum Cancer

1. A, D. A soft tissue mass is seen inferior to the bladder with heterogenous enhancement on postcontrast images and restriction on the diffusion weighted images (DWI) suggesting urethral or bladder carcinoma. Presence of abnormal lymph node in the right groin also suggests presence of malignancy.
2. A, B, C. Urethral diverticulum carcinomas are rare and adenocarcinomas are the most common lesion seen. Transitional cell and squamous cell carcinomas can also be seen in urethral diverticulum carcinomas. Sarcomas are usually not seen in urethral diverticula.
3. C. Malignancy arising in a urethral diverticulum is seen as enhancing soft tissue mass within the diverticulum. Evaluation of urethral diverticulum should include postcontrast imaging if areas of wall thickening or soft tissue masses are seen within the diverticulum.
4. B, D. Urethral diverticulum carcinomas can be asymptomatic in the early stages or manifest nonspecific symptoms. Postvoid dribbling, dysuria, and hematuria are most commonly seen. Due to the lack of or poor presence of muscle layer around the urethral diverticulum, carcinomas can extend outside the wall and present at a higher stage.

Comment

- Background: Urethral diverticulum adenocarcinoma in females is extremely rare accounting for only 0.02% of genitourinary tract malignancies.
  - Adenocarcinomas account for 75% of female urethral diverticulum cancers with the two other pathologic types (transitional cell carcinoma and squamous cell carcinoma) accounting for 15% and >10%, respectively.
  - Patients with diverticulum tumors may present with diverse symptoms, including postvoid dribbling, frequency, urgency, voiding difficulties, urinary retention, stress incontinence, microscopic hematuria, recurrent urethritis or cystitis, dysuria, vaginal pain, and dyspareunia.
  - Pelvic examination reveals a palpable mass in the anterior vaginal wall.
  - The median age of presentation is 53 years (range 14–81 years) with a higher incidence in the African American population.
- Imaging findings:
  - On ultrasound, a distended urethral diverticulum is seen posterior to the urinary bladder with a polypoid or diffuse mass lesion seen within it.
  - An enhancing mass inferior to the bladder within a cystic mass may be seen on CT scan. MRI is considered to be a definitive exam for this diagnosis.
  - On MRI, a diverticulum is seen as the hypointense area around the urethra or as a homogenous hypointense signal enlarged urethra.
    - On T2 weighted images diverticulum is seen as a hyperintense signal area around the urethra with soft tissue nodular area seen within it or as an intermediate signal intensity mass seen inferior to the bladder.
  - Heterogenous enhancement is seen within the mass with enhancing thickened walls on contrast administration.

- Management: mainstay of treatment is surgical with options:
  - Urethral diverticulectomy alone or with adjuvant radiotherapy or chemotherapy
  - Urethrectomy +/− pelvic or inguinal lymph node dissection +/− adjuvant therapy
  - Anterior exenteration (excision of the urethra, bladder, anterior vaginal wall, uterus, and pelvic lymph nodes) +/− inguinal lymph node dissection +/− adjuvant therapy
  - Radiotherapy +/− adjuvant chemotherapy alone

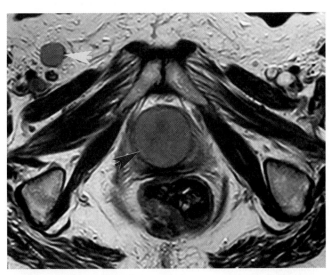

Fig. 87.1 Axial T2 weighted magnetic resonance imaging (MRI) shows intermediate mass *(red arrow)* in the region of the urethra, anterior to the vagina and rectum. This was consistent with urethral diverticulum carcinoma. Note a similar signal intensity lymph node in the right groin region *(yellow arrow)* suggesting metastasis.

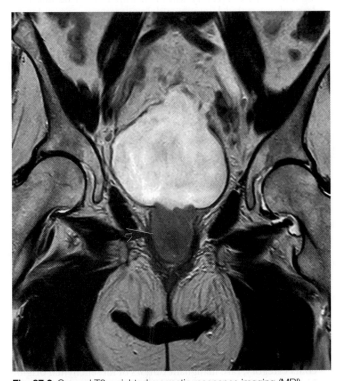

Fig. 87.2 Coronal T2 weighted magnetic resonance imaging (MRI) shows intermediate mass *(red arrow)* in the region of the urethra, anterior to the vagina and rectum and inferior to the bladder. This was consistent with a urethral diverticulum carcinoma.

REFERENCE

O'Connor, E., Iatropoulou, D., Hashimoto, S., Takahashi, S., Ho, D. H., & Greenwell, T. (2018). Urethral diverticulum carcinoma in females-a case series and review of the English and Japanese literature. *Translational Andrology and Urology*, 7(4), 703–729. doi:10.21037/tau.2018.07.08.

CASE 88

Bladder Rupture

1. C. Extravasated contrast material is seen within the perivesical space in the pelvis representing extraperitoneal bladder rupture. Air is also seen to track along the properitoneal space in the abdominal wall.
2. A. Prevesical space, also known as retropubic space or space of Retzius, is the extraperitoneal space between the pubic synthesis and urinary bladder. In extraperitoneal bladder rupture, contrast material may accumulate within the space.
3. C. CT cystography is performed by instilling a minimum of 300 mL of dilute sterile contrast material (20–30 mL 60% water-soluble contrast agent into a 500-mL back of saline) into the bladder with the low-gravity drip infusion.
4. D. Traumatic extraperitoneal bladder ruptures are nearly always (89%–100%) associated with pelvic fractures.

Comment

- Bladder rupture is most commonly due to abdominal and/or pelvic trauma but may be spontaneous or iatrogenic, an association with surgical or endoscopic procedures.
- Blunt force trauma in association with motor vehicle crashes accounts for most cases of bladder rupture.
- Bladder injuries occur in about 1.6% of patients with blunt abdominal trauma. Approximately 60% of bladder injuries are extraperitoneal, 30% are intraperitoneal, and the remaining 10% are both.
- CT cystographic technique: after Foley catheter insertion, adequate bladder distention is achieved by instilling at least 350 mL of a diluted mixture, 50 mL of 60% water-soluble contrast material in 450 to 500 mL of normal saline solution into the bladder under gravity control.
- Types of bladder injury:
  - Type 1: contusion. Bladder contusion is defined as an incomplete or partial tear of the bladder mucosa. Conventional and CT cystography may be normal in these patients.
  - Type 2: intraperitoneal rupture. Intraperitoneal bladder rupture occurs in approximately 10% to 20% of major bladder injuries. CT cystography demonstrates intraperitoneal contrast material around bowel loops, between mesenteric folds, and in the paracolic gutters.
  - Type 3: interstitial injury. Interstitial bladder injuries are rare and are defined as an intramural or partial thickness laceration with intact serosa.
  - Type 4: extraperitoneal rupture. Extraperitoneal ruptures are the most common type of bladder injury (80%–90% of cases) and are usually caused by penetrating trauma. In blunt trauma the presumed mechanism is direct laceration of the bladder by bone fragments from the pelvic fracture. Extravasation is confined to the perivesical space in simple extraperitoneal ruptures. In complex extraperitoneal ruptures, contrast material extends beyond the perivesical space and may dissect into a variety of fascial planes and spaces.
  - Type 5: combined rupture. Combined bladder rupture consists of simultaneous intraperitoneal and extraperitoneal injury. CT cystography demonstrates extravasation patterns that are typical for both types of injury.

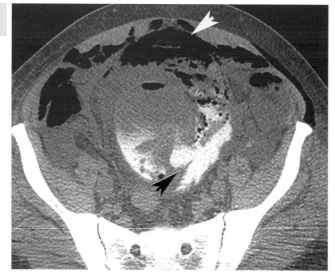

Fig. 88.1 Axial computed tomography (CT) cystography image shows extravasation of contrast into the perivesical space *(red arrow)* suggestive of extraperitoneal rupture. Note presence of air along the properitoneal space *(yellow arrow)* and lateral abdominal wall suggesting complicated extraperitoneal rupture of the bladder.

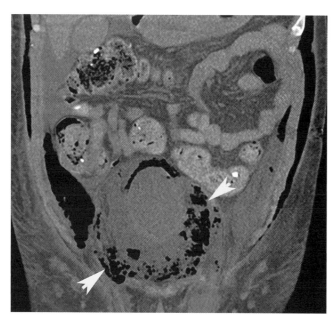

Fig. 88.2 Coronal computed tomography (CT) cystography image shows extravasation of air into the perivesical space *(red arrow)* suggestive of extraperitoneal rupture. Note presence of air along the lateral abdominal wall *(yellow arrow)* suggesting complicated extraperitoneal rupture of the bladder.

- American Association for the Surgery for Trauma bladder organ injury scale:

Bladder Injury Description

Grade	Injury	Description
I	Hematoma	Contusion, intramural hematoma
	Laceration	Partial thickness
II	Laceration	Extraperitoneal bladder wall laceration <2 cm

Grade	Injury	Description
III	Laceration	Extraperitoneal ≥2 cm or intraperitoneal <2 cm bladder wall laceration
IV	Laceration	Intraperitoneal bladder wall laceration ≥2 cm
V	Laceration	Laceration extending into bladder neck or urethral orifice (trigone)

- Management: American Urological Association (AUA) guidelines recommend that intraperitoneal bladder ruptures be surgically repaired. AUA guidelines recommend that uncomplicated extraperitoneal bladder injuries be managed conservatively with catheter placement. Standard therapy involves leaving the catheter in place for 2 to 3 weeks. Extraperitoneal ruptures that do not heal after 4 weeks of catheter drainage should be considered for surgical repair. Complicated extraperitoneal bladder ruptures, such as those associated with bone fragments within the bladder and those associated with vaginal or rectal injuries, often require operative repair.

REFERENCES

Mahat, Y., Leong, J. Y., & Chung, P. H. (2019). A contemporary review of adult bladder trauma. *Journal of Injury and Violence Research, 11*(2), 101–106. doi:10.5249/jivr.v11i2.1069.

Vaccaro, J. P., & Brody, J. M. (2000). CT cystography in the evaluation of major bladder trauma. *Radiographics, 20*(5), 1373–1381. doi:10.1148/radiographics.20.5.g00se111373.

CASE 89

Leiomyosarcoma

1. A, B, C. The images show a large mass in the uterus with significant heterogeneity within it, which could be due to a large degenerated leiomyoma, leiomyosarcoma, or endometrial carcinoma.
2. A, B, C, D. Leiomyomas can undergo degeneration—hyaline, cystic, or myxoid; large fibroids can also undergo torsion.
3. D. US is always the first-line modality for imaging fibroids.
4. D. Leiomyosarcomas are difficult to diagnose by imaging, and diagnosis is based on rate of growth, presence of metastasis, and histopathology.

Comment

- Introduction: Uterine leiomyosarcoma (LMS) is the most common type of uterine sarcoma.
  - Low annual incidence at 0.8 per 100,000 with women representing just 1% to 2% of all uterine malignancies.
  - Extremely aggressive malignancy associated with a poor overall prognosis.
  - 5-year survival between 25% and 76%, with survival for women with metastatic disease at time of initial diagnosis approaching only 10% to 15%.
  - Women affected may vary in age most often diagnosed in their perimenopausal years.
  - The most common presenting symptoms for women with leiomyosarcoma include abnormal uterine bleeding (56%), palpable pelvic mass or enlarged uterus (54%), and pelvic pressure or pain (22%).
- Pathology: Uterine LMSs are a member of the uterine sarcoma category, rare malignant tumors of mesenchymal origin. Uterine LMSs are diagnosed on histology based on hypercellularity, severe nuclear atypia, and high mitotic rate (>15 mitotic figures per 10 high-power fields).

- Imaging: Transvaginal ultrasound is usually the first imaging modality employed for the detection of uterine myometrial pathology.
  - US: leiomyomas typically appear as well-defined hypoechoic masses, with possible calcifications resulting in acoustic shadowing. However, it has a limited role in the accurate diagnosis of LMS since both LMS and leiomyomas can demonstrate similar heterogeneous echogenicity and central necrosis, especially in cases of atypical benign lesions.
  - CT: primarily used for staging purposes and to exclude distant recurrence posttherapy (LMS tends to metastasize to the lungs and liver).

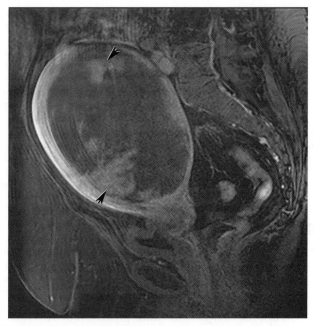

Fig. 89.3 Sagittal T1 weighted postcontrast magnetic resonance imaging (MRI) showing heterogenous nodular enhancement *(arrows)* within the large mass within the uterus. This mass was shown to be a leiomyosarcoma on surgical resection.

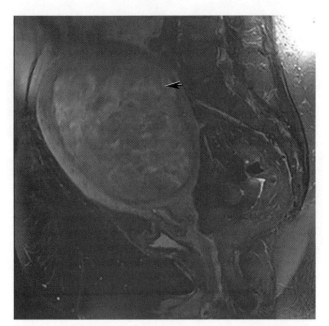

Fig. 89.1 Sagittal T2 weighted magnetic resonance imaging (MRI) showing a large heterogenous mildly T2 hyperintense mass *(arrow)* in the uterus at the fundus. The mass appears to be confined within the uterus on these images.

- MRI: LMSs usually present as solitary heterogeneous and poorly demarcated masses.
  - Lesions ≥10 cm have been found to be associated with a worse prognosis.
  - T1 weighted images: appearance is variable. They may show low or intermediate signal intensity like leiomyomas, but frequently demonstrate areas of high signal intensity on T1 weighted images, corresponding to hemorrhage or necrosis, therefore favoring malignancy.
  - T2 weighted images: LMSs show intermediate to high signal on T2 weighted images
  - Diffusion: low ADC values, ranging from 0.79 ± 0.21 [SD] $\times 10^{-3}$ mm²/s to 1.17 ± 0.15 [SD] $\times 10^{-3}$ mm²/s
  - Postcontrast: tend to enhance early and heterogeneously, often demonstrating nonenhancing areas of central necrosis
- Differential diagnosis: differentiation of LMS from large leiomyomas is difficult on any imaging modality.

REFERENCES

Lakhman, Y., Veeraraghavan, H., Chaim, J., Feier, D., Goldman, D. A., ... Moskowitz, C. S. (2017). Differentiation of uterine leiomyosarcoma from atypical leiomyoma: Diagnostic accuracy of qualitative MR imaging features and feasibility of texture analysis. *European Radiology,* *27*(7), 2903–2915. doi:10.1007/s00330-016-4623-9.

Tanaka, Y. O., Nishida, M., Tsunoda, H., Okamoto, Y., & Yoshikawa, H. (2004). Smooth muscle tumors of uncertain malignant potential and leiomyosarcomas of the uterus: MR findings. *Journal of Magnetic Resonance Imaging,* *20*(6), 998–1007. doi:10.1002/jmri.20207.

CASE 90
Cervical Carcinoma

1. A, D. Imaging illustrates a cervical mass with intermediate signal intensity appearance on T2 weighted MRI, which is centered at the cervix and hence differential includes two main histologic types of cervical cancer, squamous cell cancer (90%) and adenocarcinoma (10%). Cervical leiomyomas typically have hypointense well-circumscribed appearance

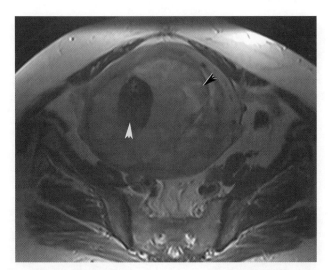

Fig. 89.2 Axial T2 weighted magnetic resonance imaging (MRI) showing a large heterogenous T2 hyperintense mass *(arrow)* in the uterus with a hypointense area *(yellow arrow)* within it, which may be due to prior hemorrhage or calcification. The mass appears to have a lobulated margin posteriorly.

on T2 weighted images, similar to fibroids in the uterine corpus. Nabothian cysts are typically small, well-circumscribed round or ovoid T2 hyperintense cystic lesions.

2. D. A recent study found that women who had ever used an IUD had a lower risk of cervical cancer. The effect on risk was seen even in women who had an IUD for <1 year and the protective effect remained after the IUDs were removed. The risk of developing cervical cancer increases with long-term use of oral contraceptives, smoking, and HIV infection.

3. A. HPV is detected in 99.7% of cervical cancers.

4. B. MRI is an adjunct to the clinical examination to assess important prognostic factors such as tumor size, parametrial and pelvic sidewall invasion, and lymph node metastasis. The accuracy of MRI for depicting tumor size is 93% and 90% for determining disease stage.

Comment

- Background and epidemiology: Cervical carcinoma is the fourth most common gynecologic malignancy worldwide. Approximately 90% of the cervical cancer occurs in low-income and middle-income countries where the mortality is 18 times higher than that in developed countries.
  - High-risk subtypes of the human papillomavirus (HPV) cause almost all cervical cancers, and HPV screening and vaccination programs are effective strategies in disease prevention.
  - Risk factors for cervical carcinoma include:
    - Early age of sexual activity
    - Multiple sexual partners or a high-risk sexual partner
    - Immunosuppression (e.g., after organ transplantation or immune deficiency disorders such as HIV)
    - History of sexually transmitted infection
    - History of HPV-related vulvar or vaginal dysplasia
    - Lack of screening and underscreening in countries with established cervical screening program
  - Squamous cell carcinoma and adenocarcinoma are the most common histologic subtypes accounting for approximately 70% and 25% of all cervical carcinomas, respectively.
  - The median age at diagnosis is 47 years in the United States, with almost 50% of all cases diagnosed under age 35 years.
- Clinical presentation and diagnosis: In its early stages, cervical carcinoma is often asymptomatic and is usually diagnosed following routine screening or pelvic examination.
  - Symptoms include postcoital or abnormal vaginal bleeding.
  - Diagnosis is based on histopathologic assessment of cervical biopsy.
  - Cervical cytology (Pap smear) has been a mainstay of cervical cancer screening and could include cytology alone or cytology with HPV testing for identification of HPV DNA.
- Imaging: Although the International Federation of Gynecology and Obstetrics (FIGO) staging system is clinically based, the revised 2009 FIGO staging encourages imaging as an adjunct to clinical staging.
  - Helps evaluate significant prognostic factors such as lesion volume, pelvic wall involvement, and nodal metastasis.
  - MRI is imaging modality of choice to depict the primary tumor and assess the local extent.
  - Distant metastasis is best assessed with CT or PET where available.
  - Ultrasound is typically the first imaging modality to evaluate women with pelvic pain or bleeding.
    - May show a hypoechoic heterogenous mass involving the cervix with increased vascularity on color Doppler
    - Frequently cervical carcinoma is isoechoic with that of the normal cervical tissue, and enlargement of the cervix may be the only sign of cancer on ultrasound exam.
  - MRI: multiplane T2 weighted MRI is the basis for cervical cancer staging. Axial oblique and sagittal high resolution T2 weighted images are essential.

- Cervical carcinoma has intermediate signal intensity on T2 weighted MRI, which distinguishes it from surrounding low-signal-intensity fibrous stroma and allows for evaluation of parametrial invasion. The intermediate signal intensity on T2 weighted imaging also helps assess for invasion of hypointense tissues of the vagina, rectum, and bladder.
- Contrast enhanced imaging depicts cervical cancers as infiltrative lesions enhancing to a lesser degree than myometrium.

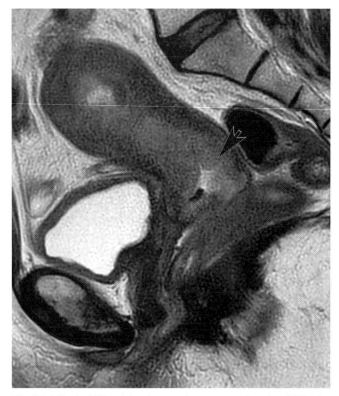

Fig. 90.1 Sagittal T2 weighted magnetic resonance imaging (MRI) of the uterus shows intermediate-signal-intensity cervical mass (arrow) replacing the expected T2 dark cervical fibrous stroma consistent with cervical carcinoma.

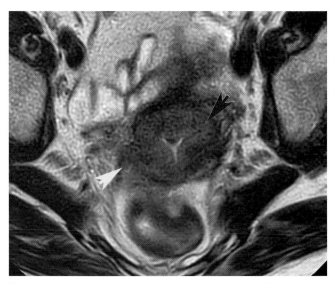

Fig. 90.2 Axial T2 weighted magnetic resonance imaging (MRI) of the uterus shows intermediate-signal-cervical mass (red arrow) invading the right lateral parametrium (yellow arrow) suggesting a stage III cancer per the FIGO staging system.

- Treatment: Radical hysterectomy could be the treatment of choice for young healthy patients with early stage disease because it preserves ovarian function. Radiotherapy is thought to be equally effective for patients with early stage disease.

REFERENCES

Hricak, H., & Yu, K. K. (1996). Radiology in invasive cervical cancer. *American Journal of Roentgenology, 167*(5), 1101–1108. doi:10.2214/ajr.167.5.8911159.

Nicolet, V., Carignan, L., Bourdon, F., & Prosmanne, O. (2000). MR imaging of cervical carcinoma: A practical staging approach. *Radiographics, 20*(6), 1539–1549. doi:10.1148/radiographics.20.6.g00nv111539.

CASE 91

Endometriosis With Adenomyosis

1. B, C. T2 weighted MR images show hyperintense foci in the myometrium, with intervening dark signal, representing adenomyosis. T1 weighted image shows hyperintense signal in the cyst in the right adnexa compatible with hemorrhage as seen in endometriomas. Hemorrhage is unlikely in an abscess, and infected debris is usually isointense and not intensely bright in T1 signal. Ovarian carcinomas present as cystic masses with solid nodular areas and thick septations, which are not seen on these images.
2. A. The prevalence of adenomyosis has been reported to range from 8.8% to 31%. Around 27% to 40% of women with endometriosis have concomitant adenomyosis. Incidence of adenomyosis among infertile women with endometriosis is up to 70%.
3. D. The junctional zone is a distinctly low signal intensity on T2-weighted images separating the high-signal-intensity endometrium from the intermediate-signal-intensity outer myometrium. Histologically, this zone corresponds to the innermost layer of the myometrium.
4. C. The threshold for junctional zone thickness for the diagnosis of adenomyosis is 12 mm.

Comment

- Introduction: Endometriosis and adenomyosis are two different but closely related conditions involving the presence of endometrial glands and stroma outside the endometrium. Approximately 27% to 40% of women with endometriosis have concomitant adenomyosis.
- Junctional zone: The term describes the interface between the endometrium and myometrium observed on T2 weighted MRI.
  - Normal values of junctional zone: 5 to 8 mm is considered to be the maximum threshold for a normal junctional zone thickness.
  - Physiologic variations of junctional zone:
    - According to patient age: during menarche, pregnancy, and postmenopausal status, junction and anatomy of the uterine muscle is often less distinct on MRI.
      - Postmenopausal status: due to atrophy of the uterine muscle, hormone-related changes, and involution of the extracellular components of the outer myometrium, junctional zone cannot be delineated in about 30% of patients.
      - Premenarchal female: junctional zone may be detectable as a faint line but is not measurable or discernible from the outer myometrium.
      - Pregnancy: junctional zone is poorly visualized as its signal is augmented and approaches the signal of the outer myometrium.
    - According to cycle: changes in the thickness of the junctional zone parallel changes in endometrial thickness

but to a lesser degree. Maximal thickness of the junctional zone is reached during the menstrual phase.

- Junctional zone in adenomyosis: junctional zone >12 mm is the most widely accepted criteria in establishing the diagnosis of adenomyosis. When the junctional zone thickness is >12 mm, adenomyosis can be diagnosed with a diagnostic accuracy of 85% and specificity of 96%.
- Diffuse involvement of the junctional zone suggests diffuse adenomyosis; however, if only a part of the junctional zone is involved, this would suggest focal adenomyosis.
- Junctional zone differential: calculated by measuring the difference in maximal and minimal thickness in both the anterior and posterior portions of the uterus. A junctional zone differential of >5 mm is also considered a reliable measurement of diagnosing adenomyosis.
- Ratio of junctional zone thickness and myometrium thickness: a ratio >40% between the thickness of the junctional zone and the thickness of the entire myometrium has a sensitivity of 65% and specificity of 92% for diagnosis of adenomyosis.
- Link between adenomyosis and endometriosis: a common pathogenesis for adenomyosis and endometriosis has been hypothesized.
  - Among infertile women with endometriosis, up to 70% also have adenomyosis.
  - Two main theories have been proposed to explain the origin of adenomyosis and endometriosis:
    - Sampson theory: implantation of normal endometrial cells, either from retrograde menstruation, neonatal menstruation, or after metaplasia of one of the following cell types: peritoneal mesenchymal cells, peritoneal or endometrial stem cells, or bone marrow cells.
    - Endometriotic disease theory: presence of a genetic and/or epigenetic incident leading to development of adenomyosis and endometriosis.

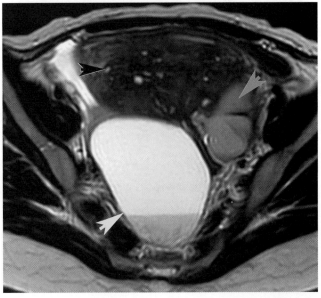

Fig. 91.1 Axial T2 weighted magnetic resonance imaging (MRI) of the uterus shows focal masslike thickening in the posterior myometrium with internal cystic foci (*red arrow*), characteristic for adenomyosis. Note that the junctional zone in the margins of the myometrial lesion is not well defined. Bilateral cystic adnexal masses are seen, with a fluid-fluid level in the right adnexa (*yellow arrow*) and T2 shading in the left adnexa (*green arrow*), consistent with bilateral endometriomas.

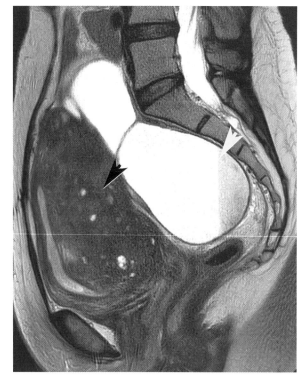

Fig. 91.2 Sagittal T2 weighted magnetic resonance imaging (MRI) of the uterus shows focal masslike thickening in the posterior myometrium with internal cystic foci *(red arrow)*, characteristic for adenomyosis. Note that the junctional zone in the margins of the myometrial lesion is not well defined. Large cystic masses are seen with a fluid-fluid level in one mass posterior to the uterus *(yellow arrow)*, consistent with endometriomas.

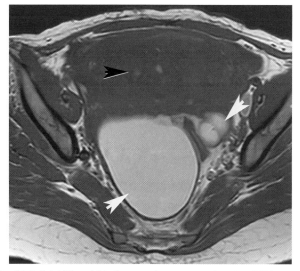

Fig. 91.3 Axial T1 weighted magnetic resonance imaging (MRI) of the uterus shows hyperintense foci within the posterior myometrium *(red arrow),* which is thickened and is characteristic for adenomyosis. Bilateral hyperintense cystic adnexal masses are seen *(yellow arrows)* consistent with bilateral endometriomas.

REFERENCES

Leyendecker, G., Wildt, L., & Mall, G. (2009). The pathophysiology of endometriosis and adenomyosis: Tissue injury and repair. *Archives of Gynecology and Obstetrics, 280*(4), 529–538. doi:10.1007/s00404-009-1191-0.

Novellas, S., Chassang, M., Delotte, J., Toullalan, O., Chevallier, A., ... Bouaziz, J. (2011). MRI characteristics of the uterine junctional zone: From normal to the diagnosis of adenomyosis. *American Journal of Roentgenology, 196*(5), 1206–1213. doi:10.2214/AJR.10.4877.

Takeuchi, M., & Matsuzaki, K. (2011). Adenomyosis: Usual and unusual imaging manifestations, pitfalls, and problem-solving MR imaging techniques. *Radiographics, 31*(1), 99–115. doi:10.1148/rg.311105110.

Tamai, K., Togashi, K., Ito, T., Morisawa, N., Fujiwara, T., & Koyama, T. (2005). MR imaging findings of adenomyosis: Correlation with histopathologic features and diagnostic pitfalls. *Radiographics, 25*(1), 21–40. doi:10.1148/rg.251045060.

CASE 93

Abdominal Wall Endometrioma

1. A, B. Endometrioma and desmoid should be included in the differential diagnosis for the mass shown. Abscess would have fluid content within it with peripheral vascularity, and lipoma has a characteristic mildly echogenic appearance compared to the adjacent subcutaneous fat and hence should not be included in the differential diagnosis.
2. C. 25% of patients with abdominal wall scar endometriosis have concomitant pelvic endometriosis.
3. A. Scar endometriosis typically appears as a hyperintense heterogenous nodule associated with anterior abdominal or pelvic wall scarring on both T1 (both with and without fat suppression) and T2 weighted images.
4. A, B, C. Surgery is the preferred treatment; however, progestogens or gonadotropin-releasing hormone (GnRH) analogs are also used.

Comment

- Endometrial implants within abdominal and pelvic wall scars are uncommon and most commonly develop after cesarean section or hysterectomy.
- Estimated incidence is approximately 0.03% to 0.4% among all women.
- Scar endometriosis may be confined to the superficial layers of the abdominal or pelvic wall, but it often infiltrates the deeper layers, commonly the rectus muscle.
- Only 25% have concomitant pelvic endometriosis.
- Pathogenesis: two theories have been proposed:
  - Specialized differentiation of primitive pluripotent mesenchymal cells to form endometriomas
  - Endometrial cells may be transported to ectopic sites, including during surgical procedures, and may proliferate into implants in surgical scars.
- Women present with small tender abdominal or pelvic wall mass associated with the previous surgical incision site. Typically, clinical symptoms occur at the time of menstruation and include abdominal or pelvic wall pain and swelling.
- Imaging:
  - US: findings of scar endometriosis vary, and other nonspecific lesions may be single or multicystic, solid or mixed cystic, and solid.
    - Scar endometriosis may demonstrate irregular often speculated margins with infiltration of the adjacent tissues. Cystic changes can be seen from recent hemorrhage associated with menstruation.
    - Vascularity is seen on color Doppler, which may be in the form of a single vascular pedicle entering the

Case 92 is online only and accessible at www.expertconsult.com.

periphery of the mass or dilated feeding vessels at the periphery of the mass.

- CT: imaging may be nonspecific but typically appears as a solid soft tissue mass directly associated with an area of surgical scarring. It may be hyperattenuating compared with muscle, and mild to moderate enhancement is seen after administration of intravenous contrast agent.
- MRI: provides better contrast resolution than CT or ultrasound
  - Scar endometriosis typically appears as a hyperintense heterogenous nodule associated with anterior abdominal or pelvic wall scarring on both T1 (both with and without fat suppression) and T2 weighted images, due to subacute hemorrhage within the endometriotic crypts.
- Treatment: Preferred treatment is wide surgical excision with clear margins to prevent local recurrence. Other therapeutic options include pharmacologic therapy with hormonal suppression agents, such as progestogens or gonadotropin-releasing hormone (GnRH) analogs.

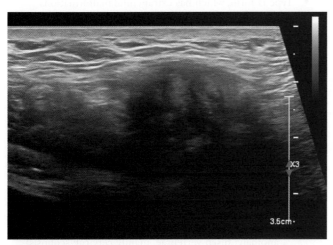

Fig. 93.1 Sagittal ultrasound image of the anterior abdominal wall showing a heterogenous hypoechoic mass *(red arrows)* involving the right rectus abdominis muscle. This was consistent with an endometrioma on percutaneous biopsy.

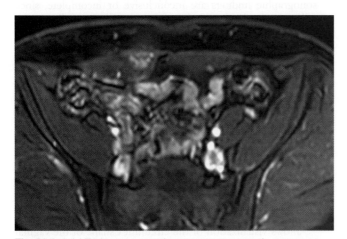

Fig. 93.2 Axial T1 fat suppressed postcontrast magnetic resonance imaging (MRI) shows enhancing mass *(red arrow)* in the right rectus muscle. This was consistent with an endometrioma on percutaneous biopsy.

REFERENCE

Gidwaney, R., Badler, R. L., Yam, B. L., Hines, J. J., Alexeeva, V., ... Donovan, V. (2012). Endometriosis of abdominal and pelvic wall scars: Multimodality imaging findings, pathologic correlation, and radiologic mimics. *Radiographics, 32*(7), 2031–2043. doi:10.1148/rg.327125024.

CASE 94

Acute Ovarian Torsion

1. C. Images show enlarged ovary with a hypoechoic appearance and absence of blood supply within it suggestive of ovarian torsion. This could also be an ovarian fibroma; however, patient age and presentation do not suggest a fibroma.
2. A, C. Ovary receives dual blood supply from the ovarian artery and uterine artery.
3. A, B, C. Twisting pedicle sign, follicular ring sign, and whirlpool sign are imaging signs seen on ultrasound with Doppler. String of pearl sign is not described in ovarian torsion.
4. C. In ovarian torsion there is enlargement of the entire ovary. The peripheral follicles are separated by edematous stroma.

Comment

- Ovarian torsion can be intermittent or sustained and requires surgical intervention to prevent ovarian necrosis.
- Risk factors include adnexal masses and cysts, polycystic ovarian syndrome, ovarian hyperstimulation syndrome, history of adnexal torsion, and previous tubal ligation.
- Blood supply: ovary receives dual blood supply from the ovarian artery and uterine artery. Ovarian artery arises from the abdominal aorta below the renal artery and travels in the infundibulopelvic ligament. Uterine artery is a branch of the internal iliac artery and bifurcates in the tuboovarian artery traveling in the ovarian ligament, which anastomoses with the ovarian artery.
- Pathophysiology: severity of vascular impairment is variable depending on degree of rotation causing varying degrees of partial to complete obstruction.
  - Initially twisted vascular pedicle in the suspensory ligament induces ovarian edema due to venous and lymphatic outflow compromise. Then arterial ischemia and ultimately necrosis ensue.
- Imaging findings: US with Doppler remains the initial study of choice
  - US: increased size of the ovary, >4 cm with hyperechoic stromal edema and peripherally displaced follicles
  - Ovarian enlargement is the key diagnostic feature early in the diagnosis
  - Other direct signs:
    - Twisting of the ovarian pedicle: round hypoechoic structure with multiple inner concentric hypoechoic broad rings
    - Follicular ring sign: hyperechoic ring around the antral follicles compatible with perifollicular edema
  - Color and spectral Doppler US: whirlpool sign—ellipsoid or spiral vascularization within the twist, decreased or interrupted intraovarian venous flow, and absence of arterial flow
    - Persistence of arterial flow does not rule out adnexal torsion, which may be due to dual blood supply, intermittent or partial torsion, or venous occlusion occurring before arterial obstruction
- CT: common findings include displacement of adnexa to the contralateral side or midline position, deviation of uterus to the side of involved ovary and adnexal enlargement. Other features include twist of the ovarian pedicle, infiltration of pelvic fat, and pelvic ascites.
- MRI: not commonly employed as a first line imaging study in suspected torsion. Findings are similar to those reported for US and CT, but MRI offers better soft tissue contrast. Ovarian masses may show specific signal characteristics that allow definitive diagnosis

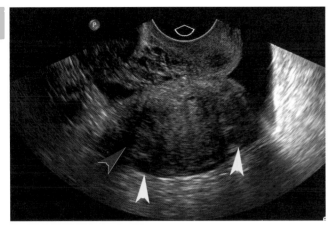

Fig. 94.1 Transvaginal B-mode ultrasound shows enlarged right ovary *(red arrow)*, which is located in the cul-de-sac. Note the small peripheral small cysts in the right ovary *(yellow arrows)*. Free fluid is seen in the pelvis.

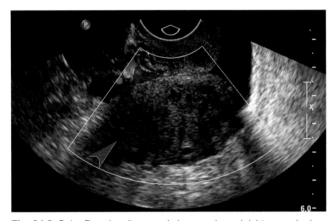

Fig. 94.2 Color Doppler ultrasound shows enlarged right ovary *(red arrow)*, which is located in the cul-de-sac with no vascularity seen in the right ovary. Note the small peripheral small cysts in the right ovary. Free fluid is seen in the pelvis.

REFERENCES

Lourenco, A. P., Swenson, D., Tubbs, R. J., & Lazarus, E. (2014). Ovarian and tubal torsion: Imaging findings on US, CT, and MRI. *Emergency Radiology, 21*, 179–187.

Ssi-Yan-Kai, G., Rivain, A. L., Trichot, C., Morcelet, M. C., Prevot, S., … Deffieux, X. (2018). What every radiologist should know about adnexal torsion. *Emergency Radiology, 25*, 51–59.

CASE 95

Mayer-Rokitansky-Küster-Hauser (MRKH) Syndrome

1. A, C, D. Mayer-Rokitansky-Küster-Hauser (MRKH) syndrome is a congenital disorder characterized by uterovaginal agenesis and can be associated with renal, skeletal, and cardiac malformations. Most cases are sporadic. Patients with MRKH syndrome usually have a normal 46,XX karyotype and have primary amenorrhea and abnormalities of internal genitalia, absence of the uterus and upper two-thirds of the vagina. These patients usually appear to have normal secondary sexual characteristics.

2. A. MRKH is a class I müllerian anomaly related to uterovaginal agenesis. As a complete failure of müllerian duct development, müllerian agenesis, MRKH is the most severe form because it shows the absence of fallopian tubes, uterus, cervix, and the upper two-thirds of the vagina. Because gonads are developed in these patients, the endocrine functions of affected women are normal.

3. B. MRKH is associated with agenesis of the uterus and upper vagina and may be associated with renal anomalies. Ovaries and the lower vagina are not derived from the müllerian system. Ovaries are derived from germ cells that migrate from the primitive yolk sac into the mesenchyme of the peritoneal cavity and subsequently into the supporting cells.

4. C. MRI is the most effective modality for detection of ovaries, which are found in 97% of patients.

Comment

- Introduction: The Mayer-Rokitansky-Küster-Hauser (MRKH) syndrome is characterized by the congenital absence of the uterus and the upper two-thirds of the vagina in 46,XX females with mostly normal ovarian function and therefore normal breast and pubic hair development.
- MRKH can be subdivided into two subtypes:
  - Isolated, type I form
  - Type II form, which has extragenital malformations
- The MRKH syndrome affects at least 1 in 4000 to 5000 female newborns.
  - Most of the cases are sporadic, familial clustering has also been described with an autosomal dominant inheritance.
  - Clinical presentation is with primary amenorrhea.
  - Clinical examination typically reveals a normal female phenotype with breast development, axillary and pubic hair, and normal external genitalia.
  - Differential diagnosis includes isolated vaginal atresia, androgen insensitivity syndrome caused by mutations of the androgen receptor gene *(AR)* in XY individuals and *WNT4* defects characterized by MRKH and hyperandrogenism.
  - Other associated malformations include (type II or MURCS association):
    - Renal (unilateral agenesis, ectopia of kidneys or horseshoe kidney)
    - Skeletal and, in particular, vertebral (Klippel-Feil anomaly; fused vertebrae, mainly cervical; scoliosis)
    - Hearing defects
    - More rarely, cardiac and digital anomalies (syndactyly, polydactyly)
- Diagnosis: MRI is more sensitive and more specific means of diagnosis than ultrasonography and is performed when ultrasonographic findings are inconclusive or incomplete, since failure to clearly identify the uterus or müllerian rudiments or ovaries does not necessarily imply their absence.
- Uterine aplasia is best characterized on sagittal images, while vaginal aplasia is best evidenced on transverse images.
- MRI can also be used at the same time to search for associated renal and skeletal malformations.
- Ovaries can be ectopic in location and are usually located in lateral pelvic walls, anteriorly to the ovarian fossa or sometimes in front of the inguinal canal.
  - They may be absent in up to 23% of cases and in 16% of cases they will be extrapelvic in location, either in the iliac fossa or in the abdomen, anterior to the psoas muscle.
- Vagina is best depicted on sagittal and axial T2 weighted images as a structure between the urethra and the bladder neck anteriorly and the rectum posteriorly.
  - In cases of complete vagina agenesis, the sagittal plane allows visualization of the circumflex shape of the vaginal cupola, between the urethra and the perineum.
  - Above the incomplete vagina, either venous plexuses between the bladder and rectum or the fibrous median structure forming the inferior border of the vestigial uterine structure is found.

- Differential diagnosis: includes congenital absence of uterus and vagina (aplasia or agenesis), isolated vaginal atresia, and androgen insensitivity.

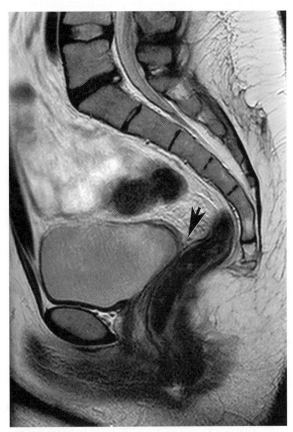

Fig. 95.1 Sagittal T2 weighted magnetic resonance imaging (MRI) shows absence of the uterus and vagina (red arrow).

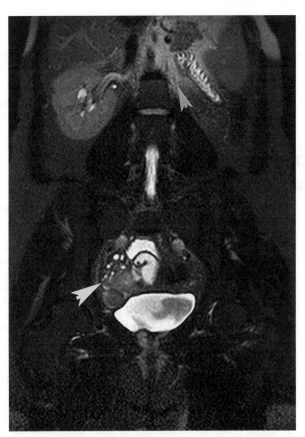

Fig. 95.3 Coronal T2 weighted fat-saturated magnetic resonance imaging (MRI) shows absence of the left kidney (blue arrowhead); and the right ovary is visualized in its normal location (yellow arrow).

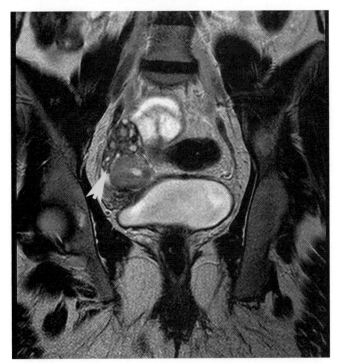

Fig. 95.2 Coronal T2 weighted magnetic resonance imaging (MRI) shows normal location and appearance of the right ovary (yellow arrow) with a hemorrhagic corpus luteum cyst in it.

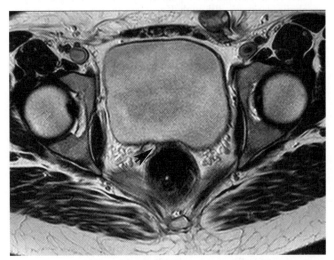

Fig. 95.4 Axial T2 weighted magnetic resonance imaging (MRI) shows absence of the uterus and vagina (red arrow).

REFERENCES

Carrington, B. M., Hricak, H., Nuruddin, R. N., Secaf, E., Laros, R. K., & Hill, E. C. (1990). Müllerian duct anomalies: MR imaging evaluation. *Radiology, 176*(3), 715–720. doi:10.1148/radiology.176.3.2202012.

Ledig, S., & Wieacker, P. (2018). Clinical and genetic aspects of Mayer-Rokitansky-Küster-Hauser syndrome. *Medizinische Genetik, 30*(1), 3–11. doi:10.1007/s11825-018-0173-7.

Maubon, A., Ferru, J. M., Courtieu, C., Mares, P., & Rouanet, J. P. (1996). Gynecological malformations. Classification and contribution of different imaging methods. *Journal de Radiologie, 77*(7), 465–475.

Rousset, P., Raudrant, D., Peyron, N., Buy, J. N., Valette, P. J., & Hoeffel, C. (2013). Ultrasonography and MRI features of the Mayer-Rokitansky-Küster-Hauser syndrome. *Clinical Radiology, 68*(9), 945–952. doi:10.1016/j.crad.2013.04.005.

Troiano, R. N., & McCarthy, S. M. (2004). Mullerian duct anomalies: Imaging and clinical issues. *Radiology, 233*(1), 19–34. doi:10.1148/radiol.2331020777.

CASE 96

Retroperitoneal Mass

1. A, B, C, D. Retroperitoneal lymphadenopathy is the most common mass seen in the retroperitoneum. Lymphadenopathy at the level of the renal hilum in a young man is typical for metastasis from a testicular germ cell tumor. Other possible ideologies of retroperitoneal lymphadenopathy include lymphoma and infection such as *Mycobacterium tuberculosis* and *Mycobacterium avium* intracellular (MAI), which are common in immunocompromised patients. Primary retroperitoneal neoplasm suggests sarcoma is also considered as a differential diagnosis.
2. B. The discovery of lymphadenopathy at the level of the renal hilum in a young man should raise the possibility of a testicular germ cell tumor, and testicular neoplasm as a possible primary site should be looked for. Ultrasonography is the primary imaging modality for investigating testicular lesions.
3. D. Ipsilateral retroperitoneal lymph nodes in the region of the renal vessels is the initial site of metastasis from testicular germ cell tumors.
4. A. Serum tumor markers including alpha-fetoprotein, HCG, and LDH have a well-established role in the diagnosis, staging, prognosis, and follow-up of testicular germ cell tumors.

Comment

- Testicular tumors most commonly metastasize gland lymphatic drainage, although Korea carcinoma can also spread hematogenously.
- Retroperitoneal nodes are the first landing site of metastatic disease with tumors originating from the right testes often spreading to the interaortocaval lymph nodes while tumors originating in the left testes will spread to the paraaortic lymph nodes.
- Crossover drainage from right-sided tumors to left-sided lymph node groups has been recorded; however, drainage from left to right has not been reported.
- Tumor markers: three well-established markers are alpha-fetoprotein (AFP), human chorionic gonadotropin (HCG), and lactate dehydrogenase (LDH).
  - AFP is never present in seminoma or pure carcinoma.
  - HCG is always elevated in the presence of choriocarcinoma and can also be elevated in the presence of embryonic carcinoma, teratoma, and up to 10% of pure seminomas.
  - LDH can be elevated in both seminoma and nonseminomatous germ cell tumor. Elevation is typically an indication of bulky or extensive disease.
- Imaging findings: Ultrasonography is the primary imaging modality for investigating testicular lesions. CT scan remains the imaging technique of choice in staging testicular germ cell tumors and assessing response to treatment.
- Staging: The tumor-node-metastasis-serum markers (TNMS) staging system from the American Joint Committee on Cancer is widely used in staging of testicular cancers. The system considers local lymph nodes to be located in the retroperitoneum and all others (e.g., supraclavicular or chest) to be distant metastasis.

T: Primary tumor staging

PTx	Primary tumor cannot be assessed
pT0	No evidence of primary tumor
pTis	Intratubular germ cell neoplasia (carcinoma in situ)
pT1	Tumor limited to testes and epididymis without lymphovascular invasion (LVI): tumor may invade tunica albuginea but not tunica vaginalis
pT2	Tumor limited to testes and epididymis with LVI: tumor extending through tunica albuginea with involvement of the tunica vaginalis
pT3	Tumor invades the spermatic cord with or without LVI
pT4	Tumor invades the scrotum with or without LVI

N: regional lymph node clinical staging

NX	Regional lymph nodes cannot be assessed
N0	No regional lymph node metastasis
N1	Lymph node mass ≤2 cm in greatest dimension or multiple LN, none ≥2 cm
N2	Lymph node mass >2 cm but not >5 cm in greatest dimension or multiple LNs, any mass >2 cm but not >5 cm
N3	LN mass >5 cm in greatest dimension

M: metastatic disease staging

Mx	Distant metastasis cannot be assessed
M0	No distant metastasis
M1	Nonregional lymph nodes or pulmonary metastasis
M1b	Nonpulmonary visceral metastasis

S: serum tumor marker staging

Sx	Markers not available or not performed
S0	Marker levels normal
S1	LDH <1.5 × upper limit of normal and HCG <5000 and AFP <1000
S2	LDH 1.5–10 × upper limit of normal or HCG 5000–50,000 or AFP 1000–10,000
S3	LDh >10 × upper limit of normal or HCG >50,000 or AFP >10,000

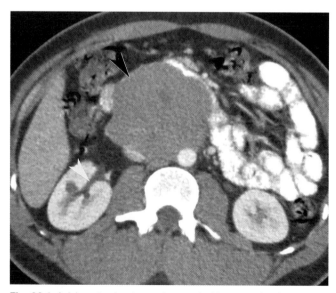

Fig. 96.1 Axial contrast-enhanced computed tomography shows a large interaortocaval mass *(red arrow)* at the level of the right renal hilum. There is mild right hydronephrosis *(yellow arrow)* that is due to the compressive effects of the mass.

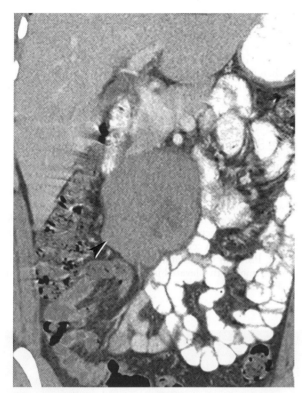

Fig. 96.2 Coronal contrast enhanced computed tomography shows a large interaortocaval *mass (red arrow)*.

REFERENCE

Kreydin, E. I., Barrisford, G. W., Feldman, A. S., & Preston, M. A. (2013). Testicular cancer: What the radiologist needs to know. *American Journal of Roentgenology, 200*(6), 1215–1225.

CASE 98

Prostate Abscess

1. D. The low-attenuation fluid collection on CT and T2 hyperintense collection on axial and sagittal MRI represents a prostate abscess. Utricle cyst is a midline cystic mass in the prostate that represents a focal dilation of the utricle. The lesion is too large, irregular, and heterogeneous to represent a glandular BPH nodule. It is not located in the seminal vesicle.
2. A. Prostate abscess is an increasingly rare but potential complication of acute bacterial prostatitis (typically due to *E. coli* or *Staphylococcus* infection). Abscess is not a complication of BPH or carcinoma.
3. A, B. Prostate abscess most commonly occurs in diabetic or immunosuppressed patients. It is not more common in patients with underlying prostate or bladder cancer.
4. C. Percutaneous transperineal or transrectal drainage is the treatment of choice for prostate abscess. Conservative therapy +/− IV antibiotics is insufficient to adequately treat the abscess. Surgery is a potential intervention but is accompanied by higher complication rates.

Comment

- Prostate abscess is a rare potential complication of acute prostatitis. It is becoming even more uncommon due to early antibiotic administration in patients with prostatitis.

Case 97 is online only and accessible at www.expertconsult.com.

- Prostate abscess most commonly occurs in diabetic and/or immunosuppressed patients.
- Affected patients typically present with signs and symptoms of acute bacterial prostatitis: dysuria, fever, suprapubic pain, and urinary retention.
- The most common culprits in acute bacterial prostatitis are *E. coli* and *Staphlococcus* organisms. Gonococcus also rarely occurs.
- The treatment of choice for prostate abscess is percutaneous transperineal or transrectal drainage with IV antibiotic administration. Surgery involves higher complication rates.
- Imaging findings of pancreatic prostate abscess:
  - US: transrectal ultrasound is high yield in diagnosis; ill-defined hypoechoic collection with internal echoes in the background of an enlarged, distorted prostate gland
  - CT: enlarged prostate gland with low-attenuation fluid collection
  - MRI: T1 hypointense, T2 hyperintense collection within the prostate demonstrating peripheral enhancement and restricted diffusion

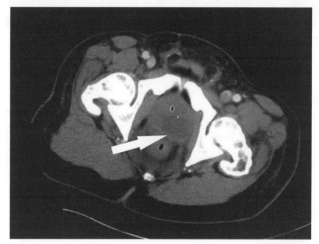

Fig. 98.1 Contrast-enhanced axial computed tomography (CT) image of the pelvis showing a low-density fluid collection in the prostate *(arrow)*, compatible with an abscess.

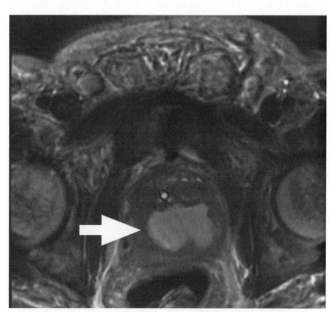

Fig. 98.2 Axial magnetic resonance imaging (MRI) through the prostate demonstrates the poorly marginated and heterogeneous appearance of the prostatic abscess *(arrow)*.

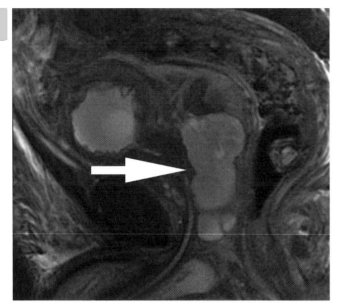

Fig. 98.3 Sagittal magnetic resonance imaging (MRI) showing the craniocaudal extent of the prostate abscess *(arrow)*.

REFERENCES

Aphinives, C., Pacheerat, K., Chaiyakum, J., Laopaiboon, V., Aphinives, P., & Phuttharak, W. (2004). Prostatic abscesses: Radiographic findings and treatment. *Journal of the Medical Association of Thailand, 87*(7), 810–815.

Barozzi, L., Pavlica, P., Menchi, I., De Matteis, M., & Canepari, M. (1998). Prostatic abscess: Diagnosis and treatment. *American Journal of Roentgenology, 170*(3), 753–757.

CASE 100

Prostatitis

1. B. The abnormality shown on the images localizes to the peripheral zone.
2. A. While prostatitis may mimic prostate malignancy and vice versa, in the provided clinical scenario of a young man with local and systemic symptoms of prostatitis, the most likely diagnosis is acute prostatitis.
3. B. When used for biochemical screening of prostate cancer, PSA is most commonly considered abnormally elevated at the threshold of 4 ng/mL.
4. D. PSA can be falsely suppressed by finasteride.

Comment

Prostatitis

- Acute:
  - More common in young men; presents with local and systemic symptoms
  - Via intraprostatic reflux of urine infected with gram-negative bacteria, or after instrumentation
- Chronic:
  - More common in older men; indolent, and often with only lower urinary tract symptoms
  - Can occur without prior history, such as with lower urinary tract obstruction
- PSA levels may fluctuate (see prostate specific antigen, later)

Case 99 is online only and accessible at www.expertconsult.com.

- MRI appearance may mimic prostate cancer
  - Can be focal or diffuse
  - T2: hypointense
  - DWI: degree of diffusion restriction is less in prostatitis than in cancer
  - DCE: increased, early enhancement compared to normal prostate
  - May be seen with enlarged, reactive pelvic lymph nodes

Prostate Specific Antigen (PSA)

- Protein produced by both normal and abnormal prostate glandular tissue
- Serum PSA typically measured in nanograms per milliliter of blood (ng/mL)
- Can be used toward screening for prostate cancer; test performance is imperfect, and wide variation exists in the clinical application of PSA screening
- While PSA can be elevated due to prostate cancer, PSA can also be transiently elevated in a variety of benign conditions:
  - Prostatitis

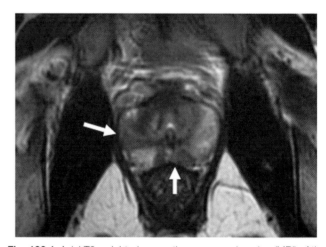

Fig. 100.1 Axial T2 weighted magnetic resonance imaging (MRI) of the prostate demonstrates multifocal wedge-shaped T2 hypointensity of the peripheral zone *(arrows)*.

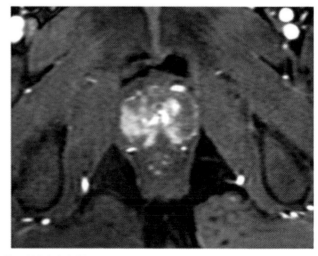

Fig. 100.2 Axial T1 weighted fat-suppressed postcontrast magnetic resonance imaging (MRI) demonstrates enhancement in the corresponding areas.

- Acute urinary retention
- Urethral or prostate instrumentation (catheterization, biopsy, resection)
- PSA can be falsely suppressed by finasteride (5-alpha-reductase inhibitor)
  - Can reduce PSA by 50% after 12 months of therapy
  - PSA is not impacted by alpha-blocker medications (e.g., tamsulosin, terazosin, doxazosin)
- A PSA level ≥4.0 ng/mL is a commonly utilized standard
  - For detection of any prostate cancer, sensitivity 21%, specificity 91%
  - For detection of high-grade cancer, sensitivity 51%

REFERENCES

Kitzing, Y. X., Prando, A., Varol, C., Karczmar, G. S., Maclean, F., & Oto, A. (2016). Benign conditions that mimic prostate carcinoma: MR imaging features with histopathologic correlation. *RadioGraphics*, *36*, 162–175.

Rosenkrantz, A. B., & Taneja, S. S. (2014). Radiologist, be aware: Ten pitfalls that confound the interpretation of multiparametric prostate MRI. *American Journal of Roentgenology*, *202*, 109–120.

Yu, J., Fulcher, A. S., Turner, M. A., Cockrell, C. H., Cote, E. P., & Wallace, T. J. (2014). Prostate cancer and its mimics at multiparametric prostate MRI. *British Journal of Radiology*, *87*, 20130659.

CASE 101

Prostate Adenocarcinoma

1. C. There is an ill-defined lesion centered in the left peripheral zone, where there is abnormal restricted diffusion (hyperintense on DWI, hypointense on ADC) and abnormal T2 hypointense signal.
2. E. As the lesion demonstrates focal markedly hyperintense diffusion abnormality on high b-value (≥1400) DWI, and focal markedly hypointense signal on ADC, and is larger than the 1.5-cm scale bar on the ADC image, the most appropriate assessment is PI-RADS 5.
3. C. According to PI-RADS v2.1, the dominant signal sequence for characterization of a peripheral zone finding is diffusion weighted imaging.
4. B. According to PI-RADS v2.1, the dominant signal sequence for characterization of a peripheral zone finding is T2 weighted imaging.

Comment

Prostate Cancer

- Most commonly adenocarcinoma arising from the glandular prostate
- Worldwide, most commonly diagnosed malignancy; sixth leading cause of cancer death among men
- Majority of cancers grow slowly, are low grade, with limited aggressiveness
- Risk factors: older age, positive family history, obesity, hypertension
- In 2012, the US Preventive Services Task Force (USPSTF) recommended against routine serum PSA screening

Histopathology

- Gleason scoring system reports two numbers from 1 to 5 (e.g., A + B)
- The first number represents the predominant histologic pattern
- The second number represents the secondary or minor pattern
- 5 = the most histologically abnormal; 1 = normal pattern
- Thus Gleason 3+4 represents less aggressive histology than Gleason 4+3

Role of MRI

- MRI can augment risk assessment strategies for the detection of prostate cancer
  - PRECISION trial (*NEJM*, 2018)
    - Prebiopsy MRI and MRI-targeted biopsy found to be superior to transrectal ultrasound-guided biopsy for the detection of clinically significant prostate cancer, and low rate of diagnosis of clinically insignificant prostate cancer

MRI Appearance of Prostate Cancer

- 70% to 75% of prostate cancer occurs in the peripheral zone
- Multiparametric MRI (mpMRI) for prostate cancer:
  - T2: prostate cancer is T2 hypointense in the peripheral zone
  - DWI: restricted diffusion (hyperintense of DW images, hypointense on ADC maps)
  - DCE: early enhancement of prostate cancer relative to normal prostate
- Prostate Imaging Reporting and Data System (PI-RADS)
  - Seeks to improve patient outcomes by improving detection, characterization, and risk stratification in treatment-naïve patients with suspected prostate cancer
  - PI-RADS v2.1 published in 2019 by American College of Radiology (ACR)
  - Lesion-based reporting based on mpMRI findings; uses a 5-point scale to assign the likelihood of clinically significant prostate cancer
    - Ranges from 1 (very low probability) to 5 (very high probability)
  - Peripheral zone:
    - DWI is the dominant factor for PI-RADS assessment
    - DCE abnormality, if present, may upgrade a PI-RADS 3 lesion to PI-RADS 4
  - Transitional zone
    - T2 is the dominant factor for PI-RADS assessment
    - DWI abnormality, if present, may upgrade classification

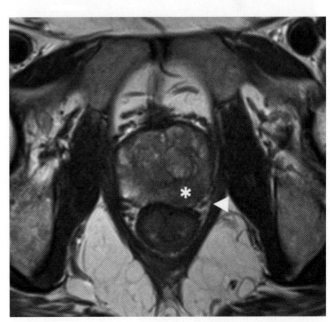

Fig. 101.1 Axial images from magnetic resonance imaging (MRI) centered on the prostate, at the level of the midgland. T2 weighted image demonstrates abnormal T2 hypointensity (*) at the left peripheral zone. The adjacent left neurovascular bundle (*arrowhead*) is not involved.

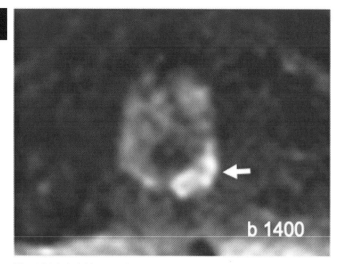

Fig. 101.2 Axial images from magnetic resonance imaging (MRI) centered on the prostate, at the level of the midgland. High b-value diffusion weighted imaging demonstrates markedly hyperintense diffusion abnormality *(arrow)*.

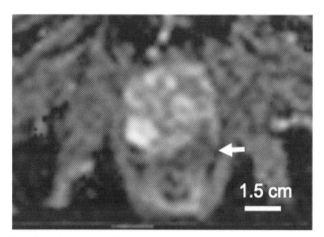

Fig. 101.3 Axial images from magnetic resonance imaging (MRI) centered on the prostate, at the level of the midgland. Corresponding ADC map demonstrates corresponding markedly hypointense signal of restricted diffusion, with size in excess of the 1.5-cm scale bar, meeting PI-RADS 5 criteria *(arrow)*.

REFERENCES

Kasivisvanathan, V., Rannikko, A. S., Borghi, M., Panebianco, V., Mynderse, L. A., ... Vaarala, M. H. (2018). MRI-targeted or standard biopsy for prostate-cancer diagnosis. *New England Journal of Medicine, 378,* 1767–1777.

Turkbey, B., Rosenkrantz, A. B., Haider, M. A., Padhani, A. R., et al. (2019). Prostate Imaging Reporting and Data System Version 2.1: 2019 update of Prostate Imaging Reporting and Data System Version 2. *European Urology, pii,* S0302-2838(19)30180-0.

CASE 102

Gastric Emphysema

1. A, C, D. The imaging appearance shown is unlikely to be from normal air in the stomach, since air is seen in the wall of the stomach in a nondependent location. Etiology for this appearance could be due to gastric emphysema, emphysematous gastritis, or trauma, which could be iatrogenic from nasogastric tube placement, laparoscopic gastric band erosion, and motor vehicle accidents.

2. C. Clinical picture primarily differentiates between gastric emphysema and emphysematous gastritis. Patients with gastric emphysema will often be asymptomatic and hemodynamically stable while patients with emphysematous gastritis often present with nausea, vomiting, mild to severe abdominal pain, hematemesis, and/or melena.

3. A, B, C. Gastric outlet obstruction, vomiting, and endoscopy are risk factors for development of gastric emphysema.

4. A, B, C, D. Predisposing factors for emphysematous gastritis are gastroduodenal surgery, ingestion of corrosive materials, gastroenteritis or gastrointestinal infarction, alcohol abuse, abdominal surgery, diabetes, and immunosuppression.

Comment

- Gastric emphysema or gastric cystic pneumatosis, defined as air in the gastric wall without an underlying infection, is a rare radiologic finding.
  - First described by Brouardel in 1895.
  - Caused by a disruption in gastric mucosal integrity leading to the entry of air into the wall.
    - Various causes for this phenomenon:
      - Raised intragastric pressure (i.e., gastric outlet obstruction)
      - Trauma (e.g., endoscopy and instrumentation)
      - Severe vomiting
      - Dissection of air from the mediastinum (e.g., chronic obstructive pulmonary disease or pneumothorax)
      - Ischemia
  - Gastric ischemia has been reported as etiology for gastric emphysema and hepatic portal venous gas.
  - Most patients usually have mild or no symptoms apart from those patients presenting with gastric ischemia, who may present with an acute abdomen.
  - The prognosis of this condition is excellent. The treatment is directed toward the precipitating etiology.

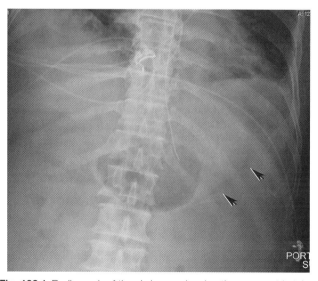

Fig. 102.1 Radiograph of the abdomen showing the nasogastric tube with the tip seen in the body of the stomach. Note air outlining the wall of the stomach *(arrows)*.

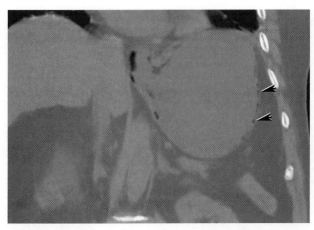

Fig. 102.2 Coronal reformat in lung kernel from a postcontrast computed tomography (CT) scan showed small air droplets *(arrows)* within the stomach wall along the greater gastric curvature. Since the patient did not have any other symptoms, this was most consistent with gastric emphysema.

- Emphysematous gastritis is an acute infection of the stomach wall with gas-forming organisms associated with systematic toxicity. *Escherichia coli, Streptococcus* spp, *Enterobacter* spp, and *Pseudomonas aeruginosa* are the usual causative agents.
  - Predisposing factors for this condition are gastroduodenal surgery, ingestion of corrosive materials, gastroenteritis or gastrointestinal infarction, alcohol abuse, abdominal surgery, diabetes, and immunosuppression.
  - Usually has a fulminant course with a mortality rate of 60% and gastric strictures are as common as 25%.
  - Usually present with severe abdominal pain, nausea, vomiting, hematemesis, low-grade fevers, and tachycardia.
  - Surgery should be avoided during the acute phase of emphysematous gastritis in the absence of bowel perforation, necrosis, or ischemia owing to friability of the mucosa and the delay in healing of the sutured margins.
  - A gastrectomy is often necessary when expectant medical management fails. Late surgical intervention is preferred due to tissue friability, as mentioned earlier.

REFERENCE
Matsushima, K., Won, E. J., Tangel, M. R., Enomoto, L. M., Avella, D. M., & Soybel, D. I. (2015). Emphysematous gastritis and gastric emphysema: Similar radiographic findings, distinct clinical entities. *World Journal of Surgery, 39*(4), 1008–1017. doi:10.1007/s00268-014-2882-7.

CASE 103

Slipped Gastric Band

1. C. A gastric band is depicted.
2. B. The typical appearance is a rectangular appearance of the band in profile; the O-shaped appearance of the band indicates slipped malposition.
3. D. The phi angle is typically measured as the acute angle formed between a line drawn through the longitudinal axis of the band and the longitudinal axis of the adjacent vertebral column.
4. D. While band slippage is associated with cessation of weight loss and gastroesophageal reflux, the O sign of slippage as depicted is a specific finding associated with posterior band slippage.

Comment

Diagnosis and Imaging Findings

Gastric banding is a less invasive surgical treatment for morbid obesity and is typically performed laparoscopically. Gastric band devices typically consist of three components:
1. Radiopaque, inflatable silicone band
2. Connector tubing
3. Subcutaneous reservoir port at the abdominal wall, by which the band can be adjusted when further insufflation or deflation is indicated

Complications

- Acute complications are rare.
- Late complications include:
  - Intragastric erosion, plateau in weight loss, and band slippage
- Band slippage
  - Associated with cessation of weight loss, gastroesophageal reflux, and nocturnal vomiting
  - Assessment for band slippage:
    - Qualitative assessment of the appropriately positioned band should demonstrate a rectangular appearance, resulting from the superimposition of the anterior and posterior aspects.
      - In contrast, if the band shows an O configuration, posterior slippage should be suspected.
  - Quantitative assessment of the phi angle can be assessed as follows on a frontal abdominal radiograph:
    - Draw a line indicating the long axis of the thoracic spine.

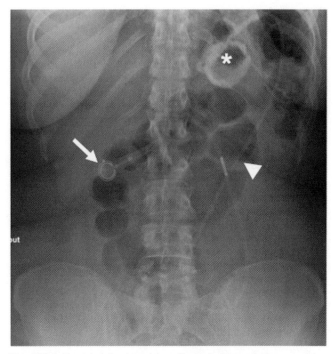

Fig. 103.1 Frontal abdominopelvic radiograph demonstrates a gastric band. The gastric band is shown in the left upper quadrant, oriented in an O configuration *(asterisk).* This is connected via radiopaque tubing *(arrowhead)* to the reservoir port in the right midabdomen *(arrow).*

- Draw a line through the longitudinal axis of the gastric band.
- The acute/superior angle between these two lines is the phi angle, and should be between 4 and 58 degrees.

Treatment

A gastric band can be insufflated or deflated via the subcutaneous reservoir port, depending on the status of weight loss, and relevant symptomatology. Alternatives to gastric banding include surgical revision or removal, or conversion to other bariatric surgical approaches to weight loss.

REFERENCE

Sonavane, S. K., Menias, C. O., Kantawala, K. P., Shanbhogue, A. K., Prasad, S. R., ... Eagon, J. C. (2012). Laparoscopic adjustable gastric banding: What radiologists need to know. *Radiographics, 32,* 1161–1178.

CASE 104

Roux-en-Y Gastric Bypass; Gastrogastric Fistula

1. C. The relative positions of the gastric fundus and vertebral column identify the prone and supine positioning of the images.
2. B. Images demonstrate a gastric pouch and gastrojejunostomy, typical of Roux-en-Y gastric bypass.
3. D. Gastric rugal folds are shown extending from the gastric pouch, in an orientation of the typical position expected of the gastric body and greater curvature, indicating gastrogastric fistula.
4. A. The typical sign of gastrogastric fistula is weight regain.

Comment

Diagnosis and Imaging Findings

Roux-en-Y gastric bypass is a bariatric surgery, performed laparoscopically or open, for the treatment of morbid obesity. The stomach is divided, resulting in a gastric pouch and the excluded stomach. The gastric pouch is received by a gastrojejunal anastomosis; the excluded stomach empties physiologically into the duodenum and proximal jejunum, ultimately joining the gastrojejunal limb at a jejunojejunal anastomosis.

Complications

- Acute
  - Fluoroscopic evaluation is performed in the early postoperative setting to assess for leak
  - Other acute complications include bleeding/hematoma and anastomotic ischemia resulting in anastomotic breakdown
- Delayed
  - Anastomotic stricture or ulcer
  - Gastrogastric fistula typically results in gradual regain of weight lost during the initial postoperative period
  - Small bowel obstruction may result from either adhesions or internal hernia

Treatment

Upon detection of gastrogastric fistula, endoscopic evaluation may be indicated, particularly if there is concern for accompanying anastomotic ulcer. Treatment considerations include surgical revision.

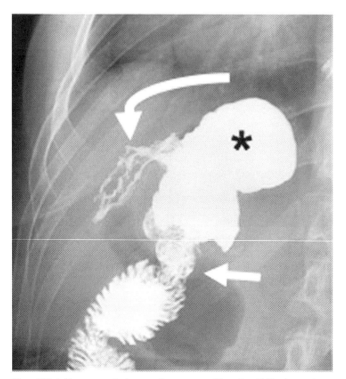

Fig. 104.1 Fluoroscopic images from upper GI series. With the patient in prone position, contrast is shown in the gastric pouch *(asterisk)* and gastrojejunostomy *(straight arrow).* Contrast additionally opacifies gastric rugal folds extending from the gastric pouch *(curved arrow),* representing gastrogastric fistula.

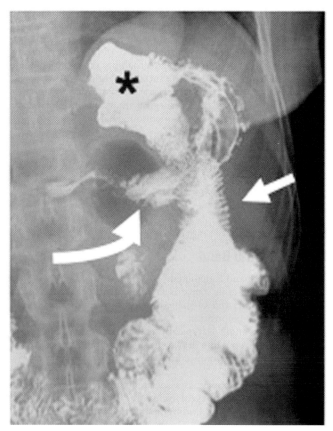

Fig. 104.2 Fluoroscopic images from upper gastrointestinal (GI) series. Correlative findings are shown with the patient in supine position.

REFERENCES

Blachar, A., Federle, M. P., Pealer, K. M., Ikramuddin, S., & Schauer, P. R. (2002). Gastrointestinal complications of laparoscopic Roux-en-Y gastric bypass surgery: Clinical and imaging findings. *Radiology, 223,* 625–632.

Levine, M. S., & Carucci, L. R. (2014). Imaging of bariatric surgery: Normal anatomy and postoperative complications. *Radiology, 270,* 327–341.

Scheirey, C. D., Scholz, F. J., Shah, P. C., Brams, D. M., Wong, B. B., & Pedrosa, M. (2006). Radiology of the laparoscopic Roux-en-Y gastric bypass procedure: Conceptualization and precise interpretation of results. *Radiographics, 26,* 1355–1371.

CASE 105

Nissen Fundoplication

1. B. The relative position of the gastric fundus and vertebral column indicate that these images were acquired in the prone position; the displaced position of the esophagus, away from the vertebral column, indicates that the patient is in right anterior oblique position.
2. E. The esophagus is anatomically positioned left anterolaterally relative to the thoracic vertebral column; supine and prone imaging results in projectional overlap of the esophagus on the vertebral column. To minimize projectional overlap, both the upright left posterior oblique and the prone right anterior oblique position can be employed.
3. D. The appearance is that of Nissen fundoplication.
4. A. The imaging findings show the normal appearance after Nissen fundoplication.

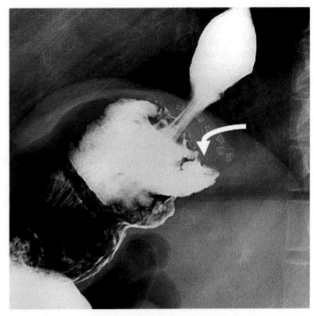

Fig. 105.2 Fluoroscopic spot images from a contrast esophagogram, in prone right anterior oblique position. Magnified image shows a broad filling defect impressing upon the gastric fundus *(curved arrow)*, representing the impression of the intact Nissen fundoplication wrap.

Comment

Diagnosis and Imaging Findings

Surgical approaches for the treatment of gastroesophageal reflux disease (GERD) refractory to medical management include Dor, Watson, Toupet, and Nissen fundoplication. The first three are noncircumferential wraps; the Nissen fundoplication is a 360-degree wrap of the gastric fundus to augment the function of the lower esophageal junction.

Nissen fundoplication typically appears as focal, circumferential smooth narrowing of the gastroesophageal junction.

Acute complications include:
- Edema, may result in delayed transit
- Bleeding/hematoma, may result in outlet obstruction
- Perforation
  Delayed complications include:
- Dysphagia
- Esophageal/gastric dysmotility
- Loosening
- Recurrent GERD symptoms

REFERENCE

Carbo, A. I., Kim, R. H., Gates, T., & D'Agostino, H. R. (2014). Imaging findings of successful and failed fundoplication. *Radiographics, 34,* 1873–1884.

CASE 107

Gastrointestinal Stromal Tumor (GIST) With Metastasis to Liver

1. A, B, C, D. Imaging findings show a mass in the stomach along the lesser curvature with liver lesions. The mass in the stomach could be a gastric malignancy or GIST with liver lesions representing benign or metastatic lesions.
2. B. GISTs are most commonly located in the stomach (50%–60%), followed by small intestine (30%–35%) and less

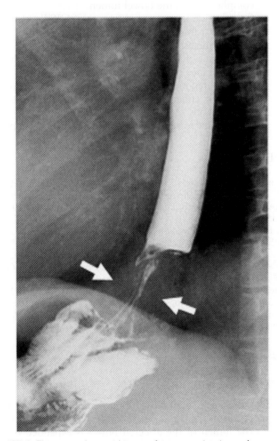

Fig. 105.1 Fluoroscopic spot images from a contrast esophagogram, in prone right anterior oblique position. At the gastroesophageal junction there is focal circumferential narrowing *(arrows).*

Case 106 is online only and accessible at www.expertconsult.com.

frequently in the colon and rectum (5%) and the esophagus (<1%).

3. D. GISTs are most commonly seen as large exophytic masses, homogenous, and appearance with a smooth wall and moderate to heterogenous contrast enhancement.

4. B. GISTs spread is hematogenous with metastasis most commonly seen in the liver.

Comment

- Gastrointestinal stromal tumors (GISTs) are the most common tumors of the gastrointestinal tract with incidence of 14 to 20 cases per million.
- They originate from interstitial cells of Cajal, which are located in the myenteric plexus of the gastrointestinal tract being responsible for its peristaltic contractions.
- GISTs may occur anywhere along the gastrointestinal tract; they are most commonly located in the stomach (50%–60%) and the small intestine (30%–35%) and less frequently in the colon and rectum (5%) and the esophagus (<1%).
- Most patients show symptoms or a palpable tumor at presentation, ~25% are discovered incidentally at imaging or surgery. Frequent symptoms are bleeding into the bowel or abdominal cavity, anemia, and abdominal pain.
- GISTs show a wide spectrum of radiologic appearances depending on imaging technique and tumor size, site of origin, and growth pattern.
  - CT: able to characterize and delineate the full extension of large exophytic masses, detect local invasion and distant metastasis, and guide tissue biopsy.
    - Typically the masses of soft tissue density with central areas of low density when necrosis is present
    - Small tumors typically appear as sharply marginated, smooth wall, homogenous, soft tissue masses but attenuation similar to muscle with moderate contrast enhancement
    - Large tumors tend to have mucosal ulceration, central necrosis and cavitation, and heterogenous enhancement.
  - Large GISTs may also present with a dumbbell-like appearance, with masses protruding both into the lumen and growing exophytically from the serosa of the bowel wall.
    - Peripheral contrast enhancement represents viable tumor whereas the central low attenuation corresponds to cystic changes, necrosis, and hemorrhage.

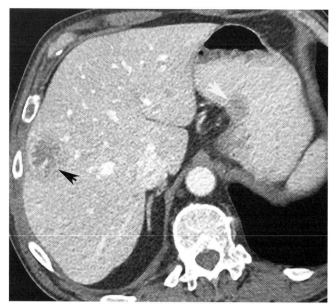

Fig. 107.2 Axial postcontrast computed tomography (CT) image at a lower level showing a mass like thickening *(yellow arrow)* seen in the stomach with a hypodense mass in the liver with heterogenous peripheral enhancement *(red arrow).* This was consistent with a gastrointestinal stromal tumor (GIST) in the stomach with metastasis to the liver.

- Air fluid levels and oral contrast media can be seen within the tumor if necrotic cavities within the tumor complicate with the bowel lumen.
- Calcification is an unusual feature of GISTs.
- GISTs rarely metastasize on the lymphatic route. Hepatic metastasis is common.
- MRI: presence of necrosis, hemorrhage, and cystic changes make appearance of GIST variable.
  - T1 weighted images: low-signal-intensity solid component with enhancement, predominantly peripheral in larger lesions
  - T2 weighted images: high-signal-intensity solid component

REFERENCES

Hong, X., Choi, H., Loyer, E. M., Benjamin, R. S., Trent, J. C., & Charnsangavej, C. (2006). Gastrointestinal stromal tumor: Role of CT in diagnosis and in response evaluation and surveillance after treatment with imatinib. *Radiographics, 26*(2), 481–495. doi:10.1148/rg.262055097.

King, D. M. (2005). The radiology of gastrointestinal stromal tumours (GIST). *Cancer Imaging, 5,* 150–156. doi:10.1102/1470-7330.2005.0109.

Lau, S., Tam, K. F., Kam, C. K., Lui, C. Y., Siu, C. W., … Lam, H. S. (2004). Imaging of gastrointestinal stromal tumour (GIST). *Clinical Radiology, 59*(6), 487–498. doi:10.1016/j.crad.2003.10.018.

Vernuccio, F., Taibbi, A., Picone, D., La Grutta, L., Midiri, M., … Lagalla, R. (2016). Imaging of gastrointestinal stromal tumors: From diagnosis to evaluation of therapeutic response. *Anticancer Research, 36*(6), 2639–2648.

CASE 108

Small Bowel Lymphoma

1. B. The thickened small bowel loop demonstrates the "aneurysmal dilation" appearance of small bowel lymphoma, in which the lumen of the affected bowel is expanded but the upstream bowel is not dilated. This appearance is not seen in Crohn's disease, which is usually characterized by luminal narrowing. Infectious and radiation enteritis presents with bowel

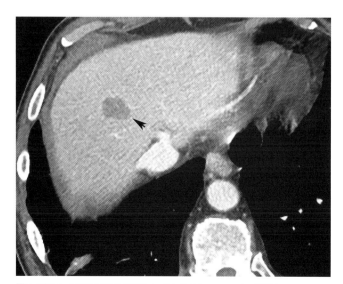

Fig. 107.1 Axial postcontrast computed tomography (CT) image showing a hypodense mass in the liver *(red arrow).*

wall thickening but usually involves a longer segment of bowel and do not show this expanded appearance of the lumen.

2. A, B, C. Small bowel lymphoma most commonly involves distal loops of small bowel (i.e., ileum), while adenocarcinoma typically occurs more proximally. Small bowel lymphoma can present with both regional and/or retroperitoneal adenopathy and splenomegaly. Concentric bowel wall thickening occurs in both malignancies.

3. D. While patients with AIDS, lupus, and celiac disease all have higher risks of developing small bowel lymphoma than the general population, transplant patients have the highest risk (50 to 100 times more likely than the general population).

4. A. Perforation is a rare complication of small bowel lymphoma, but can occur, especially in the setting of recent chemotherapy induction. Hemorrhage can also occur but is more common than perforation. Obstruction and diarrhea are not expected findings related to lymphoma.

Comment

- Lymphomas occur most commonly in the distal small bowel (compared to adenocarcinoma, which is proximal), but occur infrequently in other parts of the small bowel.
- They are often multicentric in location.
- The majority of small bowel lymphomas are of the non-Hodgkin type; Hodgkin disease of the small bowel is considered rare.
- Variable morphologic appearance. Imaging features include multiple nodules, solitary masses with an excavated cavity that acts as the bowel lumen, infiltrating tumors, and predominant mesenteric masses.
- The infiltrating or endoexenteric mass is believed to be the most common type.
- The excavating form, or aneurysmal dilation, is produced when lymphoma infiltrates, replaces the muscular layer, and destroys the nerves in this area. This results in bulging of the bowel wall, with resultant dilation.
- The bowel wall can become completely replaced by tumor with a persistent irregular lumen. Because of this unusual scenario, large masses of the small bowel show no evidence of bowel obstruction. However, perforation is a possibility.

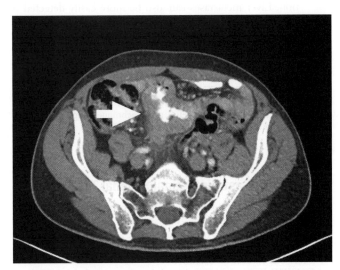

Fig. 108.1 Axial computed tomography (CT) of the abdomen with IV and PO contrast demonstrates marked circumferential wall thickening of a loop of small bowel with dilation of the bowel lumen but no obstruction *(arrow)*. This so-called aneurysmal dilation of the bowel is a characteristic appearance of small bowel lymphoma.

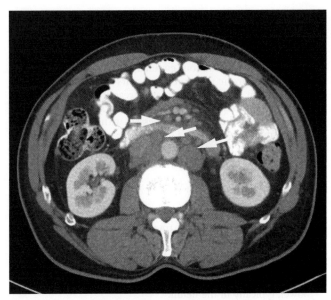

Fig. 108.2 Axial computed tomography (CT) of the abdomen with IV and PO contrast showing diffuse mesenteric and retroperitoneal adenopathy *(arrows)*.

- The bowel lumen and various layers of the bowel wall can grow back with therapy.
- A variety of conditions can lead to the development of lymphoma. Any type of immunosuppression, such as that associated with AIDS, can lead to lymphoma.
- Transplant recipients are 50 to 100 times more likely to develop lymphoma than the general population. Many of these patients have an associated infection with Epstein-Barr virus.
- Other conditions that increase the incidence of small bowel lymphoma include celiac disease and systemic lupus erythematosus.
- Imaging findings of small bowel lymphoma:
  - CT: wall thickening of a short segment of small bowel (most commonly ileum), potentially with aneurysmal dilation of the lumen. Other findings may include regional adenopathy, retroperitoneal adenopathy, and splenomegaly.
  - MRI: same as CT; would most likely be an incidental finding if encountered on MRI.

REFERENCES

Ghai, S., Pattison, J., Ghai, S., O'Malley, M. E., Khalili, K., & Stephens, M. (2007). Primary gastrointestinal lymphoma: Spectrum of imaging findings with pathologic correlation. *Radiographics, 27*(5), 1371–1388.

Ghimire, P., Wu, G. Y., & Zhu, L. (2011). Primary gastrointestinal lymphoma. *World Journal of Gastroenterology, 17*(6), 697–707.

CASE 109

Small Bowel Carcinoid

1. C. Carcinoids most commonly occur in the appendix. However, small bowel carcinoids are more likely to be symptomatic and to metastasize. Carcinoids can also occur in the bronchi because they are an embryonic bud of the intestinal tract.

2. A. Serotonin is the major by-product released by hormonally active carcinoids. Serotonin is converted in the liver and lungs to 5-hydroxyindoleacetic acid (5-HIAA), which is excreted in the urine and easily detected. Histamine and 5-HIAA can also be secreted by carcinoids. Epinephrine is not.

3. A, B, C, D. Flushing, wheezing, bronchospasm, and diarrhea are all symptoms that can occur in carcinoid syndrome. Carcinoid syndrome occurs when liver metastases excrete hormonally active substances that cannot be metabolized by the liver directly into a venous circulation.

4. C, D. The fibrotic reaction that occurs in the mesentery is a consequence of the desmoplastic reaction associated with carcinoid tumors. This results in a characteristic spokelike appearance of the mesenteric vessels with associated tethering of small bowel loops. These are the most common imaging findings in patient with small bowel carcinoid tumors, as the primary lesion is often small and difficult to detect.

Comment

- Carcinoid tumors are unusual neoplasms that arise in various structures of the intestinal tract and bronchi (an embryonic bud of the intestinal tract).
- The most common location in which carcinoids occur is the appendix.
- However, most symptomatic carcinoids arise in the small bowel, typically in the ileum.
- Carcinoids are slow-growing tumors that can progressively invade over time. They are multiple in ~20% of cases.
- All carcinoids are considered premalignant, but those of the small bowel are most likely to metastasize. Appendiceal carcinoids rarely do.
- Carcinoids belong to the group of lesions called APUD (amine precursor uptake and decarboxylation) lesions. They are hormonally active, with serotonin being the major by-product that is released.
- Secretion of histamine, 5-hydroxytryptophan, and other hormones scan also occur. Serotonin is converted in the liver and lungs to 5-HIAA, which is excreted in the urine and easily detected.
- Carcinoid syndrome occurs when liver metastases excrete hormonally active substances that cannot be metabolized by the liver directly into a venous circulation. This action produces vasomotor changes of flushing and vasodilation. Bronchospasm and wheezing can occur. Intestinal hypermotility, with diarrhea and cramping, is another symptom. With time, right-sided endocardial fibrosis and valve problems occur in the heart.

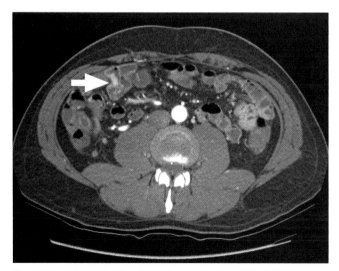

Fig. 109.1 Axial contrast enhanced computed tomography (CT) of the abdomen in the late arterial phase shows a small hyperenhancing mass (arrow) in the lumen of a small bowel loop.

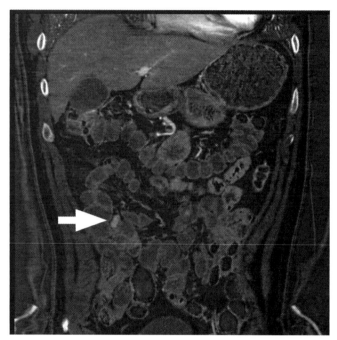

Fig. 109.2 Coronal reformatted subtraction postcontrast computed tomography (CT) of the abdomen in the late arterial phase better demonstrates the hyperenhancing small bowel mass (arrow) in the right abdomen.

- The serotonin secreted by the tumor incites an intense desmoplastic reaction in the mesentery, producing a typical fibrotic response with tethering of small bowel loops. Bowel obstruction and even vascular obstruction are possible complications of this fibrosis.
- Imaging findings of small bowel carcinoid:
  - CT: the primary lesion in the small bowel is hyperenhancing but is often not seen due to its small size. Mesenteric metastases can be well defined or spiculated, causing the characteristic spokelike appearance of mesenteric vessels. Liver metastases are hypervascular in the arterial phase.
  - MRI: as on CT, the primary lesion is usually very difficult to detect but may be seen due to improved contrast resolution. Liver metastases can also be more easily detected if subtle on CT.

REFERENCES

Ganeshan, D., Bhosale, P., Yang, T., & Kundra, V. (2013). Imaging features of carcinoid tumors of the gastrointestinal tract. *American Journal of Roentgenology, 201*(4), 773–786.

Horton, K. M., Kamel, I., Hofmann, L., & Fishman, E. K. (2004). Carcinoid tumors of the small bowel: A multitechnique imaging approach. *American Journal of Roentgenology, 182*(3), 559–567.

CASE 110

Small Bowel Gastrointestinal Stromal Tumor (GIST)

1. A, B, C, D. Imaging findings show an enhancing exophytic mass in the small bowel with smooth margins and a hypodense core. This is more likely to be a small bowel GIST or carcinoid; however, leiomyosarcoma or lymphoma are less likely but cannot be excluded.

2. C. GISTs have no sex predilection, are usually benign, and are most commonly diagnosed in the sixth or seventh decade of life.

3. A, B. Successful response to imatinib on CT scan is characterized by rapid transition to a homogeneously cystic pattern,

with resolution of the enhancing tumor. Tumor size does not predict response, and development of enhancing components within the treated tumor would suggest recurrence.
4. A, B, C, D. All the features mentioned suggest malignancy in GIST.

Comment

- Gastrointestinal stromal tumors (GISTs) are rare mesenchymal tumors ranking third in prevalence behind adenocarcinomas and lymphomas.
- GISTs may occur anywhere along the gastrointestinal tract; they are most commonly located in the stomach (50%–60%) and the small intestine (30%–35%) and less frequently in the colon and rectum (5%) and the esophagus (<1%).
- GISTs have no racial prevalence, no sex predilection, and are most commonly diagnosed in the sixth or seventh decade of life.
- GISTs are submucosal lesions, which can grow endophytically, although most of the time they manifest as an exophytic extraluminal mass.
- These tumors are usually benign (70%–90%) and can often grow quite large before they are discovered.
- GISTs show a wide spectrum of radiologic appearances depending on imaging technique and tumor size, site of origin, and growth pattern.
  - CT: able to characterize and delineate the full extension of large exophytic masses, detect local invasion and distant metastasis, and guide tissue biopsy.
    - Appear as solid, large, and well-circumscribed masses arising from the gastrointestinal tract
    - Enhance moderately, with a heterogeneously enhancing rim, surrounding low-attenuation areas in the center (necrosis, hemorrhage, or cystic formation)
    - Calcifications in GIST occur in 10% of the cases.
    - CT features that may suggest malignancy include diameter >5 cm, ill-defined margins, heterogeneous attenuation before and after contrast administration, central necrosis, invasion of surrounding structures, hepatic metastasis, and peritoneal dissemination.

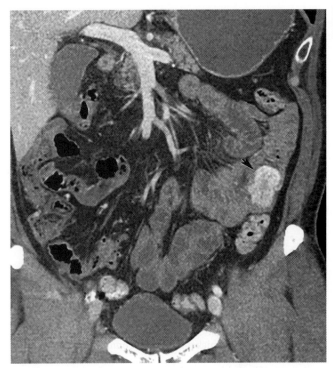

Fig. 110.2 Coronal reformat from a postcontrast computed tomography (CT) image showing a hyperdense mass in the small bowel, likely ileum *(red arrow)*. This was consistent with a gastrointestinal stromal tumor (GIST).

- Metastatic lymphadenopathy is uncommon.
- Successful response to imatinib is characterized by rapid transition to a homogeneously cystic pattern, with resolution of the enhancing tumor.
- Development of an enhancing nodule within the treated tumor indicates recurrence, regardless of changes in tumor size.

REFERENCES

Cai, P. Q., Lv, X. F., Tian, L., Luo, Z. P., Mitteer, R. A., … Fan, Y. (2015). CT characterization of duodenal gastrointestinal stromal tumors. *American Journal of Roentgenology, 204*(5), 988–993. doi:10.2214/AJR.14.12870.

Hong, X., Choi, H., Loyer, E. M., Benjamin, R. S., Trent, J. C., & Charnsangavej, C. (2006). Gastrointestinal stromal tumor: Role of CT in diagnosis and in response evaluation and surveillance after treatment with imatinib. *Radiographics, 26*(2), 481–495. doi:10.1148/rg.262055097.

Vernuccio, F., Taibbi, A., Picone, D., La Grutta, L., Midiri, M., … Lagalla, R. (2016). Imaging of gastrointestinal stromal tumors: From diagnosis to evaluation of therapeutic response. *Anticancer Research, 36*(6), 2639–2648.

CASE 111
Acute Mesenteric Ischemia

1. A, B, C. Images show dilated bowel loops with nonenhancement of small bowel wall consistent with acute mesenteric ischemia. Small bowel obstruction and volvulus could also be causes for acute mesenteric ischemia.
2. C. Superior mesenteric artery occlusion is the common cause of acute mesenteric ischemia.
3. A. The commonest feature of bowel ischemia seen on CT is bowel wall thickening.
4. A, B, C. Mural edema, hemorrhage, or associated infection are the reasons for bowel wall thickening seen on CT in acute mesenteric ischemia.

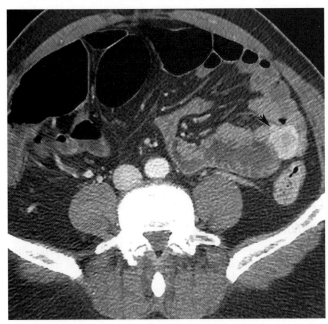

Fig. 110.1 Axial postcontrast computed tomography (CT) image showing a hyperdense mass in the small bowel, likely ileum *(red arrow)*.

Comment

- Background: Acute mesenteric ischemia (AMI) is a rare life-threatening condition.
  - The mortality rate for AMI is as high as 50% to 69% due to the difficulty of early detection and subsequent delays in appropriate management.
- Can be acute or chronic
- Acute:
  - Occlusive mesenteric ischemia
    - Superior mesenteric artery occlusion (75% of cases)
    - Superior mesenteric vein occlusion (5%–10% of cases)
  - Nonocclusive mesenteric ischemia
    - Systemic hypotension
    - Blunt abdominal trauma
    - Medication induced from vasoconstrictors
  - Small vessel involvement
  - Small bowel obstruction
- Chronic:
  - Atherosclerotic stenosis of SMA
  - Chronic radiation enteritis
- Imaging: CT is the most sensitive and specific diagnostic tool for AMI and is the first-line imaging modality
  - Imaging findings:
    - Bowel wall thickening: most common but nonspecific finding
      - Caused by mural edema, hemorrhage, or associated infection
      - May show target or halo appearance at contrast enhanced CT (CECT)
    - High attenuating bowel wall due to hemorrhagic infarction
    - Hyperattenuating bowel wall at CECT caused by congestion or reperfusion
    - Filling defects in the mesenteric arteries and veins indicate emboli or thrombi
    - Absence of wall enhancement indicates cessation of arterial flow
    - Paper-thin bowel wall due to thinning of the wall from volume loss of the tissues and vessels and by the loss of

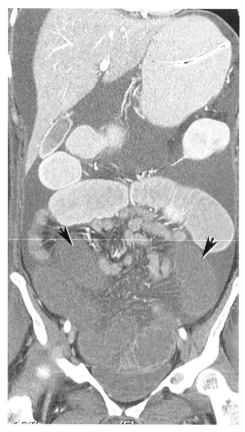

Fig. 111.2 Coronal reformat from postcontrast computed tomgraphy (CT) image shows bowel dilatation with nonenhancement of the central small bowel loops *(red arrow)*. This is consistent with acute mesentric ischemia. Note the wall thickening seen in the central bowel loops.

intestinal muscular tone (adynamic ileus) in arterial occlusive ischemia and bowel infarction
- Mesenteric stranding and ascites are nonspecific findings due to congestive or reperfusion mesenteric edema
- Pneumatosis, portomesenteric venous gas, and free peritoneal gas due to transmural infarction of the bowel, with or without perforation

REFERENCES

Kanasaki, S., Furukawa, A., Fumoto, K., Hamanaka, Y., Ota, S., ... Hirose, T. (2018). Acute mesenteric ischemia: Multidetector CT findings and endovascular management. *Radiographics, 38*(3), 945–961. doi:10.1148/rg.2018170163.

Rha, S. E., Ha, H. K., Lee, S. H., Kim, J. H., Kim, J. K., ... Kim, P. N. (2000). CT and MR imaging findings of bowel ischemia from various primary causes. *Radiographics, 20*(1), 29–42. doi:10.1148/radiographics.20.1.g00ja0629

CASE 112

Epiploic Appendagitis

1. D. The images demonstrate findings of epiploic appendagitis.
2. C. Pain management with NSAIDs is the typical therapy for epiploic appendagitis.
3. A. Epiploic appendagitis is most prevalent at the rectosigmoid colon.
4. E. Omental infarction is most prevalent in the right colon: anterior to the transverse colon or anteromedial to the ascending colon.

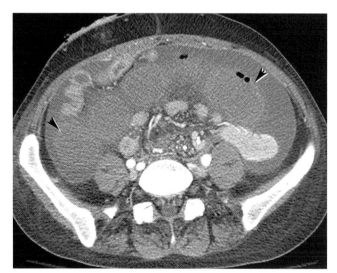

Fig. 111.1 Axial postcontrast computed tomography (CT) image shows bowel dilatation with nonenhancement of the central small bowel loops *(red arrow)*. This is consistent with acute mesenteric ischemia. Note the wall thickening seen in the central bowel loops.

Comment

Epiploic Appendagitis

- Epiploic appendages are fatty excrescences distributed along the length of the colon.
- Epiploic appendagitis most commonly results from spontaneous torsion of one (or more) of these, causing vascular/venous occlusion.
- Clinical presentation of abdominal pain and guarding is similar to acute diverticulitis, appendicitis, or other acute abdominal pathology.
- Most common location: rectosigmoid colon > descending colon > right colon.

Imaging Appearance

- On CT, epiploic appendagitis typically presents as a 1.5- to 3.5-cm ovoid lesion of fat attenuation in a pericolonic distribution.
- Often accompanied by adjacent fat stranding and peritoneal thickening
- May feature a central or linear focus of hyperattenuation representing venous thrombosis
- On US, oval noncompressible hyperechoic pericolonic mass, without central Doppler flow
- On MRI, pericolonic lesion of fat signal; postcontrast imaging with rim enhancement

Mimics

- Omental infarction
  - Uncommon; omentum is perfused by numerous collateral vessels
  - Nontorsion omental infarction results from trauma or thrombosis of omental veins
  - In contrast to epiploic appendagitis, right-sided distribution is more common than left sided
  - On CT, solitary nonenhancing omental mass, relatively large, most often in right lower quadrant; must be distinguished from inflammatory stranding of acute appendicitis or diverticulitis

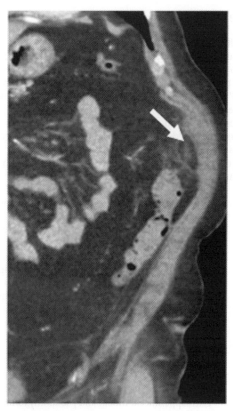

Fig. 112.2 Contrast enhanced computed tomography (CT) image. Coronal image shows a central linear hyperdensity within the fat-density structure *(arrow)* typical of epiploic appendagitis.

- Acute diverticulitis
  - Common; affected patients are typically older than those with epiploic appendagitis or omental infarction
  - On CT, colonic diverticulae are shown at the epicenter of acute inflammatory fat stranding
  - Complications include extraluminal air or abscess from focal perforation, or fistulous tracts to adjacent organs
- Peritoneal metastasis
  - Peritoneal or omental metastases are distinguished from epiploic appendagitis by their diffuse or multifocal peritoneal distribution, or by their infiltrative or poorly marginated lesional appearance.

REFERENCE

Singh, A. K., Gervais, D. G., Hahn, P. F., Sagar, P., Mueller, P. R., & Novelline, R. A. (2005). Acute epiploic appendagitis and its mimics. *Radiographics, 25,* 1521–1534.

CASE 113

Epithelial Appendiceal Neoplasm

1. D. Images demonstrate cystic, lobulated structure in the right lower quadrant, with cystic expansion of the right mesentery, and trace perihepatic fluid, likely mucin. The most likely diagnosis is mucinous appendiceal neoplasm.
2. D. A pattern of disease extension associated with appendiceal epithelial neoplasms is pseudomyxoma peritonei.
3. C. The next best step in the management of this patient is surgical oncologic consultation. None of the other choices have a role in the treatment of mucinous appendiceal neoplasm.
4. A. Appendiceal neuroendocrine tumor has the typical imaging appearance of a small enhancing mass at the appendiceal tip.

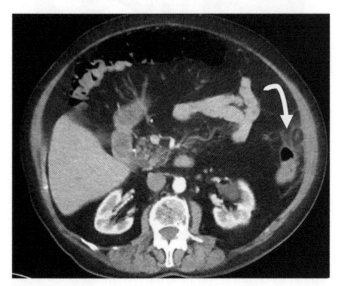

Fig. 112.1 Contrast-enhanced computed tomography (CT) image. Axial image demonstrates inflammatory fat stranding *(curved arrow)* adjacent to a small ovoid fat-density structure arising from the sigmoid colon.

Comment

Appendiceal Neoplasm

- Primary and secondary neoplasms of the appendix are found in 1% of appendectomy specimens.
- Most common presenting manifestation is acute appendicitis.
  - 30% to 50% of cases (more common with NETs than epithelial neoplasms)
- Represents a group of histologically distinct entities
  - Histologic type predicts imaging features, patterns of disease spread, and clinical course
- Epithelial neoplasms (peak incidence in fifth to sixth decade)
  - Mucinous neoplasm (70% of epithelial tumors)
    - Adenoma
      - Confined to appendiceal mucosa; no extraappendiceal mucin
      - Appendix may appear normal, or distended by mucin
    - Appendiceal mucinous neoplasm
      - Designated as low grade (LAMN) or high grade (HAMN) by the degree of cytologic atypia
      - Mucin-distended appendix, with or without wall calcification
      - Extraappendiceal mucin and pseudomyxoma peritonei may be shown
    - Mucinous adenocarcinoma
      - Mucin-distended appendix
      - Periappendiceal fat stranding and/or soft tissue is present
      - Extraappendiceal mucin and pseudomyxoma peritonei may be shown
  - Nonmucinous adenocarcinoma (peak incidence in sixth to seventh decade)
    - Soft tissue infiltration or mass +/− regional lymphadenopathy
    - May have peritoneal or extraperitoneal metastases (liver, lung)
  - Goblet-cell carcinoma
- Neuroendocrine tumors (NETs; peak incidence in young adults)
  - Typically shown as enhancing submucosal mass or nodular thickening of the appendiceal tip, <1 cm
- Lymphoma
  - Primary: diffuse wall thickening, with preservation of the vermiform appendiceal contour; no luminal obstruction
  - Secondary: regional lymphadenopathy and adjacent bowel involvement

Imaging Appearances

Mucocele
- Macroscopic description of an appendix that is abnormally distended by mucin
- Appearance can result from nonneoplastic luminal obstruction (e.g., by mucous retention cyst) or by mucin-secreting epithelial neoplasm
- On CT, in patients with symptoms of appendicitis, appendiceal diameter >15 mm, or cystic appendiceal dilatation has 95% sensitivity for underlying appendiceal tumor
- Typical appearance:
  - Right lower quadrant ovoid cystic mass/fluid-filled dilated appendix
  - May have peripheral calcification
  - Mural nodularity and irregular wall thickening create an appearance that favors underlying adenocarcinoma
  - Finding of appendiceal mucocele should trigger search for extraluminal mucin in either the adjacent right lower quadrant or other peritoneal interfaces

Pseudomyxoma Peritonei

- Clinical syndrome indicated by the presence of mucin within the peritoneum and on serosal surfaces of abdominopelvic organs
- Most common underlying primary pathology is appendiceal; others may include ovarian, colonic, pancreatic, and urachal primaries

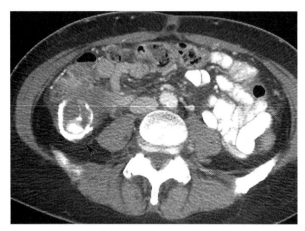

Fig. 113.1 Axial contrast-enhanced computed tomography (CT) image demonstrates a mixed solid and cystic mass *(arrow)* in the right lower quadrant with calcifications within it. This was considered to be either of colonic or appendiceal origin.

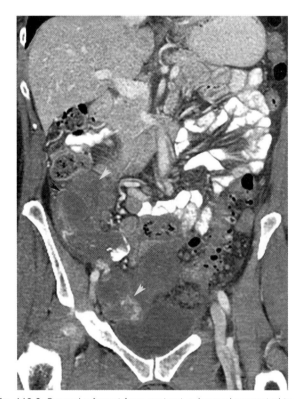

Fig. 113.2 Coronal reformat from contrast-enhanced computed tomography (CT) shows a tubular structure *(red arrow)* in the right lower quadrant surrounded by mixed solid and cystic masses *(yellow arrow)* in the right lower quadrant with calcifications in it. This was shown to be an epithelial appendiceal neoplasm—mucinous adenocarcinoma on histopathology.

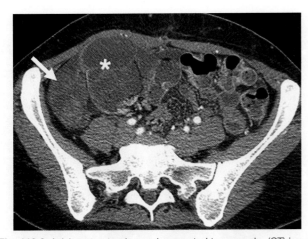

Fig. 113.3 Axial contrast-enhanced computed tomography (CT) image in a different patient demonstrates lobulated cystic structure in the right lower quadrant *(arrow),* with cystic expansion of the right mesentery *(asterisk),* representing likely appendiceal mucinous neoplasm.

- Fluidlike/hypoattenuating deposits on CT in peritoneal distribution:
  - Ascites, peritoneal soft tissue, omental caking, diaphragms, involvement of GI tract and ovaries
  - Scalloped appearance interface with solid abdominal organs; hollow visceral organs are displaced or distorted
- Comprehensive imaging assessment is essential to surgical planning for cytoreductive surgery (CRS) with hyperthermic intraperitoneal chemotherapy (HIPEC)
  - Peritoneal cancer index (PCI): scoring system based on volume and extent of peritoneal tumor at laparoscopy

REFERENCES

Leonards, L. M., Pahwa, A., Patel, M. K., Petersen, J., Nguyen, M. J., & Jude, C. M. (2017). Neoplasms of the appendix: Pictorial review with clinical and pathologic correlation. *Radiographics, 37,* 1059–1083.

Pickhardt, P. J., Levy, A. D., Rohrmann, C. A., & Kende, A. I. (2003). Primary neoplasms of the appendix: Radiologic spectrum of disease with pathologic correlation. *Radiographics,* 23:645–662.

CASE 114

Diaphragmatic Herniation

1. B, D, E. Morgagni hernia is herniation through the foramen of Morgagni, which is right sided. Spigelian hernias occur along the semilunar line, which is herniation between the muscles of abdominal wall. The defect shown is left sided and along the diaphragm, hence Bochdalek hernia, diaphragmatic herniation, and traumatic diaphragmatic herniation are possibilities in this case.
2. A. Most common injuries associated with left-sided diaphragmatic rupture are splenic injuries.
3. A. Stomach is the most common organ that hernias in a left-sided diaphragmatic rupture.
4. D. Segmental diaphragmatic defect or discontinuity of the diaphragm is most commonly seen in patients with diaphragmatic herniation on CT.

Comment

- Diaphragmatic rupture most commonly results from blunt abdominal trauma.
  - Most common mechanism is motor vehicle collisions. Other mechanisms include penetrating trauma from knife or gunshot.

- Estimated incidence is 4.5% of patients who sustain blunt abdominal or lower thoracic trauma (range 0.8%–8%).
  - Can remain undiagnosed at initial presentation in 7% to 66% of cases.
- Left hemidiaphragm is involved three times more frequently than the right possibly because the liver has a buffering effect. Mean left-to-right ratio is approximately 3:1.
- Diaphragmatic rupture causes a loss of continuity in muscular and tendinous fibers of the membrane.
  - Most common site of rupture is the posterior lateral aspect of the hemidiaphragm between the lumbar and intercostal muscle slips. They extend centrally in a radial fashion frequently toward the angle between the pericardium and the esophageal hiatus.
  - Most tears are longer than 10 cm, but penetrating injuries to the diaphragm tend to be short (1–2 cm).
- Associated with other life-threatening injuries in 44% to 100% of cases and almost never occurs as an isolated injury. Most common injuries associated with left-sided diaphragmatic rupture are splenic injuries, with right-sided diaphragmatic rupture liver lesions most common, but renal, aortic, cardiac, and osseous (spine, pelvis, rib) lesions are also frequently encountered. Rib fractures, pneumothorax, and pleural effusion are present in 90% of cases of diaphragmatic rupture.
- Complications: spontaneous healing of ruptures has never been reported. The use of positive pressure ventilator support at the patient's admission overcomes the negative pleuroperitoneal pressure gradient and may thereby prevent or delay herniation and may account for false-negative findings at initial examination.
- Imaging findings:
  - Plain radiograph: findings may not be seen in up to 50% of cases; the following signs are helpful in making the diagnosis:
    - Inability to trace the normal hemidiaphragm contour
    - Intrathoracic herniation of a hollow viscus (stomach, colon, small bowel) with or without focal construction of the viscus at the site of the tear (collar sign)
    - Contralateral mediastinal shift if large in size
    - Visualization of a nasogastric tube about the hemidiaphragm on the left side
    - Elevated left hemidiaphragm much higher than the right hemidiaphragm
  - CT: multiple signs are described later
    - Direct signs:
      - Segmental diaphragmatic defect: abrupt discontinuity or direct visualization of injury
      - Dangling diaphragm: produced by the free edge of the torn diaphragm, which curls inward from its normal course toward the center of the body, forming a comma-shaped or curvilinear structure with soft tissue attenuation at a near right angle with the chest wall.
      - Absent diaphragm: complete absence of visualization of the diaphragm, segmental nonrecognition of the diaphragm, indistinct hemidiaphragm
    - Indirect signs related to herniation:
      - Herniation through a defect
      - Collar sign: hourglass construction sign, mushroom sign (in hepatic herniation): a waistlike constriction of the herniating hollow viscus from the abdomen into the chest at the site of the diaphragmatic tear
      - Dependent viscera: when a patient with a ruptured diaphragm lies supine at CT examination, the herniated viscera (bowel or solid organs) are no longer supported posteriorly by the injured diaphragm and fall to a dependent position against the posterior ribs.

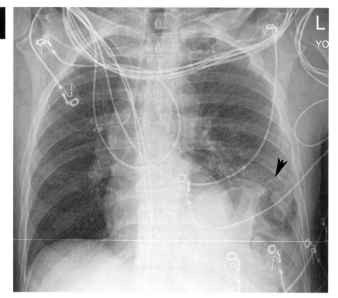

Fig. 114.1 Plain radiograph showing elevation of the left hemidiaphragm with the hollow viscus *(arrow)* seen in the lower thorax.

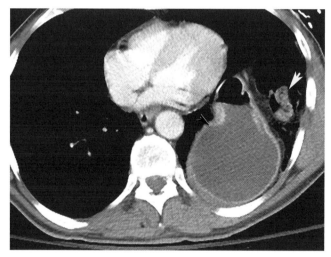

Fig. 114.2 Axial computed tomography (CT) image showing location of the stomach *(red arrow)* and colon *(yellow arrow)* in the lower left hemithorax in close approximation to the lung suggesting presence of diaphragmatic herniation.

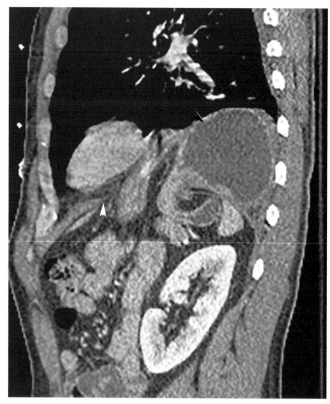

Fig. 114.3 Sagittal computed tomography (CT) image showing location of the stomach *(red arrow)* in the lower left hemithorax in close approximation to the lung suggesting presence of diaphragmatic herniation. Note the discontinuity in the diaphragm *(white arrow).*

- Abdominal content peripheral to the diaphragm or lung
- Elevated abdominal organs: apparent elevation of the hemidiaphragm
- Indirect signs related to loss of border between thorax and abdomen
  - Abdominal fluid abutting a thoracic structure
  - Abdominal viscera abutting thoracic fluid or a thoracic organ
  - Pneumothorax and pneumoperitoneum
  - Hemothorax and hemoperitoneum
- Other signs:
  - Focal diaphragmatic thickening

REFERENCE

Desir, A., & Ghaye, B. (2012). CT of blunt diaphragmatic rupture. *Radiographics, 32*(2), 477–498. doi:10.1148/rg.322115082.

Challenge

CASE 115

MRI Safety

1. B. Zone II serves as the interface between publicly accessible, uncontrolled Zone I, and strictly controlled Zones III and IV; functions in Zone II include patient waiting and reception, patient interview and screening, and toilet facilities and changerooms.
2. A. In Zone III, free access by unscreened non-MR personnel or equipment can result in serious injury or death. Zone III is a three-dimensional space related to the strength of the magnetic field, and hence its boundaries may include adjacent rooms or floors. Access to Zone III is strictly restricted, such as by standard key or electronic passkey locking mechanisms.
3. D. All of the statements accurately apply to MR Zone IV.
4. C. In the event of an emergency, MR personnel should initiate basic life support while the patient is removed from the scanner magnet room to a magnetically safe location.

Comment

Safe operation of MRI requires the coordination of numerous professionals of diverse training and backgrounds, along with dedicated planning of physical spaces and human resources, as well as vigilant adherence to policies and procedures. The following represent a focused introduction regarding MR zoning and personnel, excerpted from the 2013 American College of Radiology Guidance Document on MR Safe Practices.

MR Safety: Zoning

- Zone I
  - All areas that are freely accessible to the general public
  - Typically outside the MR environment
- Zone II
  - Interface between publicly accessible, uncontrolled Zone I and strictly controlled Zones III and IV
  - Patient movement through Zone II is supervised by MR personnel
  - Functions in Zone II include patient waiting and reception, patient interview and screening, and facilities for toilet, patient changing and gowning, and storage of patient possessions
- Zone III
  - Access to Zone III is strictly restricted, such as by standard key or electronic passkey locking mechanisms; free access by unscreened non-MR personnel or equipment can result in serious injury or death
  - Magnetic fields encompass three-dimensional spaces; Zone III designations may apply beyond walls, floors, and ceilings
- Zone IV
  - Represents physical space of the MR scanner magnet room
  - By definition, always located within Zone III
  - Should be clearly marked as being potentially hazardous due to the presence of very strong magnetic fields
  - Should be clearly marked with a red lighted sign indicating "The Magnet is On," preferably with accompanying signage that the magnetic field is active even when electric power to the facility is deactivated
  - Access to Zone IV is directly observed by level 2 MR personnel

- In the event of a medical emergency:
  - MR personnel should initiate basic life support while the patient is removed from the scanner magnet room to a predetermined magnetically safe location
  - Quenching the magnet is not routinely advised in case of a medical emergency; the quenching process is not immediate, and may additionally pose its own hazards to the occupants of the magnet room
  - For the protection of all involved, Zone III and IV site access restrictions must be maintained during a medical emergency and resuscitation

MR Personnel

- Non-MR personnel
  - Have not undergone or not successfully complied with MR safety instruction guidelines
  - All non-MR personnel must first pass an MR safety screening process prior to entering Zone III
  - Non-MR personnel should be either accompanied or immediately supervised by one specific level 2 MR person for the duration of their time in Zone III or IV
- Level 1 MR personnel
  - Have passed minimal safety education standards to work within Zone III
  - Are permitted unaccompanied access to Zone III and IV
  - May accompany non-MR personnel throughout Zone III, but not Zone IV
- Level 2 MR personnel
  - Have been more extensively trained in broader MR safety issues

REFERENCE
Expert Panel on MR Safety. (2013). ACR guidance document on MR safe practices: 2013. *Journal of Magnetic Resonance Imaging, 37*, 501–530.

CASE 116

Iron Overload

1. B. Images show drop in signal in the liver on the in-phase image (Fig. 116.1) compared to the opposed-phase image (Fig. 116.2) and hence is consistent with iron overload.
2. B, C. T2 relaxometry and signal intensity ratio (SIR) imaging are used for iron quantification on MRI.
3. A, C, D. MR features of increased iron content in the liver include decreased liver attenuation on in-phase images, low signal in the liver on T2 weighted images compared to spleen, and hypointense liver compared to paraspinous muscle on gradient recalled echo (GRE) sequence.
4. B, C, D. Iron overload, Wilson disease, and amyloidosis can cause an increase in attenuation on nonenhanced CT scan.

Comment

- Background: MR liver iron quantification is a noninvasive means of measuring liver iron concentration.
  - Helpful in management of patients with hemochromatosis (primary or secondary)
  - Advantage: noninvasive and sampling of a large cross section of the liver

- Two methods of liver iron quantification
  - T2 relaxometry
    - Due to paramagnetic properties: results in decrease in T2 relaxation times
    - Proportional to iron content
    - Acquisition sequences with several different echo times are acquired
    - T2 parametric map is then obtained by displaying signal intensity as a function of echo time
  - Signal intensity ratio (SIR)
    - Ratio between signal intensity of the liver and that of paraspinal muscle can be used to determine liver iron concentration
    - Signal intensity of normal liver parenchyma (i.e., without iron overload) should always be higher than that of the paraspinal muscles
    - A hypointense liver relative to the paraspinal muscles indicates iron overload
  - SIR is easier than T2 relaxometry; however, less accurate at iron concentration of >350 micromol Fe/g
  - T2 relaxometry is more accurate but not yet standardized and needs offsite processing
- Other imaging techniques
  - In-phase and opposed-phase images:
    - Iron leads to decreased signal intensity on in-phase images compared with the opposed-phase
    - Fast spin echo (FSE) T2 weighted imaging leads to low liver signal intensity, relative to that of the spleen due to T2 shortening
  - CT: at nonenhanced CT normal hepatic parenchyma usually ranges between 55 and 65 HU
    - Hepatic iron overload >65 HU value in the liver
    - Not specific to iron overload
- Other pathologic conditions can manifest with increased liver attenuation
  - Wilson disease
  - Glycogen storage diseases
  - Long-term amiodarone administration

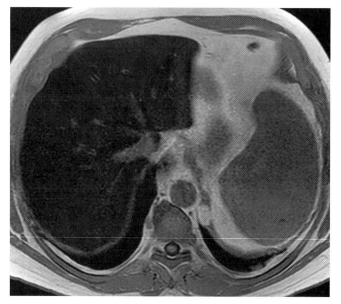

Fig. 116.2 Axial T1 weighted magnetic resonance imaging (MRI) in-phase image showing drop in signal in the liver compared to the spleen and compared to the liver images in Fig. 116.1.

REFERENCES

Henninger, B., Alustiza, J., Garbowski, M., & Gandon, Y. (2020). Practical guide to quantification of hepatic iron with MRI. *European Radiology, 30*, 383–393.

Hernando, D., Levin, Y. S., Sirlin, C. B., & Reeder, S. B. (2014). Quantification of liver iron with MRI: State of the art and remaining challenges. *Journal of Magnetic Resonance Imaging, 40*(5), 1003–1021. doi:10.1002/jmri.24584.

Labranche, R., Gilbert, G., Cerny, M., Vu, K. N., Soulières, D., ... Olivié, D. (2018). Liver iron quantification with MR imaging: A primer for radiologists. *Radiographics, 38*(2), 392–412.

CASE 117

Inflammatory Pseudotumor

1. A, B, C, D. Metastasis, posttransplant lymphoproliferative disease, inflammatory pseudotumor, and abscess should be included in the differential diagnosis of the mass shown. The patient in this case had an inflammatory pseudotumor on biopsy.
2. D. Biopsy is necessary for definitive diagnosis of this disease.
3. B. Lung is the most common location of IPT.

Comment

- Inflammatory pseudotumor (IPT) is also known as an inflammatory myofibroblastic tumor or plasma cell granuloma, a xanthomatous pseudotumor, and inflammatory fibrosarcoma.
- Hepatic IPT is a rare benign lesion characterized by chronic infiltration of inflammatory cells and an area of fibrosis that sometimes mimics a malignant tumor.
- IPT most commonly occurs in the lung but can be found in the central nervous system, major salivary glands, kidneys, liver, omentum, ovaries, larynx, urinary bladder, breasts, pancreas, spleen, lymph nodes, skin, soft tissues, and orbit of the eye. IPT in the liver (IPTL) is quite rare and accounts for 8% of extrapulmonary IPTs.
- Etiology and pathogenesis of IPTL remain unknown but thought to involve an inflammatory reaction.
- Imaging appearance: US and CT scans are not specific, revealing variable patterns of echogenicity or a liver mass

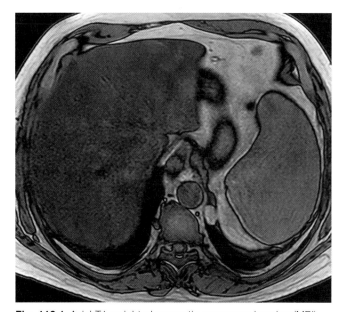

Fig. 116.1 Axial T1 weighted magnetic resonance imaging (MRI) opposed-phase image showing low signal intensity in the liver compared to the spleen.

mimicking hepatocellular cancer or an abscess. The lesion can manifest itself as single or multiple masses.

- On unenhanced CT, the lesions are low in attenuation relative to the surrounding liver. CT scan usually shows lesions with variable contrast enhancement, including a hypovascular pattern because of fibrosis with delayed enhancement, similar to metastatic liver tumors and cholangiocarcinomas.
- MRI shows low signal intensity on T1 weighted images with moderate to high signal intensity (hyperintensity) on a T2 sequence with heterogenous enhancement.

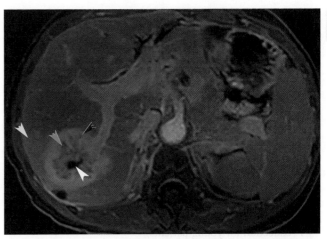

Fig. 117.3 Axial T1 weighted postcontrast magnetic resonance image (MRI) during the delayed phase shows heterogenous enhancement in the mass with central hypovascularity and peripheral hypervascular rim *(red arrow)*. The internal part of the mass did not show washout but was isointense to the adjacent liver *(green arrow)*. The washout appearance is a pitfall due to the peripheral rim enhancement. The absolute central part of the mass remained hypointense on all postcontrast sequences and was likely an area of necrosis *(white arrowhead)*. Note the wedge-shaped peripheral hyperenhancement *(yellow arrow)* in normal adjacent liver tissue from hyperperfusion in the edematous region remaining persistent though decreased from the portal venous phase.

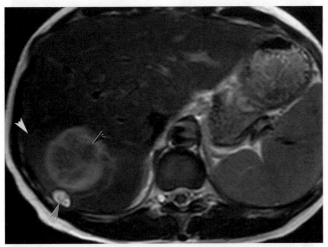

Fig. 117.1 Axial T2 weighted magnetic resonance image (MRI) shows a heterogenous mass *(red arrow)* in the right lobe of the liver with central hypointense area surrounded by a hyperintense rim. Note the edema *(yellow arrow)* in the surrounding normal liver tissue seen as mildly hyperintense area surrounding the lesion. Also note a small cyst with a hypointense rim adjacent to the large mass, which was a small area of hematoma *(green arrow)* from prior biopsy.

- Definitive diagnosis of IPT can be made based on liver biopsy findings.
- If an atypical solid mass is found in the liver, IPTL should be considered as a potential diagnosis, particularly if the mass is accompanied by clinical evidence of an inflammatory process.
- IPTL may spontaneously regress or regress following antibiotic treatment; however, the treatment of choice is still surgical resection, and this is especially true for patients with severe symptoms or an indeterminate diagnosis.

REFERENCES

Patnana, M., Sevrukov, A. B., Elsayes, K. M., Viswanathan, C., Lubner, M., & Menias, C. O. (2012). Inflammatory pseudotumor: The great mimicker. *American Journal of Roentgenology, 198*(3), W217–W227. doi:10.2214/AJR.11.7288.

Zhang, Y., Lu, H., Ji, H., & Li, Y. (2015). Inflammatory pseudotumor of the liver: A case report and literature review. *Intractable & Rare Diseases Research, 4*(3), 155–158. doi:10.5582/irdr.2015.01021.

CASE 119

Fibrolamellar Hepatocellular Carcinoma

1. C. The provided images show a large, heterogeneously hyperattenuating liver mass with a subtly enhancing central scar on delayed imaging; the most likely diagnosis is fibrolamellar hepatocellular carcinoma. Hemangioma typically shows peripheral discontinuous arterial enhancement with delayed central enhancement. Heptatocellular carcinoma typically shows more homogeneous arterial enhancement, delayed hypoenhancement (washout), and does not demonstrate a central scar. Liver abscess is not typically a hyperattenuating liver lesion at postcontrast imaging.

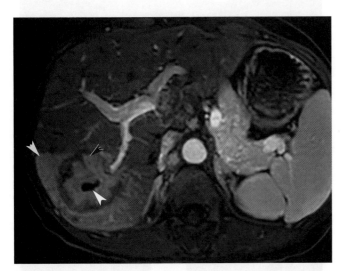

Fig. 117.2 Axial T1 weighted postcontrast magnetic resonance image (MRI) during the portal venous phase shows heterogenous enhancement in the mass with central hypervascularity and peripheral hypointense rim *(red arrow)*. The central part of the mass remained hypointense on all postcontrast sequences and was likely an area of necrosis *(white arrowhead)*. Note the wedge-shaped peripheral hyperenhancement *(yellow arrow)* in normal adjacent liver tissue from hyperperfusion in the edematous region.

Case 118 is online only and accessible at www.expertconsult.com.

2. A. Unlike patients with hepatocellular carcinoma, patients with fibrolamellar hepatocellular carcinoma are typically younger than 40 years of age and do not have history of hepatitis/cirrhosis.

3. A. Unlike in hepatocellular carcinoma, patients with fibrolamellar hepatocellular carcinoma typically have normal serum alpha-fetoprotein levels.

4. B. Fibrolamellar hepatocellular carcinoma does not typically demonstrate intralesional fat.

Comment

Fibrolamellar Hepatocellular Carcinoma

- Rare liver mass; in the United States, represents <1% of hepatocellular carcinoma (HCC)
- Predilection for young patients
  - 65% to 85% of cases occur in patients <40 years old
  - Compared to 2% to 4% of HCC occurring in patients <40 years old
- While chronic liver disease is a major risk factor for HCC, 95% of fibrolamellar HCC occurs in patients without hepatitis or cirrhosis.
- Unlike HCC, only 7% of fibrolamellar HCC have elevated serum alpha-fetoprotein (AFP).

Imaging Features

US
- Well-defined liver mass
- Nonspecific sonographic features
- Characterization typically by multiphasic contrast enhanced CT or MRI

CT
- Large, heterogeneous liver mass (mean diameter, 13 cm)
- Well-defined, lobulated margin
- May have few, small calcifications (35%–68%)
- Heterogeneous enhancement at arterial phase with hyperattenuating regions
- Variable appearance at portal venous phase, 50% are isoatteunating to liver
- Variable appearance at delayed phase
- Central stellate scar (65%–70%), with variable enhancement
- Portal vein thrombosis and biliary obstruction are uncommon.

MRI
- Usually T1 hypointense, T2 hyperintense
- Central scar is typically hypointense on both T1 and T2 weighted imaging.
  - Central scar in FNH is typically T2 hyperintense
- Postcontrast appearance, similar to that described earlier
- Intralesional fat is not typically shown.

Mimics

- Differential diagnosis of other hypervascular liver masses
- Focal nodular hyperplasia (FNH)
  - Calcification rare in FNH
  - Central scar in FNH typically T2 hyperintense
  - FNH retains liver-specific contrast at hepatobiliary phase imaging
- Hepatocellular carcinoma
  - Arterial phase contrast imaging is typically more homogeneously hyperenhancing than with the heterogeneous appearance of fibrolamellar hepatocellular carcinoma

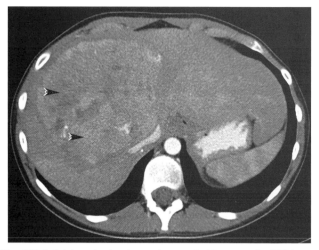

Fig. 119.1 Axial contrast-enhanced computed tomography (CT) image in the late arterial phase demonstrates a large, heterogeneously enhancing right liver mass with hyperattenuating and hypoattenuating regions *(arrows)*.

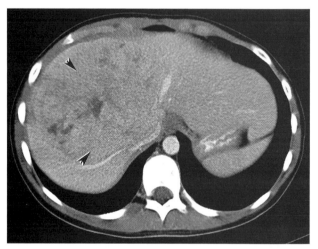

Fig. 119.2 Axial contrast-enhanced computed tomography (CT) image in the portal venous phase shows persistent enhancement in the lesion predominantly isoattenuating to normal left liver *(arrow)*.

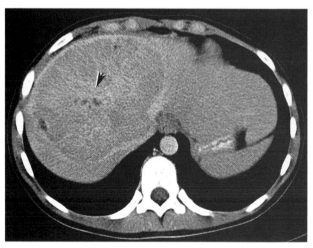

Fig. 119.3 Axial contrast-enhanced computed tomography (CT) image in the delayed phase shows subtle contrast enhancement of a central scar *(red arrow)*.

- Hepatocellular carcinoma more typically demonstrates washout at delayed-phase imaging
- Intralesional fat seen in 10% to 40% of hepatocellular carcinoma; not reported in fibrolamellar hepatocellular carcinoma
- Hemangioma
  - Peripheral discontinuous contrast enhancement at arterial-phase imaging typical of hemangioma
- Hepatic adenoma
  - Arterial-phase contrast imaging is typically more homogeneously hyperenhancing than with the heterogeneous appearance of fibrolamellar hepatocellular carcinoma

REFERENCES

Ganeshan, D., Szklaruk, J., Kundra, V., Kaseb, A., Rashid, A., & Elsayes, K. M. (2014). Imaging features of fibrolamellar hepatocellular carcinoma. *American Journal of Roentgenology, 202*, 544–552.

Smith, M. T., Blatt, E. R., Jeflicka, P., Strain, J. D., & Fenton, L. Z. (2008). Fibrolamellar hepatocellular carcinoma. *Radiographics, 28*, 609–613.

CASE 120

Perforated Peptic Ulcer

1. D. The provided images demonstrate findings of hollow viscus perforation, with intraperitoneal free air and fluid, and focal enhancement abnormality of the gastric antrum, representing gastric ulcer.
2. A. While the majority of peptic ulcers are related to *H. pylori* infection, based on the history of chronic osteoarthritis, the most likely associated risk factor is NSAID-induced peptic ulcer.
3. D. The next best step in the management of this patient is surgical consultation. There is no indication for further imaging evaluation or corticosteroid therapy.
4. A. Graham patch represents surgical repair of perforated gastric or duodenal ulcer, by securing a piece of healthy omentum to the site of disease. Whipple resection is performed for pancreatic cancer, Nissen fundoplication for the treatment of gastroesophageal reflux disease, and Hartmann procedure for diverting distal colorectal resection.

Comment

Gastrointestinal Perforation

- CT plays an important role in identifying the presence, site, and cause of GI tract perforation.
- Accuracy of CT for site of bowel perforation reported between 82% and 90%.

Imaging Findings

- Detection of extraluminal free air is the major imaging finding of GI tract perforation.
  - Utilize wide CT viewing windows (e.g., lung windows) to enhance detection of free air
  - Extraluminal free air may be present in intraperitoneal, extraperitoneal, or retroperitoneal distribution
- Amount and location of free air differs among perforation sites.
  - Stomach/duodenum: can have abundant free air around liver and stomach
  - Small bowel: small amount of free air among mesentery and around liver
  - Appendix: can have absent intraperitoneal free air
  - Colon: variable free air; mostly common in mesenteric folds or extraperitoneal space of the pelvis secondary to perforated diverticulitis

- Direct findings:
  - Bowel wall discontinuity with adjacent extraluminal air; uncommonly seen (<50% of cases) due to frequently small size of defect
- Ancillary findings:
  - Segmental bowel wall thickening
  - Abnormal bowel wall enhancement
  - Free air bubbles in close proximity to perforation site
  - Focal inflammatory change adjacent to bowel

Peptic Ulcer Disease

- Major cause of gastroduodenal perforation
  - Other etiologies include malignant ulcer, traumatic injury, iatrogenic injury
- Peptic ulcers are distributed primarily at gastric antrum and duodenal bulb
- Risk factors:
  - *Helicobacter pylori* infection: associated with 95% of duodenal ulcers, 70% of gastric ulcers
  - NSAIDs
  - Corticosteroids
  - Acute/severe illness
  - Zollinger-Ellison syndrome
- Treatment
  - Diagnosis of *H. pylori* infection may involve urea breath test, serologic testing, and/or endoscopy
  - A number of combination medication regiments are used for the treatment of *H. pylori* infection
- Complications and management
  - Upper GI tract bleeding
    - Most common cause of upper GI tract bleeding
    - May present acutely with hematemesis, melena, or both
    - Endoscopic intervention for diagnosis/identification, and therapeutic endoscopic intervention (ulcer coagulation, injection, and/or clipping)
  - Perforation
    - Urgent/emergent surgical consultation for repair
  - Gastric outlet obstruction
    - Gastric decompression and endoscopic management

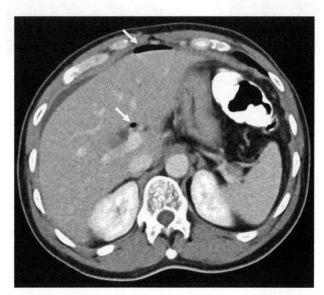

Fig. 120.1 Axial contrast-enhanced computed tomography (CT) image shows intraperitoneal free air at the upper abdomen and periportal region *(arrows)*.

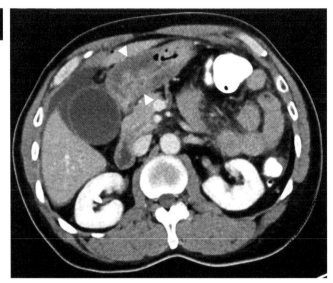

Fig. 120.2 Axial computed tomography (CT) image shows distal gastric wall thickening *(arrowheads)*.

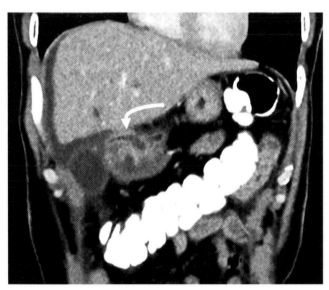

Fig. 120.3 Coronal computed tomography (CT) image shows right perihepatic free fluid and focal rim-enhancing wall abnormality at the gastric antrum *(curved arrow),* representing the site of gastric ulcer with associated findings of perforation.

REFERENCES

ASGE Standards of Practice Committee. (2010). The role of endoscopy in the management of patients with peptic ulcer disease. *Gastrointestinal Endoscopy, 71,* 663–668.

Fashner, J., & Gitu, A. C. (2015). Diagnosis and treatment of peptic ulcer disease and *H. pylori* infection. *American Family Physician, 91,* 236–242.

Hainaux, B., Agneessens, E., Bertinotti, R., De Maertelaer, V., Rubesova, E., … Capelluto, E. (2006). Accuracy of MDCT in predicting site of gastrointestinal tract perforation. *American Journal of Roentgenology, 187,* 1179–1183.

Kim, S. H., Shin, S. S., Jeong, Y. Y., Heo, S. K., Kim, J. W., & Kang, H. K. (2009). Gastrointestinal tract perforation: MDCT findings according to the perforation sites. *Korean Journal of Radiology, 10,* 63–70.

CASE 121

Biliary Cystadenoma

1. A, B, C. Images show a cystic mass with enhancing septations within it. This appearance will not be seen in a simple cyst but will be seen in the other lesions mentioned.
2. B. High signal intensity in the cyst on T1 weighted images helps differentiate between hemorrhagic cyst and biliary cystadenoma on MRI.
3. D. Due to the high risk of malignant transformation (20%), surgical resection is the preferred treatment in these cases. Percutaneous aspiration, ethanol injection, and fenestration are unnecessary and generally inappropriate.
4. A. Aspiration of biliary cystic tumor often demonstrates bile-tinged mucin and can allow differentiation from parasitic cysts, hematoma, or hemorrhagic cysts.

Comment

- Cystic diseases of the liver occur in 5% to 10% of the population; however, most of these are simple cysts, and biliary cystic tumors (BCTs) are uncommon and comprise <5% of all liver cysts.
- Biliary cystadenomas (BCAs) occur predominantly in females (90%), and biliary cystadenocarcinomas (BCAC) are distributed equally among men and women.
- BCAs present at approximately 45 years of age while BCACs present a decade later.
- Imaging appearances: Sonography is more sensitive at detecting septa in cystic lesions whereas CT more accurately demonstrates size and anatomic extent of these lesions.
  - US: BCTs are anechoic with thickened irregular walls and internal septations. Septal thickening, papillary infolding, and mural nodules are characteristic of BCTs. BCAC is more likely to contain mural or septal nodules and papillary projections.
  - CT: BCT lesions are isodense to water (<30 HU) with nodular areas enhancing with intravenous contrast. Biliary duct dilatation, single cysts, and lesions in the left lobe of the liver can be predictive of BCT on CT.
  - MRI: BCTs appears as multilocular with irregular thick walls. A homogeneous low-intensity T1 signal and high-intensity T2 signal are characteristic.

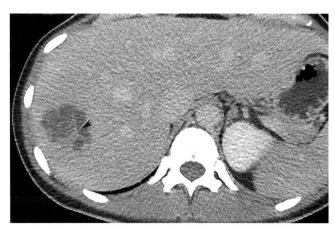

Fig. 121.1 Axial image from contrast-enhanced computed tomography shows a cystic mass in the right lobe of the liver with thick enhancing septations *(red arrow)* within it. This mass was suspected to be a biliary cystic tumor and was resected and found to be a biliary cystadenoma.

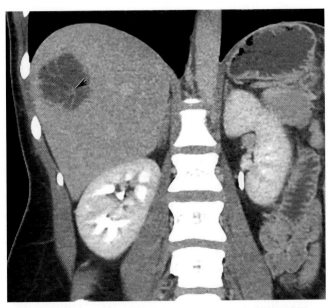

Fig. 121.2 Coronal reformat from contrast-enhanced computed tomography shows a cystic mass in the right lobe of the liver with thick enhancing septations *(red arrow)* within it. This mass was suspected to be a biliary cystic tumor and was resected and found to be a biliary cystadenoma.

- BCA and BCAC cannot be reliably differentiated with preoperative imaging. Mural nodule and irregular cyst wall thickness on CT may suggest a higher likelihood of malignancy, but these features are not pathognomonic for BCAC.
- Aspiration of BCT often demonstrates bile-tinged mucin and can allow differentiation from parasitic cysts, hematoma, or hemorrhagic cysts.
- The risk of malignant transformation of BCA to BCAC can be as high as 20%, and hence formal surgical resection with negative margins is recommended.

REFERENCES

Lewin, M., Mourra, N., Honigman, I., Fléjou, J. F., Parc, R., ... Arrivé, L. (2006). Assessment of MRI and MRCP in diagnosis of biliary cystadenoma and cystadenocarcinoma. *European Radiology, 16*(2), 407–413. doi:10.1007/s00330-005-2822-x.

Soares, K. C., Arnaoutakis, D. J., Kamel, I., Anders, R., Adams, R. B., ... Bauer, T. W. (2014). Cystic neoplasms of the liver: Biliary cystadenoma and cystadenocarcinoma. *Journal of the American College of Surgeons, 218*(1), 119–128. doi:10.1016/j.jamcollsurg.2013.08.014.

Xu, H. X., Lu, M. D., Liu, L. N., Zhang, Y. F., Guo, L. H., ... Liu, C. (2012). Imaging features of intrahepatic biliary cystadenoma and cystadenocarcinoma on B-mode and contrast-enhanced ultrasound. *Ultraschall in Der Medizin, 33*(7), E241–E249. doi:10.1055/s-0031-1299276.

CASE 122

Biliary Stricture Post Liver Transplantation

1. A and B. Images show intrahepatic biliary dilatation with cystic fluid collection, which can be seen with bilomas and biliary dilatation.
2. D. Biliary strictures are the most commonly seen biliary complications after 3 months in post–liver transplant patients.
3. A, B, C. MRI features of malignant strictures include irregular, asymmetric strictures with a shouldered margin, longer strictures (>30 mm), and abrupt narrowing (less reliable sign).
4. A, B, C, D. Treatment options for biliary stricture include all of the options mentioned.

Comment

- Background: Biliary strictures are one of the most common complications following liver transplantation.
  - Incidence is 5% to 15% following deceased donor liver transplantations and 28% to 32% following living donor liver transplantations.
- Most common biliary complications
  - Bile leaks: early posttransplant period (<3 months)
  - Anastomotic (most frequent type of late biliary complication [>3 months]) and intrahepatic strictures
    - Due to ischemia/reperfusion injury, vascular insufficiency, or fibrotic healing caused by improper technique
  - Stones
  - Ampullary dysfunction
- Biliary strictures:
  - Classified as
    - Anastomotic strictures (AS): isolated 4% to 9%
      - Localized to the site of the anastomosis
      - Short in length
      - Ischemia or fibrosis following a suboptimal surgical technique or a bile leak in the postoperative period
    - Nonanastomotic strictures (NAS): 10% to 25%
      - Classified as
        - NAS secondary to macroangiopathy
        - NAS secondary to microangiopathy (preservation injury, prolonged cold and warm ischemia times, donation after cardiac death, and prolonged use of vasopressors in the donor)
        - Immunogenicity (chronic rejection, ABO incompatibility, autoimmune hepatitis, and primary sclerosing cholangitis)
- Imaging:
  - US: the initial modality in the investigation of increasing bilirubin and for detection of biliary dilatation
    - Highly sensitive for detection of biliary obstruction and level of obstruction (accuracy 90%); however, accuracy for detection of cause varies (30%–70%)
    - Highly operator dependent
    - In liver transplant patients, ultrasound is not sensitive (38%–66%) to detect biliary obstruction
      - Size of the duct has not been found to be a reliable indicator in follow-up or in accessing the response to the treatment
      - Lack of correlation between the ducal dilatation on the ultrasound and the cholangiographic and clinical feature
  - CT: helps in detection of biliary dilatation, underlying cause of obstruction, and complications such as cholangitis and cholangitic abscess
    - Multiphase CT may help in differentiating benign from malignant strictures
      - Malignant stricture: arterial and venous hyperenhancement, wall thickness >1.5 mm, longer length of stricture (>18 mm), and greater extent of proximal dilatation compared to benign strictures. Enlarged lymph nodes and metastases seen.
  - ERCP: gold standard; can obtain tissue diagnosis
  - MRCP: optimal noninvasive diagnostic tool for the assessment of biliary complications after orthotopic liver transplantation
    - Malignant strictures: irregular, asymmetric strictures with a shouldered margin, longer strictures (>30 mm), abrupt narrowing (less reliable sign)
    - Benign strictures: smooth and symmetric borders with tapered margins, shorter strictures (<13 mm)
  - PET with 18F-FDG: highly sensitive to differentiate between malignant and benign strictures
  - Endoscopic ultrasound and intraductal sonography: sensitivity -97%, specificity 88%

- Management: three therapeutic strategies
  - ERC-guided therapy: first-line approach
    - Anastomotic strictures after orthotopic liver transplant
      - Balloon dilatation alone
      - Balloon dilatation and plastic stent placement
      - Balloon dilatation and metal stent placement
    - Nonanastomotic strictures
      - Secondary to early hepatic artery thrombosis requires urgent revascularization or retransplant for irreversible diffuse bile duct injury
      - Secondary to late hepatic artery thrombosis can be managed by endoscopic means
  - PTC-guided therapy
  - Surgical revision: Roux-en-Y hepaticojejunostomy used as a rescue therapy for patients in whom ERC- or PTC-guided therapy has failed
  - Retransplant: salvage treatment of biliary strictures; is now rare and performed in fewer than 1% of cases

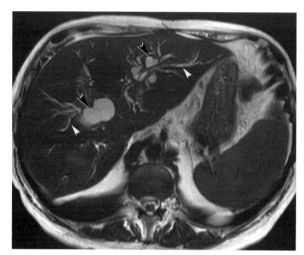

Fig. 122.1 Axial T2 weighted magnetic resonance image (MRI) shows cystic areas in the liver *(red arrows)* with biliary dilatation *(yellow arrows)*.

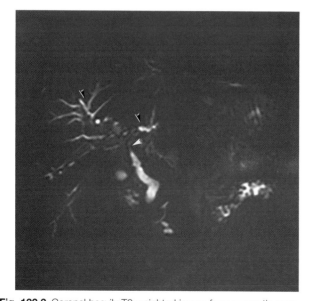

Fig. 122.2 Coronal heavily T2 weighted image from magnetic resonance cholangiopancreatography (MRCP) shows intrahepatic biliary dilatation *(red arrows)* with stricture *(yellow arrow)* seen at the anastomosis. This is consistent with an anastomotic stricture.

REFERENCES

Ryu, C. H., & Lee, S. K. (2011). Biliary strictures after liver transplantation. *Gut and Liver, 5*(2), 133–142. doi:10.5009/gnl.2011.5.2.133.

Villa, N. A., & Harrison, M. E. (2015). Management of biliary strictures after liver transplantation. *Gastroenterology & Hepatology, 11*(5), 316–328.

CASE 123

Ectopic Pancreas

1. A, B, C, D. Images show a lobulated subserosal mass in the distal duodenum. This appearance can be seen with any of the causes mentioned.
2. A. Approximately 47% of cases of heterotopic pancreas are located in the stomach. The rest of the locations mentioned are less commonly seen.
3. D. Diagnosis of heterotopic pancreas is easier in the upper gastrointestinal (GI) tract compared to lower GI tract. Imaging findings are nonspecific on both CT and MRI. CT findings are usually nonspecific; however, after intravenous contrast administration heterotopic pancreatic tissue can enhance to the same degree as orthotopic pancreas. Also, CT may show exophytic bowel wall lesions or mural wall thickening, luminal or compressive obstructions. The MRI appearance of heterotopic pancreas is similar to the normal pancreas.
4. D. Definitive diagnosis of heterotopic pancreas can only be performed with histopathology.

Comment

- Introduction: Heterotopic pancreas is a congenital anomaly, in which pancreatic tissues lacking anatomic or vascular connections with the normal pancreas may be found anywhere within the abdominal cavity other than its usual location.
  - Can be found throughout the entire gastrointestinal tract; however, studies indicate that 70% to 90% of cases are located in the upper gut, including the stomach (25%–47%), duodenum (11.7%–36.3%), and jejunum (15–35%).
  - Mainly located in submucosa (54%–75% of cases; also, it may span the submucosa and muscularis propria in 23% of cases), followed by muscular layer (muscularis propria in 8% of cases) and serous layer (11%–13% of cases).
  - Lesions located in the stomach and duodenal bulb may involve full thickness of the wall (4% of cases).
- Heterotopic pancreas is usually asymptomatic, but it may become clinically evident when complicated by inflammation, bleeding, obstruction, or malignant transformation.
  - Symptoms depend on the site where heterotopic pancreas is located
  - Abdominal pain is one of the most common symptoms
    - The most reasonable explanation is that the pain is caused by secretion of hormones and enzymes triggering the onset of spasms, chemical irritation, and inflammation of surrounding tissue
  - The incidence of malignant transformation of heterotopic pancreas is very low, occurring only in 0.7% to 1.8% of cases
- Imaging: Heterotopic pancreas has several characteristic radiographic and endoscopic features that may lead to its identification.
  - Barium swallow shows nonspecific fold thickening with rounded filling defects and sometimes a typical central indentation, which helps to differentiate it from other types of intramural masses
  - CT findings are usually nonspecific; however, after intravenous contrast administration, heterotopic pancreatic tissue can enhance to the same degree as orthotopic pancreas
    - May show exophytic bowel wall lesions or mural wall thickening, luminal, or compressive obstructions

- MRI: appearance of heterotopic pancreas is similar to the normal pancreas
- Diagnosis of heterotopic pancreas is easier in the upper GI tract, where it may present characteristic features
- During esophagogastroduodenoscopy the heterotopic pancreas classically presents as soft, rubbery, well-circumscribed broad-based yellow submucosal lesion (ranging from 1 mm to 5 cm). The characteristic central umbilication represents the orifice of the ductal system.
- Definitive diagnosis of heterotopic pancreas is possible only by histopathologic examination.

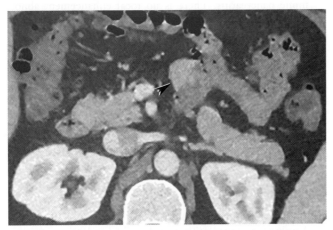

Fig. 123.1 Axial postcontrast computed tomography (CT) image showing a mass *(arrow)* along the serosal surface of the jejunum with enhancement characteristics similar to the pancreas.

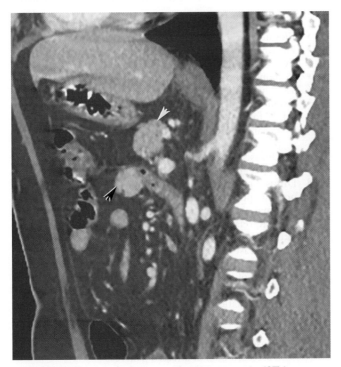

Fig. 123.2 Sagittal postcontrast computed tomography (CT) image showing a mass *(red arrow)* along the serosal surface of the jejunum with enhancement characteristics similar to the pancreas *(yellow arrow).*

REFERENCES

Mickuniene, R., Stundiene, I., Jucaitis, T., Valanciene, D., & Valantinas, J. (2019). A case of ectopic pancreas in the ileum presenting as obscure gastrointestinal bleeding and abdominal pain. *BMC Gastroenterology,* *19*(1), 57. doi:10.1186/s12876-019-0971-7.

Patel, A., Hellmann, A., Spychalski, P., Szymański, M., & Śledziński, M. (2020). Jejunal ectopic pancreas mimicking a gastrointestinal stromal tumor. *Polish Archives of Internal Medicine, 130*(1), 77–78. doi:10.20452/pamw.14992.

CASE 124

Insulinoma

1. A, B. Images show a hypervascular mass in the pancreatic neck. Though this is not a typical site for renal metastasis, hypervasuclar metastases are known to occur in the pancreas in a small number of patients. Insulinoma is seen as a hypervascular mass and can be seen in the pancreas commonly.
2. D. About 80% of insulinomas express the somatostatin receptor 2, and the ^{68}Ga-dotatate scans have a high affinity for these receptors and therefore have high sensitivity in the detection of these tumors, which has been reported in up to 90%.
3. A. Most insulinomas are benign; 90% of insulinomas have been reported to be benign, 90% are solitary, >90% occur at intrapancreatic sites, and 90% are <2 cm in diameter.
4. A. VIPoma is the most common pancreatic neuroendocrine tumor compared to the other tumors mentioned.

Comment

- Introduction: Insulinomas are the most common functioning endocrine neoplasm of the pancreas. They are insulin-secreting tumors of pancreatic origin that cause hypoglycemia.
  - Insulinomas occur in one to four people per million in the general population and represent 1% to 2% of all pancreatic neoplasms.
  - Insulinomas can occur at any age and have an equal gender distribution.
  - Insulinomas are evenly distributed over the entire pancreas. Most insulinomas are located in the pancreas or are attached directly to the pancreas.
    - Extrapancreatic insulinomas causing hypoglycemia are extremely rare (incidence <2%); extrapancreatic insulinomas are most commonly found in the duodenal wall.
  - The classical diagnosis of insulinoma depends on satisfying the criteria of Whipple triad, which remains the cornerstone of the screening process: (1) hypoglycemia (plasma glucose <50 mg/dL); (2) neuroglycopenic symptoms; and (3) prompt relief of symptoms following the administration of glucose.

Imaging

The sensitivity of transabdominal ultrasonography in the localization of insulinomas is poor (ranging from 9%–64%). However, insulinomas demonstrate characteristic features when on both CT and MRI, and the sensitivity of these techniques has been reported to be 33% to 64% and 40% to 90%, respectively.

- Insulinomas are hypervascular and hence show a greater degree of enhancement than normal pancreatic parenchyma during the arterial and capillary phases of contrast bolus.
- Atypical CT appearance of insulinomas is occasionally encountered and can include hypovascular and hypodense lesions postcontrast, hyperdense lesions precontrast, cystic masses, and calcified masses.
- Calcification, when it occurs, tends to be discrete and nodular, and is more common in malignant than benign tumors.
- ^{68}Ga-Dotate scans have high sensitivity in the detection of these tumors.

Treatment

Most patients with benign insulinomas can be cured with surgery, although other techniques for the management of insulinomas include injection of octreotide, EUS-guided alcohol ablation, radiofrequency ablation (RFA), or embolization of an insulinoma of the pancreas.

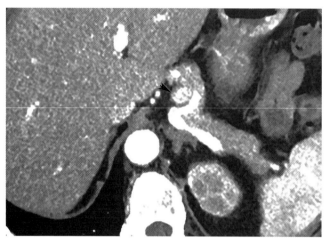

Fig. 124.1 Axial postcontrast arterial phase image showing a hypervascular mass *(arrow)* in the pancreatic neck. This patient presented with fainting episodes and had hypoglycemia, which suggests that this mass was likely an insulinoma.

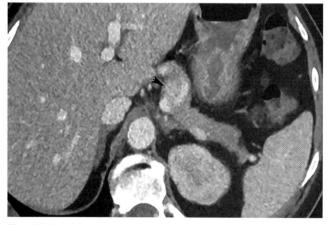

Fig. 124.2 Axial postcontrast venous phase image shows that the mass *(arrow)* in the pancreatic neck is isodense on the venous phase. This patient presented with fainting episodes and had hypoglycemia, which suggests that this mass was likely an insulinoma.

REFERENCES

Lee, L., Ito, T., & Jensen, R. T. (2018). Imaging of pancreatic neuroendocrine tumors: Recent advances, current status, and controversies. *Expert Review of Anticancer Therapy, 18*(9), 837–860. doi: 10.1080/14737140.2018.1496822

Okabayashi, T., Shima, Y., Sumiyoshi, T., Kozuki, A., Ito, S., … Hanazaki, K. (2013). Diagnosis and management of insulinoma. *World Journal of Gastroenterology, 19*(6), 829–837. doi: 10.3748/wjg.v19.i6.829

CASE 125

IgG4-Related Autoimmune Pancreatitis

1. C. From the provided images, the pancreatic parenchyma appears diffusely enlarged, without abnormal pancreatic ductal dilatation.
2. B. From the provided MRCP image, the biliary system has an abnormal beaded appearance of alternating segments of normal and diminutive caliber. There is no overt biliary ductal dilatation or cystic outpouching.
3. C. The findings of enlarged pancreatic parenchyma, enhancing rim enveloping the pancreatic body and tail, biliary ductal beading, make the most likely diagnosis of autoimmune pancreatitis. There is no focal enhancement abnormality to indicate pancreatic adenocarcinoma. There is no abnormal pancreatic ductal dilatation to represent chronic pancreatitis. There is no fluid-signal structure to represent postpancreatitis pseudocyst.
4. B. Fig. 125.4 shows relative atrophy of the pancreas compared to its pretreatment appearance. Treatment response after a trial of corticosteroids is among the diagnostic criteria of autoimmune pancreatitis. Neither antibiotics nor IVIG are typical primary therapies for autoimmune pancreatitis. Tyrosine kinase inhibitors are used for targeted treatment of various cancers.

Comment

Diagnosis and Imaging Features

- Autoimmune pancreatitis, first described in 1995, is now recognized to represent a manifestation of IgG4-related disease.
- Demographics:
  - Male to female ratio >2:1
  - Mean age of presentation >60 years old
- Symptoms:
  - Abdominal pain, weight loss, steatorrhea, obstructive jaundice
- Diagnostic criteria include:
  - Elevated serum IgG4 level
  - Histopathologic criteria for IgG+ cellular infiltrates
  - Typical radiologic findings
  - Response to corticosteroid therapy
- CT/MR appearance:
  - Extent of pancreatic involvement may be diffuse, multifocal, or focal
    - Focal appearance can be difficult to distinguish from pancreatitis or underlying malignancy
    - Diffuse or multifocal appearance overlaps with chronic pancreatitis of other etiologies
  - Diffuse pancreatic enlargement, or focal enlargement; normal appearance in a minority of patients
  - Minimal peripancreatic fat stranding, vascular encasement
  - On MR, relative T1 hypointense signal, relative T2 hyperintense signal
  - Postcontrast imaging with diminished early enhancement of the pancreas and increased delayed enhancement, including of a peripancreatic rim of enhancement
  - Pancreatic duct typically shows diffuse or segmental narrowing, not dilatation
  - Biliary system may show distal common bile duct narrowing or stricture
  - Response to corticosteroid therapy:
    - Decreased bulk of affected pancreas
    - Normalization of enhancement abnormality
    - Normalization of pancreatic ductal abnormality

IgG4-Related Disease

- A systemic inflammatory disorder, characterized by the histopathologic finding of lymphoplasmacytic cellular infiltrate, and pattern of storiform fibrosis of involved organs
- One or multiple organs may be involved:
  - Pancreaticobiliary: see earlier
  - Kidneys: renal parenchymal lesions (round or wedge shaped) or renal pelvic involvement
  - Lymph nodes: lymphadenopathy (cervical, mediastinal, hilar, mesenteric, retroperitoneal)
  - Head and neck: salivary glands, lacrimal glands, thyroid; glandular enlargement or focal lesions
  - Retroperitoneum: soft tissue encasement of abdominal aorta and branches, retroperitoneal fibrosis; may result in hydronephrosis

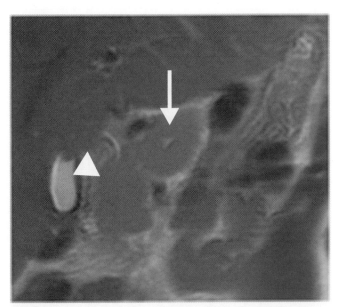

Fig. 125.1 Coronal T2 weighted magnetic resonance imaging (MRI) demonstrates diffuse pancreatic enlargement *(arrowhead)* and nondilated pancreatic duct *(arrow)*.

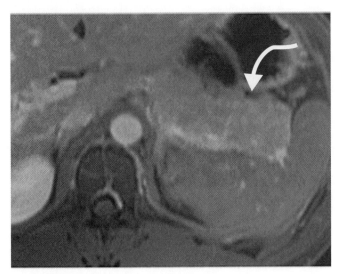

Fig. 125.2 Axial delayed T1 postcontrast image demonstrates a thin enhancing rim of tissue surrounding the pancreatic tail *(curved arrow)*.

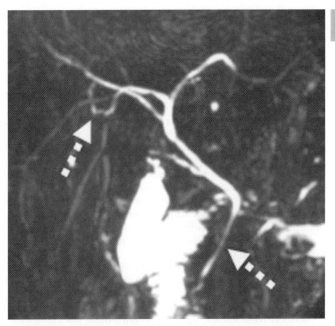

Fig. 125.3 Coronal T2 weighted three-dimensional (3D) magnetic resonance cholangiopancreatography (MRCP) maximum-intensity projection (MIP) image demonstrates distal common bile duct narrowing and mild beading of intrahepatic ducts *(dashed arrows)*.

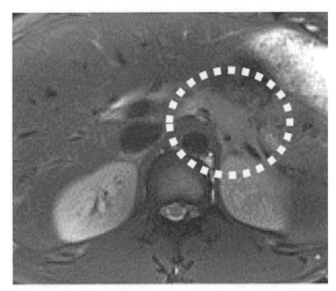

Fig. 125.4 After the patient was treated with corticosteroid therapy, follow-up T2 weighted fat-suppressed magnetic resonance imaging (MRI) demonstrates normalization of the previously expanded pancreatic contour *(dashed circle)*.

- Blood vessels: perivascular soft tissue
- Lungs: parenchymal nodules, masslike lesions, and a spectrum of airspace opacities

REFERENCES

Lee, L. K., & Sahani, D. V. (2014). Autoimmune pancreatitis in the context of IgG4-related disease: Review of imaging findings. *World Journal of Gastroenterology, 20,* 15177–15189.

Vlachou, P. A., Khalili, K., Jang, H. J., Fischer, S., Hirschfield, G. M., & Kim, T. K. (2011). IgG4-related sclerosing disease: Autoimmune pancreatitis and extrapancreatic manifestations. *Radiographics, 31,* 1379–1402.

CASE 126

Main Duct IPMN

1. C. The MRIs demonstrate diffuse main pancreatic duct dilation with solid mural nodules, compatible with main duct intraductal papillary mucinous neoplasm (IMPN). Diffuse ductal dilation as pictured is common in chronic pancreatitis, but the mural nodules favor malignant degeneration of a main duct IPMN. Pancreatic ductal adenocarcinoma will also commonly present with a dilated pancreatic duct, but usually with abrupt cutoff at the level of the tumor. There is a normal pancreaticobiliary junction with no pancreas divisum.

2. D. Dilation of the main pancreatic duct beyond 5 mm should raise concern for possible main duct IPMN. Normal pancreatic duct caliber varies with age and may be up to 3 mm, 4 mm, or 5 mm depending on the reference. Careful investigation for an obstructing mass or intraductal solid mural nodule should be performed.

3. A, B, C, D. Patients with new-onset diabetes, jaundice, acute pancreatitis, or elevated serum CA 19-9 in the setting of a dilated pancreatic duct should be worked up for malignant degeneration of a main duct IPMN with gastrointestinal and surgical consultation. Endoscopic ultrasound for fine-needle aspiration is commonly performed with potential for surgical resection depending on cytology and patient presentation.

4. B. A bulging papilla at ERCP is pathognomonic for main duct IPMN and is due to increased intraductal pressure from secreted mucin. It can rarely also be seen at MRCP. The double bubble sign is seen in neonates on radiography in the setting of duodenal atresia. The double duct sign refers to dilation of the pancreatic duct and common bile duct at CT or MRI, often due to a pancreatic head or ampullary mass. A long common channel refers to an abnormal pancreaticobiliary junction in which a common channel between the pancreatic duct and common bile duct exceeds 1.5 cm in length, predisposing to biliary carcinoma.

Comment

- Intraductal papillary mucinous neoplasm (IPMN) is a mucin-producing tumor arising from epithelial cells of the pancreatic duct.
- IPMNs occur primarily in older patients with a slight male predilection.
- IPMNs are categorized into three types:
  - Main duct: involves the main pancreatic duct, with segmental or diffuse dilation. Highest malignant potential.
  - Side branch (or branch duct): focal cystic lesions that may demonstrate ductal communication or high resolution CT or MRI. May be multifocal. Most commonly in the pancreatic head. Much more indolent behavior.
  - Mixed type: have elements of both main duct and side branch IPMNs. Prognosis and management resemble main duct IPMN.
- The most critical findings on imaging are dilation of the main pancreatic duct (>5 mm) and identification of a solid enhancing component.
- Surveillance imaging is performed in most patients to evaluate for change in size and development of duct dilation or solid mural nodules but also to evaluate for a tumor elsewhere in the pancreatic parenchyma, as these patients are thought to harbor a field defect that predisposes them to development of ductal adenocarcinoma.
- Clinical symptoms and comorbidities drive management in patients with suspected IPMN. New-onset jaundice, diabetes, and acute pancreatitis are worrisome as well as increased serum CA 19-9 levels. Key features at endoscopic ultrasound-guided fine-needle aspiration include CEA level, KRAS/GNAS mutation analysis, and cytology (identification of malignant cells, dysplasia, or atypia).

- Imaging findings of main duct IPMN:
  - US: side branch IPMNs appears as small parenchymal cysts. Main duct IPMN will show ductal dilation and parenchymal atrophy, which can mimic chronic pancreatitis or ductal adenocarcinoma.
  - CT: side branch IPMNs are cystic lesions in the pancreas, most commonly in the head. Ductal communication may be depicted on high-resolution, thin-slice imaging. Ductal dilation >5 mm is concerning for main duct IPMN.
  - MRI: current mainstay and gold standard for IPMN workup.
    - Sidebranch IPMN: one or multiple T2 hyperintense lesions. May be difficult to distinguish from other cystic lesions, including pseudocyst, serous cystadenoma, or

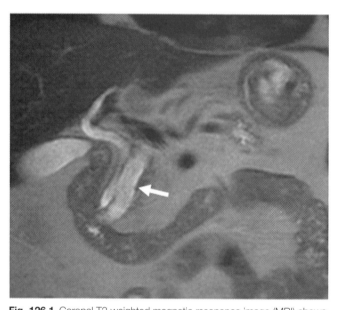

Fig. 126.1 Coronal T2 weighted magnetic resonance image (MRI) shows dilatation of the main pancreatic duct at the pancreatic head *(arrow)*.

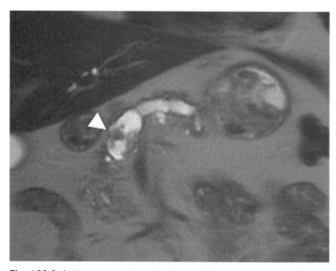

Fig. 126.2 At the pancreatic neck, there is T2 hypointense mural nodularity *(arrowhead)*.

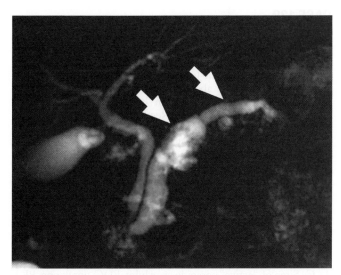

Fig. 126.3 Two-dimensional (2D) T2 weighted magnetic resonance cholangiopancreatography (MRCP) image demonstrates diffuse pancreatic ductal dilatation *(arrows)*.

mucinous cystic neoplasm. Communication with the pancreatic duct is helpful in diagnosis (but does not exclude pseudocyst—history is key).

- Main duct IPMN: segmental or diffuse dilation of the main pancreatic duct >5 mm. There may be associated parenchymal atrophy. Solid mural nodules within the duct are concerning for malignancy.
- Bulging of the papilla from secreted mucus that distends the pancreatic duct is pathognomonic but is uncommonly seen at MRI. The bulging papilla is more commonly associated as a buzzword finding with main duct IPMN at ERCP.

REFERENCES
Kawamoto, S., Horton, K. M., Lawler, L. P., Hruban, R. H., & Fishman, E. K. (2005). Intraductal papillary mucinous neoplasm of the pancreas: Can benign lesions be differentiated from malignant lesions with multidetector CT? *Radiographics, 25*(6), 1451–1468.
Silas, A. M., Morrin, M. M., Raptopoulos, V., & Keogan, M. T. (2001). Intraductal papillary mucinous tumors of the pancreas. *American Journal of Roentgenology, 176*(1), 179–185.

CASE 127

Cystic Pancreatic Lesion

1. B. Images show a multilobulated T2 hyperintense lesion at the pancreatic tail. It demonstrates a honeycombed appearance, with a central T2 hypointense scar, features of serous cystic neoplasms, which typically occur in elderly females (grandmother lesion).
2. B. Mucinous cystic neoplasms occur exclusively in women, typically in middle-aged females (mother lesion). This is thought to relate to ovarian embryologic origin of MCNs, which almost always occur in the pancreatic body or tail. Surgical resection is the treatment of choice due to malignant potential.
3. D. Solid pseudopapillary epithelial neoplasms (SPEN) occur in young females (daughter lesion). They are usually heterogeneous with both solid and cystic components. Intratumoral hemorrhage is a characteristic appearance. MCNs, SCNs, and IPMNs occur in older patient populations.

4. D. Approximately 10% of pancreatic neuroendocrine tumors present as cystic masses. In this setting, these tumors classically demonstrate early peripheral rim enhancement and may contain a solid mural nodule. Other cystic tumors such as serous cystic neoplasms demonstrate more central enhancement of internal septations.

Comment

- Cystic pancreatic lesions are encountered in increasing frequency due to the ubiquity of CT and MRI scans.
- Initial approach when a cystic pancreatic lesion is encountered is to determine whether the lesion is a pseudocyst (related to pancreatitis) versus one of a number of cystic pancreatic neoplasms:
  - Serous cystic neoplasm
    - Grandmother lesion
    - Microcystic or honeycombed lesion containing serous fluid (although can be macrocystic in a minority of cases)
    - May contain a characteristic stellate scar that can calcify
    - Delayed enhancement of septations is a distinguishing feature
    - Typically has no communication with the pancreatic duct
    - Not considered premalignant
  - Mucinous cystic neoplasm
    - Mother lesion
    - Unilocular cyst with mucin
    - May contain thickened wall or wall calcification (specific finding)
    - Seen exclusively in women
    - Almost always occurs in the pancreatic tail or body
    - Premalignant (may degenerate to mucinous cystadenocarcinoma)

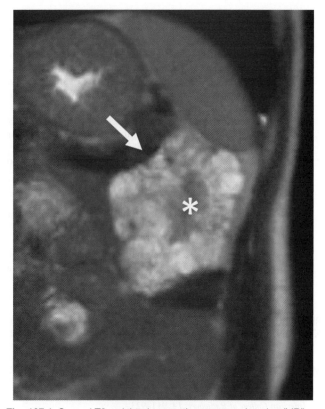

Fig. 127.1 Coronal T2 weighted magnetic resonance imaging (MRI) shows a T2 hyperintense multilobulated multicystic lesion of the pancreatic tail *(arrow)*, with a central T2 hypointense scar *(asterisk)*.

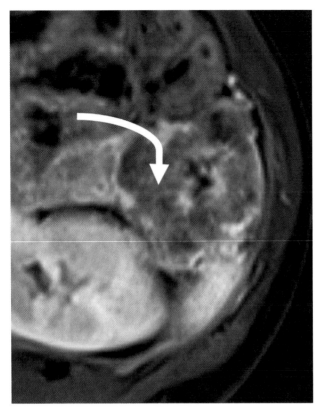

Fig. 127.2 Axial T1 weighted fat suppressed postcontrast image shows enhancement of thin septations *(curved arrow);* the imaging features are those of pancreatic serous cystadenoma.

- Intraductal papillary mucinous neoplasm
  - Mucin-producing tumor involving main pancreatic duct or side branches (or both)
  - Communication with the pancreatic duct is characteristic (seen best on MRCP)
  - Main duct IPMN carries a higher risk of malignancy; bulging papilla sign seen at ERCP due to distention of the main pancreatic duct with mucin
  - Risk factors for malignancy include pancreatic duct dilation (>8 mm) and solid mural nodule in the cyst or in the duct
- Less common cystic neoplasms of the pancreas are also encountered:
  - Solid pseudopapillary epithelial neoplasm (SPEN)
    - Daughter lesion
    - Solid and cystic tumor with capsule and early enhancement
    - May demonstrate intratumoral hemorrhage
  - Cystic neuroendocrine tumor
    - Approximately 10% of neuroendocrine tumors are cystic
    - Usually show hypervascular rim enhancement +/− a solid mural nodule

REFERENCES

Kalb, B., Sarmiento, J. M., Kooby, D. A., Adsay, N. V., & Martin, D. R. (2009). MR imaging of cystic lesions of the pancreas. *Radiographics, 29,* 1749–1765.

Megibow, A. J., Baker, M. E., Morgan, D. E., Kamel, I. R., Sahani, D. V., ... Newman, E. (2017). Management of incidental pancreatic cysts: A white paper of the ACR incidental findings committee. *Journal of the American College of Radiology, 14,* 911–923.

Sahani, D. V., Kadavigere, R., Saokar, A., Fernandez-del Castillo, C., Brugge, W. R., & Hahn, P. F. (2005). Cystic pancreatic lesions: A simple imaging-based classification system for guiding management. *Radiographics, 25,* 1471–1484.

CASE 128

Splenic Sarcoidosis

1. B. The formation of noncaseating granulomas is the hallmark of sarcoidosis. Howell-Jolly bodies are seen in various forms of hyposplenism or absent spleen. Reed-Sternberg cells are seen in patients with Hodgkin lymphoma. Owl's eye is a descriptor for the nucleoli of Reed-Sternberg cells.
2. A. The liver is the most commonly involved abdominal organ in sarcoidosis, followed by the spleen. The pancreas and testicles can also be involved. Liver involvement is usually asymptomatic, but hepatomegaly can occur. Approximately one-third of patients with liver involvement have liver enzyme abnormalities. Serious hepatic disease, including portal hypertension, occurs in a very small minority of patients.
3. B. Sarcoid nodules in the spleen are typically hypoechoic to background parenchyma. Although splenomegaly can occur, the spleen is more commonly of normal size when involved with sarcoidosis.
4. C. Sites of "active" sarcoidosis exhibit FDG uptake on PET scan. This can help guide which site of disease would provide the highest yield for tissue biopsy. Ultrasound, sulfur colloid scan, and MRI cannot distinguish active sarcoidosis.

Comment

- Sarcoidosis is a systemic inflammatory condition characterized by the presence of noncaseating granulomas. It classically affects the thorax, skin, or eyes but can present throughout the body, including solid organs of the abdominal viscera.
- The exact etiology of sarcoidosis is unknown, although some have postulated that a microorganism may incite the formation of these noncaseating granuluomas.
- Abdominal manifestations of sarcoidosis can mimic infectious or neoplastic processes (such as lymphoma). The liver and spleen are the most commonly involved abdominal organs, although the kidneys, pancreas, bowel, and testicles may also be involved.
- Abdominal sarcoidosis is usually asymptomatic. Patients with liver and spleen involvement can demonstrate hepatomegaly or, less commonly, splenomegaly.
- Patients with severe liver and splenic involvement can develop portal hypertension.

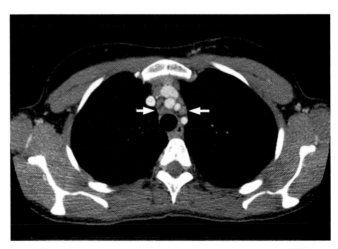

Fig. 128.1 Contrast-enhanced axial computed tomography (CT) image of the thorax demonstrates lymphadenopathy in the superior mediastinum *(arrows).*

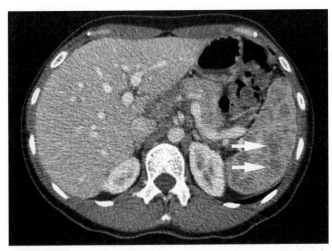

Fig. 128.2 Contrast-enhanced axial computed tomography (CT) image of the upper abdomen showing multiple small low attenuation granulomas in the spleen (arrows).

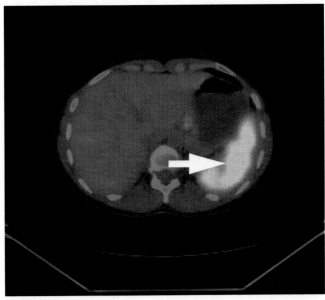

Fig. 128.3 Fused axial positron emission tomography (PET)/computed tomography (CT) demonstrating avid fluorodeoxyglucose (FDG) uptake within the splenic granulomas (arrow), compatible with active sarcoidosis.

- Imaging findings of splenic sarcoidosis:
  - US: small hypoechoic nodules relative to background splenic parenchyma
  - CT: small low attenuation nodules between 5 and 20 mm in size that are relatively hypoenhancing compared to background spleen
  - MRI: small nodules that are hypointense to the spleen on T1 and T2 weighted imaging. Hypoenhancing to background spleen.
  - PET: nodules can be FDG-avid when disease is "active," which can help guide a choice for needle biopsy when a tissue diagnosis is necessary.

REFERENCE

Warshauer, D. M., & Lee, J. K. (2004). Imaging manifestations of abdominal sarcoidosis. *American Journal of Roentgenology*, *182*(1), 15–28.

CASE 129

Splenic Rupture

1. A, C. Images show a high-density area around the spleen, which could be due to hemorrhage or less likely abscess.
2. A, B. No history of trauma or unusual effort, either prior to or on retrospect questioning after operation, and no evidence of disease that could involve the spleen are considered two of the five criteria for diagnosis of splenic rupture.
3. A, B. Subcapsular and intraparenchymal hematomas are two features seen in CT scan from splenic rupture.
4. D. Presence of vascular injury is graded as Grade IV injury on the AAST scale.

Comment

- Spontaneous rupture:
  - Spontaneous splenic rupture is rare and can be seen in diseased or normal spleen
  - Due to its vascularity, if the spleen is affected by disease, it has an increased risk of rupture after trivial stress
  - Causes of spontaneous rupture include:
    - Infective
    - Hematologic
    - Malignant
    - Metabolic
    - Infiltrative
    - Local disorders
  - Criteria for diagnosis include the following:
    - No history of trauma or unusual effort, either prior to or on retrospect questioning after operation
    - No evidence of disease that could involve the spleen
    - There should be no evidence of adhesions or scarring of the spleen to suggest trauma or previous rupture
    - Other than rupture and hemorrhage, the spleen should be normal on gross and histologic examination
    - There should be no rise in viral antibody titers in either the acute or convalescent period to suggest viral infection with the types associated with splenic involvement
  - Imaging: CT is the preferred imaging for splenic issues. CT features include
    - Subcapsular hematoma, crescentic in shape and closely applied to the splenic margin
    - Intraparenchymal hematoma: broader and more irregular with a mass effect and enlargement of the spleen
    - On contrast enhanced images: a rim of normal spleen is seen
- Splenic trauma:
  - Splenic trauma can occur after blunt or penetrating trauma or be iatrogenic.
  - Imaging:
    - CT: demonstrates laceration, hypoperfusion, subcapsular/parenchymal hematoma, active bleeding, and pseudoaneurysms in a splenic injury
      - Parenchymal hematoma: result of contusion and hemorrhage restricted in parenchyma with intact capsule
      - Subcapsular hematoma: located between the intact capsule and parenchyma with lenticular shape
      - Active hemorrhage: on contrast enhanced CT as an extravasation of intravenously introduced contrast material to the abdominal cavity
        - Can be seen as a focus of linear or nodular hyperdensity within a hematoma or into the abdominal cavity, on arterial phase images
        - Delayed phase images: accumulation of contrast is seen within or in the dependent portion of hematoma with regard to degree of clot formation

- American Association for Surgery of Trauma (AAST) grading:
  - Grade I
    - Subcapsular hematoma <10% of surface area
    - Parenchymal laceration <1 cm depth
    - Capsular tear
  - Grade II
    - Subcapsular hematoma 10% to 50% of surface area
    - Intraparenchymal hematoma <5 cm
    - Parenchymal laceration 1 to 3 cm in depth
  - Grade III
    - Subcapsular hematoma >50% of surface area
    - Ruptured subcapsular or intraparenchymal hematoma >5 cm
    - Parenchymal laceration >3 cm in depth
  - Grade IV
    - Any injury in the presence of a splenic vascular injury or active bleeding confined within splenic capsule
    - Parenchymal laceration involving segmental or hilar vessels producing >25% devascularization
  - Grade V
    - Shattered spleen
    - Any injury in the presence of splenic vascular injury with active bleeding extending beyond the spleen into the peritoneum

REFERENCES

Amonkar, S. J., & Kumar, E. N. (2009). Spontaneous rupture of the spleen: Three case reports and causative processes for the radiologist to consider. *British Journal of Radiology, 82*(978), e111–e113. doi:10.1259/bjr/81440206.

Unal, E., Onur, M. R., Akpinar, E., Ahmadov, J., Karcaaltincaba, M., … Ozmen, M. N. (2016). Imaging findings of splenic emergencies: A pictorial review. *Insights into Imaging, 7*(2), 215–222. doi:10.1007/s13244-016-0467-8.

CASE 130
Splenic Lymphangiomatosis

1. D. Each of splenic pseudocyst, lymphangiomatosis, and echinococcal disease may present with multiple hypoechoic/hypoenhancing cystic splenic lesions.
2. B. The incidental finding in an asymptomatic patient of multiple splenic cysts is most suggestive of splenic lymphangiomatosis. Abscesses and lymphoma would not be incidentally detected; there is no travel history or specific imaging features of echinococcal disease.
3. B. Secondary splenic cysts (pseudocysts) are more prevalent than primary (true) splenic cysts. Both represent benign findings and neither requires annual imaging follow-up.
4. D. Each of these statements is true, regarding imaging findings of echinococcal disease.

Comment
Splenic Lymphangiomatosis
- Benign congenital abnormality of lymphatic tissue
- Reported in pediatric case series; rarely reported in adults
- Splenic lymphangiomas may be solitary, multiple, or diffuse within the spleen.
- May be localized to the spleen, or with multiorgan/systemic involvement of head and neck, liver, kidney, and GI tract
- May represent asymptomatic finding detected incidentally, or symptoms may result from splenomegaly, if present
- Subtypes: capillary, cavernous, cystic

Imaging Features
US
- Anechoic/hypoechoic cysts; may have internal hypoechogenicity depending on the presence of protein or hemorrhage
- Septa are hyperechoic, may have vascular flow on color Doppler.

CT
- Thin-walled cystic masses without enhancement
- Peripheral calcifications may be present (most common with cystic subtype).
- Thin septa, if present, may slightly enhance.

MRI
- Hypointense to spleen on T1 weighted imaging
- Hyperintense to spleen on T2 weighted imaging
- Signal intensity may vary, depending on presence of protein or hemorrhage.
- Thin septa, if present, may slightly enhance with cystic subtype.
- Progressive sepal enhancement may be shown with cavernous and capillary subtypes.

Differential Diagnosis: Cystic Splenic Lesion
- Secondary splenic cysts/pseudocysts (80%)
  - Posttraumatic or postinfarction, after liquefactive conversion from splenic hematoma or necrosis; no epithelial lining
  - May have mural calcification in 30% to 40% of cases

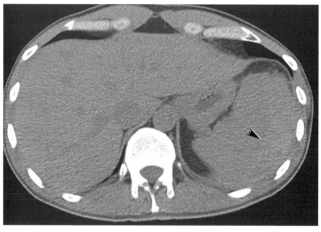

Fig. 129.1 Axial noncontrast computed tomography (CT) scan shows a high-density cresentric area *(red arrow)* around the spleen. This is consistent with a hematoma.

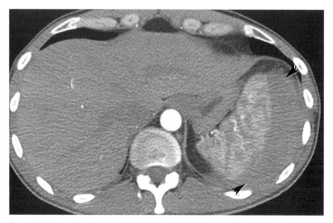

Fig. 129.2 Axial contrast computed tomography (CT) scan shows no enhancement in the high-density cresentric area *(red arrows)* around the spleen. This is consistent with a hematoma.

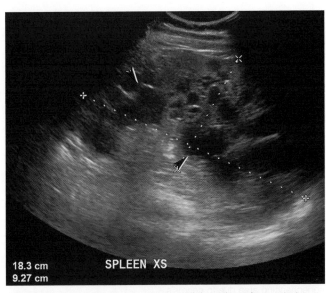

Fig. 130.1 Grayscale ultrasound image of the spleen demonstrates an enlarged spleen with multiple anechoic cysts *(arrows).*

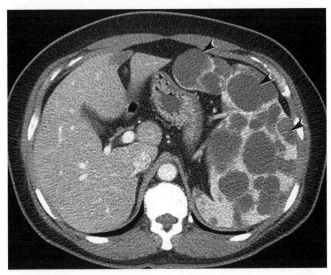

Fig. 130.2 Axial contrast-enhanced computed tomography (CT) image confirms multiple hypoenhancing cystic lesions *(arrows)* of the spleen. Splenectomy was performed, since the patient had pain and splenomegaly. This was confirmed to be due to splenic lymphangiomatosis on histopathology.

- Congenital/primary splenic cyst
  - Epithelial lining at histopathologic examination
  - Mesothelial cysts, arising from embryonic inclusions of mesothelium in the developing spleen
- Echinococcal cyst
  - Suspicion defined by history or origin or travel to endemic areas, can be confirmed with serologic testing
  - Echinococcal cysts may demonstrate daughter cyst (cyst-within-a-cyst), collapsed membranes (water lily sign), or concomitant hepatic involvement

REFERENCES

Thipphavong, S., Duigenan, S., Schindera, S. T., Gee, M. S., & Philips, S. (2014). Nonneoplastic, benign, and malignant splenic diseases: Cross-sectional imaging findings and rare disease entities. *American Journal of Roentgenology, 203,* 315–322.

Thut, D., Smolinski, S., Morrow, M., McCarthy, S., Alsina, J., ... Kreychman, A. (2017). A diagnostic approach to splenic lesions. *Applied Radiology, 46,* 7–22.

CASE 131
Adrenocortical Carcinoma

1. A, B, D. MRIs show a large heterogenous mass about the left kidney originating from the left adrenal gland. A fat plane is seen between the mass and the left kidney, and hence renal cell carcinoma is not likely. Adrenal metastasis, pheochromocytoma, and adrenocortical carcinoma are the most likely diagnosis.
2. D. Elevated ACTH levels are seen in tumors of the pituitary gland or adrenal adenomas. Adrenal metastases are known to cause a decrease in the ACTH levels. Pheochromocytomas increase the secretion of catecholamnies like norepinephrine, epinephrine and dopamine. Adrenal adenomas secrete ACTH however the imaging features do not support an adrenal adenoma in this patient. Aderenocortical carcinomas are known to secrete ACTH and the imaging features support this diagnosis.
3. C. Hormonally active adrenocortical carcinomas tend to be smaller than nonfunctioning tumors at presentation.
4. C. In adults, Cushing syndrome is the most common clinical presentation for functioning adrenocortical carcinomas and is seen in approximately 30% of the hormonally active tumors.

Comment

- Introduction: adrenocortical carcinoma (ACC) is a rare, aggressive tumor arising from the adrenal cortex.
  - ACCs account for only 0.05% to 2% of all cancers with a bimodal age distribution, with increased incidence in infants and children <5 years old and in individuals in the fourth and fifth decades of life
- Female preponderance
- Approximately 50% to 60% of adrenocortical carcinomas are hormonally active
- Hyperfunctioning tumors are more common in children than in adults
- Secrete a variety of hormones, including cortisol, androgens, estrogens, and aldosterone
- In the adults, the most common clinical presentation is Cushing syndrome
- Most ACCs in children are functional, and virilization is the most common presenting symptom
  - Feminization due to estrogen excess and hyperaldosteronism is much less common
- Nonfunctioning ACCs may be large at presentation and patients often have pain presenting from local invasion and mass effect
- Can be associated with genetic syndromes, including the following:
  - Li-Fraumeni cancer syndrome results in a familial susceptibility to a variety of cancers, including adrenocortical tumors (carcinomas, adenomas), sarcomas, leukemias, breast, brain, lung, and laryngeal cancers because of a germline *TP53* mutation
  - Carney complex consists of primary pigmented nodular adrenal dysplasia, cardiac myxomas, cutaneous myxomas, testicular tumors, and other endocrine neoplasms
  - Beckwith-Wiedemann syndrome is a congenital disorder characterized by prenatal and postnatal overgrowth, macroglossia, and anterior abdominal wall defects (most commonly exomphalos)
  - Familial adenomatous polyposis coli causes multiple adenomatous polyps and cancer of the colon and rectum, thyroid tumors, hepatoblastoma, and adrenocortical tumors (carcinomas, adenomas)
  - Multiple endocrine neoplasia, type 1 causes pituitary, parathyroid, and pancreatic tumors; adrenocortical adenomas or hyperplasia; and, very rarely, adrenocortical carcinomas

- Diagnosis:
  - Usually large at presentation, ranging from 2 to 25 cm, average size ~9 cm
  - Bilateral into 10% of cases
  - Slightly more common in the left and on the right
  - Often contain areas of cystic necrosis and hemorrhage and enhance heterogeneously
  - US: typically seen as heterogenous tumors
  - CT:
    - Large, inhomogeneous, but well-defined suprarenal mass invading into adjacent structures as it grows
    - Regions of low attenuation correspond to necrosis pathologically present when the tumors reached 6 cm in size
    - After IV contrast administration, there is inhomogenous enhancement of the tumor typically with enhancement seen mainly peripherally and little enhancement seen centrally because of central necrosis
  - MRI: has been shown to be superior to CT in the delineation of the presence and extent of IVC invasion
    - Heterogenous in signal intensity due to the presence of hemorrhage and necrosis
    - On T1 weighted imaging, typically isointense, a slightly hypointense to normal liver parenchyma
    - High T1 signal intensity can be seen in the presence of hemorrhage.
    - On T2 weighted imaging usually hyperintense to liver parenchyma and has a heterogenous texture because of the presence of intratumoral cystic regions and hemorrhage
  - Functional imaging: FDG PET can identify some malignant adrenal masses due to the increased metabolic activity within them.
    - Novel PET tracer ^{11}C metomidate, a marker of 11β-hydroxylase, is used as tracer for adrenocortical tissue and is taken up by adenomas and ACCs. This marker differentiates adrenal cortical lesions from pheochromocytomas and metastases, which are uptake negative. PET imaging is most valuable in its ability to detect distant metastasis.
- Management: surgical excision is a standard treatment of ACCs. If en bloc resection is not possible because of local extension into adjacent structures, maximum tumor bulking

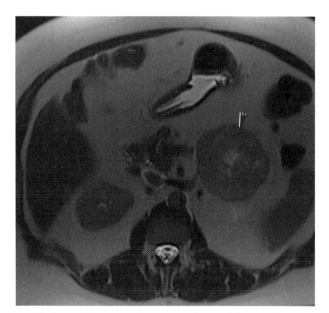

Fig. 131.1 Axial T2 weighted image showing a mildly hyperintense mass *(red arrow)* in the left upper quadrant with central cystic portion likely from necrosis.

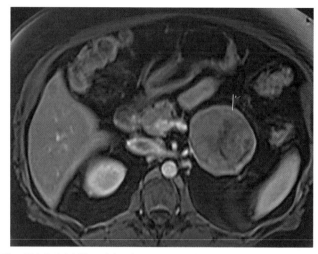

Fig. 131.2 Axial T1 weighted postcontrast image showing a heterogenously enhancing mass *(arrow)* in the left upper quadrant with central nonenhancing area due to necrosis.

surgery is indicated. Treatment with the adrenolytic drug mitotane may improve survival or at least control symptoms and is used in both primary and adjuvant therapy. It also plays a role in metastatic and recurrent disease.

REFERENCES

Bharwani, N., Rockall, A. G., Sahdev, A., Gueorguiev, M., Drake, W., ... Grossman, A. B. (2011). Adrenocortical carcinoma: The range of appearances on CT and MRI. *American Journal of Roentgenology, 196*(6), W706–W714.

Lattin Jr., G. E., Sturgill, E. D., Tujo, C. A., Marko, J., Sanchez-Maldonado, K. W., ... Craig, W. D. (2014). From the radiologic pathology archives: Adrenal tumors and tumor-like conditions in the adult: Radiologic-pathologic correlation. *Radiographics, 34*(3), 805–829.

CASE 132

Adrenal Castleman Disease

1. B, C, D. CT images show a large lobulated enhancing mass in the right suprarenal region likely involving the adrenal gland. Due to the large size of the mass and heterogenous enhancement, adrenocortical carcinoma could be a consideration. Due to the significant enhancement, pheochromocytoma should be considered as well. Considering the lobulated appearance and retroperitoneal location, a large lymph nodal mass as seen in Castleman disease should be included in the differential diagnosis.

2. B. More than 70% of cases of Castleman disease occur in the chest, and it is seen as enhancing hypervascular mediastinal or hilar mass. Multistation enhancing lymph nodes or cervical lymph nodes can also be seen; however, they are seen less often. Retroperitoneal or intraabdominal enhancing mass is seen less often in only ~15% of cases.

3. A. The classic CT appearance of Castleman disease is that of a solitary and large lymph node or localized nodal mass that demonstrates intense homogenous enhancement after contrast administration. Infiltrative mass and matted lymph nodes are less commonly seen in Castleman disease. Castleman disease does not involve the colon and originates in lymphatic tissue.

4. A, D. Both pheochromocytomas and adrenal adenoma can show enhancement after contrast administration; however, pheochromocytomas are known to show intense enhancement compared to adenomas. Adrenal myelolipoma and cyst do not show intense enhancement after contrast administration.

Comment

- Introduction: Castleman disease (giant lymph node hyperplasia) is a benign proliferation of mature lymphocytes and/or plasma cells with preservation of the lymph node architecture.
  - Poorly understood lymphoproliferative disorder
  - Occurs mainly in the mediastinum (70%)
  - Extra thoracic sites have been reported with 50% of the cases seen in the abdomen and pelvis
  - Lymphoid-hamartomatous hyperplasia, autoimmune phenomena, immunodeficiency, and chronic low-grade inflammation have been suggested as potential etiologic factors for the development of Castleman disease
- Imaging appearance: the classic imaging appearance of hyaline vascular Castleman disease is that of a solitary and large lymph node or localized nodal masses that demonstrate homogenous intense enhancement of the contrast administration.
  - Other adrenal lesions that can show intense enhancement after contrast administration include pheochromocytoma and adrenal adenoma
  - Heterogenous enhancement can be seen in larger lesions due to central necrosis
  - Approximately 10% of hyaline vascular Castleman disease have internal calcifications
    - Three patterns of involvement have been described:
      - Solitary noninvasive mass (most common: 50% of cases)
      - Dominant infiltrative mass with associated lymphadenopathy (40% of cases)
      - Matted lymphadenopathy without the dominant mass (10% of cases)
  - Hyaline vascular Castleman disease can manifest as a mesenteric or retroperitoneal mass with mild contrast enhancement, with an imaging appearance mimicking retroperitoneal adenopathy and carcinoid tumor
  - MRI: heterogenous T1 and T2 hyperintensity compared with skeletal muscle
    - Prominent flow voids may be seen due to the feeding vessels.
  - PET/CT provides information regarding metabolic status of lymph nodes involved in Castleman disease
- Differential diagnosis: nodal or extranodal masses, generalized adenopathy, hyperenhancing lymph nodes, lymphoma, and systemic infection

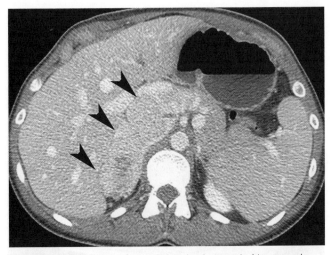

Fig. 132.2 Axial venous-phase postcontrast computed tomography after intravenous contrast administration shows strong homogenous enhancement of the right adrenal mass (arrows). The mass is displacing the surrounding structures.

REFERENCES

Bonekamp, D., Horton, K. M., Hruban, R. H., & Fishman, E. K. (2011). Castleman disease: The great mimic. *Radiographics, 31*(6), 1793–1807. doi:10.1148/rg.316115502.

Hong, S. B., Lee, N. K., Kim, S., Han, G. J., Ha, H. K., ... Ku, J. Y. (2017). Adrenal Castleman's disease mimicking other adrenal neoplasms: A case report. *Journal of the Korean Society of Radiology, 76*(1), 73–77.

CASE 133

Renal Abscess

1. B. Diabetes is a known risk factor for the development of renal abscess. Hypertension, hepatic steatosis, and hypercholesterolemia are not associated with renal abscess.
2. B. Rupture of a renal abscess into the collecting system is termed pyonephrosis, in which infected fluid, or pus, drains into the renal collecting system. Pyelonephritis typically serves as a precursor and inciting condition for renal abscess formation. Emphysematous pyelonephritis is a complication of pyelonephritis in which gas forms in the renal cortex. Pyelitis is an infection/inflammation of the collecting system that can occur independent of renal abscess.
3. A, B. Treatment for renal abscess includes intravenous antibiotic administration and image-guided percutaneous drainage (if amenable). Surgery is usually only necessary in the background of emphysematous pyelonephritis.
4. D. The presence of restricted diffusion can help identify renal abscess and distinguish it from a complex cyst. T2 hyperintensity, peripheral enhancement, and internal septations can all be seen with abscess or complex cysts.

Comment

- A renal abscess is a collection of infected fluid that usually occurs secondary to complications of acute pyelonephritis.
- Risk factors for formation of renal abscess include diabetes, nephrolithiasis, and urinary obstruction.
- Signs and symptoms of renal abscess may include fever, flank pain, chills/rigors, and dysuria.
- If untreated, a renal abscess can rupture into the collecting system (pyonephrosis), into the perinephric space (perinephric abscess), and beyond Gerota fascia (paranephric abscess).
- Treatment involves aggressive intravenous antibiotics with percutaneous drainage (if large enough).

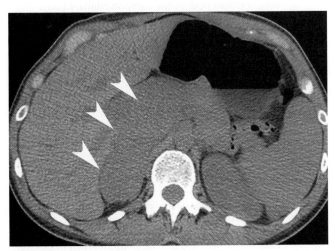

Fig. 132.1 Axial noncontrast computed tomography shows lobulated homogenous right adrenal mass (arrow).

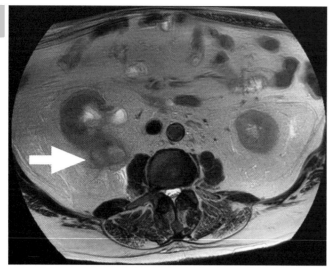

Fig. 133.1 Axial T2 weighed image at the level of the kidneys shows a heterogeneous ill-defined slightly T2 hyperintense exophytic lesion *(arrow)* at the posterior interpolar right kidney.

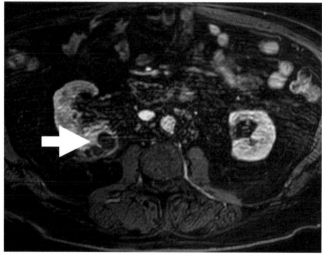

Fig. 133.2 Axial postcontrast T1 weighted image with fat saturation demonstrates irregular peripheral enhancement *(arrow)* within the poorly marginated lesion in the posterior right kidney. This is compatible with a renal abscess in this patient with flank pain and leukocytosis.

- The main differential considerations on imaging include a complex cyst and cystic renal cell carcinoma.
- Imaging findings of pelvic kidney:
  - US: hypoechoic fluid collection with internal echoes in the renal cortex and/or perinephric space
  - CT: low attenuation fluid collection, usually with thick irregular margins and peripheral enhancement. Intralesional gas is not always seen but is diagnostic. Perilesional perfusion changes are common along with inflammatory thickening of the perinephric fat and Gerota fascia.
  - MRI: T1 hypointense, T2 hyperintense heterogeneous fluid collection with thick, irregular peripheral enhancement. Should demonstrate restricted diffusion. Edematous changes in the perinephric fat on fluid sensitive sequences.

REFERENCE

Das, C. J., Zohra, A., Sharma, S., & Gupta, A. K. (2014). Multimodality imaging of renal inflammatory lesions. *World Journal of Radiology,* 6(11), 865–873.

CASE 134

Acute Cholecystitis

1. A, B. Images show a distended gallbladder, which can be seen with acute cholecystitis and gallbladder hydrops.
2. B. Papillary RCC is the most common type of RCC that can be bilateral.
3. B, C. Papillary and medullary RCCs are usually hypovascular on CT.
4. A, B, C, D. All are familial syndromes that can develop renal cell carcinomas.

Comment

- Background: Papillary RCC (chromophil RCC) is the second most common histologic subtype (10%–15% of RCCs).
  - Commonly affects end stage kidneys
  - Often contain areas of hemorrhage, necrosis, and cystic degeneration
  - Present in the third to eighth decades of life
  - Most common multifocal or bilateral renal tumor
  - Smaller mean diameter and of lower stage
  - Two types:
    - Type 1 tumors
      - Papillae covered by a single layer of cuboidal or low columnar cells with scanty cytoplasm and low-grade nuclei
      - Better prognosis
    - Type 2 tumors
      - Higher nuclear grade and contain more than one layer of cells with abundant eosinophilic cytoplasm
      - Carry a worse prognosis
    - Sarcomatoid dedifferentiation seen in ~5% of pRCCs; it has been associated with both type 1 and type 2 tumors and is associated with a worse prognosis
  - Familial forms
    - Hereditary papillary renal cell cancer syndrome
    - Hereditary leiomyomatosis
    - RCC syndrome
    - Birt-Hogg-Dubé syndrome
- Imaging:
  - US: tends to be hypoechoic
  - CT:
    - Nonenhanced CT, calcification is seen slightly more often in pRCC than in cRCC
    - pRCC are less vascular than cRCC: differences in enhancement peak in the corticomedullary phase
    - Degree of enhancement directly proportional to the MVD of the tumor
    - MVD in pRCC is less than in cRCC
    - Smaller lesions homogenous in attenuation
    - Larger lesions >3 cm are heterogenous with areas of necrosis and hemorrhage
    - Enhancement is usually >10 HU with a very small percentage of lesions showing enhancement <10 HU
    - In the absence of precontrast images, lesions show deenhancement or contrast material washout at delayed-phase imaging
  - MRI:
    - Show a pseudocapsule
    - T1 weighted images: low signal intensity
    - T2 weighted images: low signal intensity
    - cRCC has higher signal intensity on T2 weighted images
    - Enhancement is less intense in pRCC than in cRCC
    - Diffusion weighted imaging (DWI): restricted diffusion may be useful for differentiating from a hemorrhagic cyst

- Other uncommon types of RCC:
  - Multilocular cystic RCC: multiseptated cystic RCC
    - Septa contain small clusters of clear cells
    - Adults aged 20 to 76 years with a mean age of 51 years
    - Males predominate with a male to female ratio of 3:1
    - Characterized by septated, variable-sized cysts separated from the kidney by a fibrous capsule
    - Cyst fluid may be serous or hemorrhagic
    - Imaging:
      - Multilocular cystic tumors
      - Asymmetric septal thickening
      - Septal or wall calcification in 20%
  - Chromophobe RCC
    - Third most common histologic subtype
    - Mean age of incidence in the sixth decade
    - Men and women are equally affected
    - Imaging:
      - US: appears uniformly hyperechoic

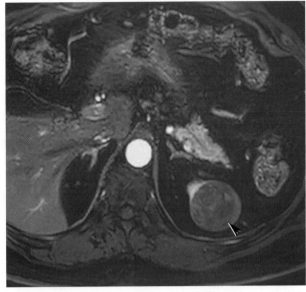

Fig. 134.3 Axial T1 weighted postcontrast image shows mild vascularity within the left renal mass *(red arrow)*. This was consistent with papillary renal cell carcinoma type 1.

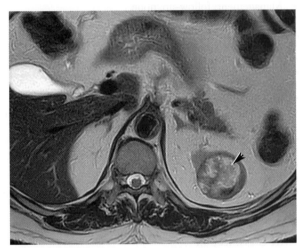

Fig. 134.1 Axial T2 weighted image with a mixed solid and cystic mass in the upper pole of the left kidney with a heterogenous appearance *(red arrow)*.

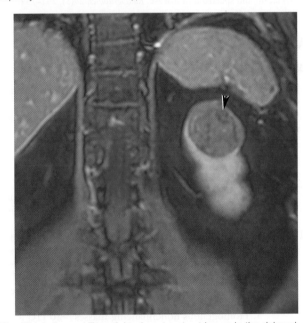

Fig. 134.4 Coronal T1 weighted postcontrast image in the delayed phase shows mild vascularity within the left renal mass *(red arrow)*. This was consistent with papillary renal cell carcinoma type 1.

- CT and MR imaging
  - Homogeneous enhancement
  - May show a spoke-wheel pattern of contrast enhancement
  - May appear hypointense on T2 weighted MRI
- Collecting duct carcinoma
  - Highly aggressive subtype
  - <1%
  - Age range 13 to 83 years (mean age, 55 years)
  - Male to female ratio ~2:1
  - Imaging:
    - An infiltrative growth pattern at imaging
    - Small lesion epicenter in the medulla
    - Larger neoplasms are indistinguishable from the more common RCC subtypes

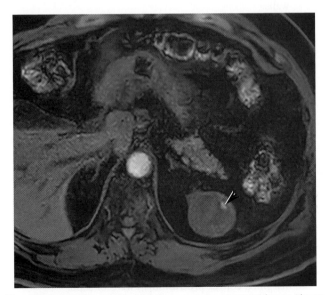

Fig. 134.2 Axial T1 weighted fat-suppressed precontrast image shows a hypointense mass in the left upper pole with an area of high signal intensity *(red arrow)* that is likely due to hemorrhage.

- US: hyperechoic, isoechoic, or hypoechoic to renal parenchyma
- CT and MRI: appears heterogeneous with areas of necrosis, hemorrhage, and calcification
- T2 weighted images: low signal intensity
- Medullary carcinoma
  - Extremely rare malignant neoplasm
  - In patients with sickle cell trait
  - Age 10 to 40 years (mean age, 22 years)
  - Male to female ratio is 2:1
  - Imaging: infiltrative, heterogeneous mass with a medullary epicenter
    - Hemorrhage and necrosis lead to heterogeneity
    - Typically associated with caliectasis
    - T2 weighted MRI: hypointense due to the presence of by-products of hemorrhage and necrosis

REFERENCES

Prasad, S. R., Humphrey, P. A., Catena, J. R., Narra, V. R., Srigley, J. R., … Cortez, A. D. (2006). Common and uncommon histologic subtypes of renal cell carcinoma: Imaging spectrum with pathologic correlation. *Radiographics, 26*(6), 1795–1806.

Vikram, R., Ng, C. S., Tamboli, P., Tannir, N. M., Jonasch, E., … Matin, S. F. (2009). Papillary renal cell carcinoma: Radiologic-pathologic correlation and spectrum of disease. *Radiographics, 29*(3), 741–754.

CASE 135

Bosniak Classification

1. D. Images show a cystic mass in the left kidney with multiple thick septations with it, which is consistent with a Bosniak III cyst.
2. C. Incidence of malignancy in Bosniak III cysts is approximately 50%.

3. B. Homogenous masses markedly hyperintense at T1 weighted imaging (approximately X2.5 normal parenchymal signal intensity) at noncontrast MRI would be classified as Bosniak II cyst.
4. D. Presence of enhancing nodule >4 mm in size would be classified as Bosniak IV cyst.

Comment

- Bosniak classification:
  - Divides renal masses into five categories based on imaging characteristics on contrast enhanced imaging
  - Helpful in predicting risk of malignancy
  - Helpful in suggesting either follow up or treatment
- Bosniak I:
  - Simple cyst
  - Management: follow-up: none
  - % malignant: 0%
- Bosniak II:
  - Minimally complex
  - Management: follow-up: none
  - % malignant: 0%
- Bosniak IIF
  - Minimally complex
  - Management: follow-up with US/CT/MRI at 6 months
  - % malignant: 5%
- Bosniak III
  - Indeterminate
  - Management: partial nephrectomy or radiofrequency ablation in elderly or poor surgical candidates
  - % malignant: 55%
- Bosniak IV
  - Malignant
  - Management: partial or total nephrectomy
  - % malignant: 100%

Class	CT Classification	MR Classification
I	Well defined, thin (<2 mm) smooth wall; homogenous simple fluid (-9 to 20 HU); no septa or calcifications, walls may enhance	Well-defined, thin (<2 mm) smooth wall; homogenous simple fluid (signal intensity similar to CSF); no septa or calcifications; walls may enhance
II	Six types, all well defined with thin (<2 mm) smooth walls 1. Cystic masses with thin (<2 mm) and few (1–3) septa; septa and wall may enhance; may have calcification of any type 2. Homogenous hyperattenuating (>70 HU) masses at noncontrast CT 3. Homogenous nonenhancing masses >20 HU at renal mass protocol CT, may have calcification of any type 4. Homogenous masses -9 to 20 HU at noncontrast CT 5. Homogenous masses 21 to 30 HU at portal venous phase CT 6. Homogenous low-attenuation masses that are too small to characterize	Three types, all well defined with thin (<2 mm) smooth walls: 1. Cystic masses with thin (<2 mm) and few (1–3) enhancing septa; any nonenhancing septa; may have calcifications of any type 2. Homogenous masses markedly hyperintense at T2 weighted imaging (similar to CSF) at noncontrast MRI 3. Homogenous masses markedly hyperintense at T1 weighted imaging (approximately X2.5 normal parenchymal signal intensity) at noncontrast MRI
IIF	Cystic masses with a smooth minimally thickened (3 mm) enhancing wall or smooth minimal thickening (3 mm) of one or more enhancing septa, or many (>4) smooth thin (<2 mm) enhancing septa	Two types: 1. Cystic masses with a smooth minimally thickened (3 mm) enhancing wall or smooth minimal thickening (3 mm) of one or more enhancing septa or many (>4) smooth thin (<2 mm) enhancing septa 2. Cystic masses that are hetergenously hyperintense at unenhanced fat-saturated T1 weighted imaging
III	One or more enhancing thick (>4 mm width) or enhancing irregular (displaying <3 mm obtusely margined convex protrusion[s]) walls or septa	One or more enhancing nodule(s) (>4 mm width) or enhancing irregular (displaying <3 mm obtusely margined convex protrusion[s]) walls or septa
IV	One or more enhancing nodule(s) (>4 mm convex protrusion with obtuse margins or a convex protrusion of any size that has acute margins)	One or more enhancing module(s) (>4 mm convex protrusion with obtuse margins or a convex protrusion of any size that has acute margins)

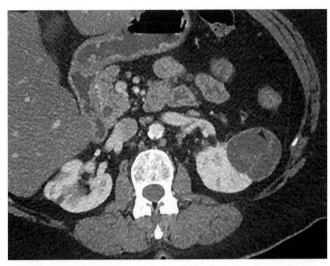

Fig. 135.1 Axial contrast-enhanced computed tomography (CT) image showing a cystic mass in the left kidney with thick septations *(arrow)* within it. This is suggestive of Bosnaik III cyst.

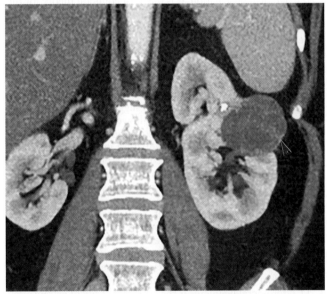

Fig. 135.2 Coronal reformat from a contrast-enhanced computed tomography (CT) image showing a cystic mass in the left kidney with thick septations *(arrow)* within it. This is suggestive of Bosnaik III cyst.

REFERENCES

Israel, G. M., & Bosniak, M. A. (2005). How I do it: Evaluating renal masses. *Radiology, 236*(2), 441–450.

Silverman, S. G., Pedrosa, I., Ellis, J. H., Hindman, N. M., Schieda, N., … Smith, A. D. (2019). Bosniak classification of cystic renal masses, version 2019: An update proposal and needs assessment. *Radiology, 292*(2), 475–488.

CASE 136

Bladder Carcinoma Staging

1. D. The muscle is seen as a hypointense band on T2 weighted imaging, and this is lost in muscle-invasive disease.
2. D. Retraction of the outer bladder wall is considered an indirect sign of muscle-invasive disease.

3. D. Invasion of lateral pelvic wall is considered to be T4 disease.
4. D. Presence of common iliac lymph nodes suggests N3 disease.

Comment

- Background: Transitional cell carcinoma of the bladder is staged using the TNM system. It has become the system of choice because it has the advantage of distinguishing nodal involvement from locally advanced tumors and distant metastatic spread.

Primary tumor (T)

TX	Primary tumor cannot be assessed
T0	No evidence of primary tumor
Ta	Noninvasive papillary carcinoma
Tis	Carcinoma in situ: flat tumor
T1	Tumor invades lamina propria (subepithelial connective tissue)
T2	Tumor invades muscularis propria
pT2a	Tumor invades superficial muscularis propria (inner half)
pT2b	Tumor invades deep muscularis propria (outer half)
T3	Tumor invades perivesical tissue
pT3a	Microscopically
pT3b	Macroscopically (extravesical mass)
T4	Tumor invades any of the following: prostatic stroma, seminal vesicles, uterus, vagina, pelvic wall, abdominal wall
T4a	Tumor invades prostatic stroma, uterus, vagina
T4b	Tumor invades pelvic wall, abdominal wall

Regional lymph nodes (N)

Regional lymph nodes include both primary and secondary drainage regions. All other nodes above the aortic bifurcation are considered distant lymph nodes.

NX	Lymph nodes cannot be assessed
N0	No lymph node metastasis
N1	Single regional lymph node metastasis in the true pelvis (perivesical, obturator, internal and external iliac, or sacral lymph node)
N2	Multiple regional lymph node metastasis in the true pelvis (perivesical, obturator, internal and external iliac, or sacral lymph node metastasis)
N3	Lymph node metastasis to the common iliac lymph nodes

Distant metastasis (M)

M0	No distant metastasis
M1	Distant metastasis
M1a	Distant metastasis limited to lymph nodes beyond the common iliacs
M1b	Non–lymph node distant metastases

- Imaging: Cystoscopy and biopsy are used at the initial examination to assess the tumor's cell type, grade, and depth of invasion.
  - Imaging primary tumor (T stage)
    - CT: primary tumor is detected either as thickening of the bladder wall or as an intraluminal mass
      - Individual bladder wall layers cannot be imaged individually on CT and hence the accuracy of T staging is limited
      - Retraction of the outer bladder wall is indirect evidence of muscle invasive disease (stage T2b)
    - MRI: T2a and T2b tumors can be differentiated using a combination of T2 weighted and contrast enhanced T1 weighted sequences
      - On T2 weighted images, the hypointense band (muscle) is preserved in T2a tumors

- Extravesical fat extension (T3) disease and invasion into adjacent organs and the abdominal and pelvic walls can be evaluated on CT and MRI
  - Seen as irregular, ill-defined outer bladder wall
  - Soft tissue nodules or fat stranding in the surrounding perivesical fat
- Imaging nodal metastases (N stage)
  - Lymphatic spread occurs contiguously by moving first into anterior and lateral perivesical lymph nodes, then to sacral and presacral nodes followed by hypogastric, obturator, and external iliac nodes
  - Common iliac and paraaortic lymph nodes are considered distant metastasis
- Imaging distant metastases (M stage)
  - TCC can spread hematogenously
  - Most common sites are liver, bones, and lungs in decreasing order of frequency
  - PET/CT is helpful in evaluating distant metastases

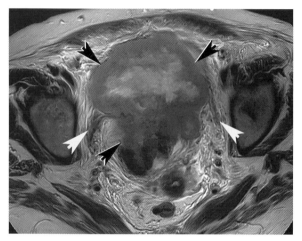

Fig. 136.1 Axial T2 weighted magnetic resonance imaging (MRI) showing large lobulated masses *(red arrows)* in the bladder with retraction of the bladder wall posteriorly and soft tissue areas seen extending into the pelvis *(yellow arrows)*. This is consistent with T4 bladder cancer.

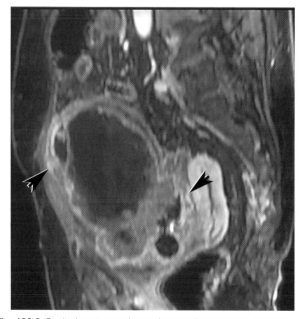

Fig. 136.2 Sagittal contrast enhanced magnetic resonance imaging (MRI) in the early phase showing enhancement in the tumor *(red arrows)* with extension posteriorly to the uterus. This suggests T4 bladder cancer.

REFERENCES
Verma, S., Rajesh, A., Prasad, S. R., Gaitonde, K., Lall, C. G., … Mouraviev, V. (2012). Urinary bladder cancer: Role of MR imaging. *Radiographics, 32*(2), 371–387. doi:10.1148/rg.322115125.
Vikram, R., Sandler, C. M., & Ng, C. S. (2009a). Imaging and staging of transitional cell carcinoma: Part 1, lower urinary tract. *American Journal of Roentgenology, 192*(6), 1481–1487. doi:10.2214/AJR.08.1318.
Vikram, R., Sandler, C., & Ng, C. (2009b). Imaging and staging of transitional cell carcinoma: Part 2, upper urinary tract. *American Journal of Roentgenology, 192*(6),1488–1493. doi:10.2214/AJR.09.2577.

CASE 138
Rectal Endometriosis

1. B, C, D. Rectal carcinoma originates from the epithelial cells of the colorectal mucosa and is seen as a lesion extending from the mucosa to the underlying layers. The lesion shown in this image is external to the rectum, serosal in location. Rectal gastrointestinal stromal tumors (GIST) are mesenchymal tumors and originate from the mesenchymal tissue. Rectal endometriosis and peritoneal metastases are serosal-based lesions that may invade into the underlying rectal wall.
2. B. The metastatic theory suggests that endometriosis results from the metastatic implantation of endometrial tissue from retrograde menstruation. It is the most common theory for the pathophysiology of endometriosis. Viable endometrial tissue refluxes through the fallopian tube during menstruation and is deposited on the peritoneal surface of pelvic organs. Iatrogenic spread of endometrial implants during needle biopsy or surgery is a rare possibility; however, endometriosis is seen in women who have never had any pelvic intervention. There have been reports of extrapelvis endometriosis, even in distant organs such as the lungs and brain suggesting vascular or lymphatic spread of endometrial cells; however, this is infrequently seen. The less common metaplastic theory suggests the possibility of peritoneal cells differentiating into functional endometrial cells, which is supported by the presence of endometriosis in women without functional endometrium due to Turner syndrome or gonadal dysgenesis as well as in men.
3. A. Fat-suppressed T1 weighted images are the most sensitive for the detection of T1 bright hemorrhagic foci, which are most conspicuous in the fat-suppressed dark background. Fat-suppressed T2 weighted images are not as sensitive for the detection of hemorrhagic foci because they appear dark on T2 and are inconspicuous. On nonfat-suppressed T1 bright hemorrhagic foci may be indistinguishable from T1 bright fat tissue.
4. D. Uterosacral ligaments is the commonest site of extraovarian involvement from endometriosis.

Comment
Introduction
- Deep infiltrating endometriosis (DIE) is defined as subperitoneal endometrial implants, >5 mm in depth affecting the gastrointestinal tract, urinary tract, and pelvic cul-de-sac and is usually associated with reactive inflammation, fibrosis, adhesions, and smooth muscle hyperplasia.
- Gastrointestinal DIE typically involves the rectosigmoid, small bowel, colon, and appendix.
- DIE of the urinary tract can affect the ureters and urinary bladder while DIE of the cul-de-sac can involve the uterosacral ligaments, vagina, and the cervix.
- The rectovaginal septum and uterosacral ligaments are commonly affected in ~69% of cases with DIE.

Case 137 is online only and accessible at www.expertconsult.com.

- The symptoms of the pelvic endometriosis include pelvic pain, dysmenorrhea, dyspareunia, dyschezia, and can be associated with infertility. Urinary symptoms may also occur.
- Pathophysiology: Different theories have been proposed as the etiology of endometriosis, including the retrograde menstruation theory and metaplasia theory.
  - Retrograde menstruation theory proposes that endometriosis occurs due to the retrograde flow of sloughed endometrial cells/debris via the fallopian tubes into the pelvic cavity during menstruation
  - The coelomic metaplasia theory postulates that endometriosis originates from the metaplasia of specialized cells that are present in the mesothelial lining of the visceral and abdominal peritoneum
  - Other theories include possibility of hormones influencing endometrial proliferation and ectopic sites, increased oxidation of lipoproteins causing DNA damage in the endometriotic cells, and possible defective immune response in patients with endometriosis
- Diagnosis: MRI is the imaging modality of choice for evaluation of DIE due to inherent high sensitivity for detecting blood products and global evaluation of structures compared to the limited reach of transvaginal ultrasound.
  - MRI has high accuracy, sensitivity of 90.3%, specificity of 91%, positive predictive value of 92.1%, and negative predictive value of 89% in the detection of the pelvic endometriosis
  - DIE of the gastrointestinal tract appears as irregular, eccentric mass/masses infiltrating into the intestinal wall causing lumen of narrowing with associated fibrosis and smooth muscle hyperplasia appearing at times as irregular, speculated, hypointense lesions on T2 weighted images
    - Fat-saturated T1 weighted images show a mass or thickening, which is isointense to muscle, possibly with interspersed hyperintense foci that reflect hemorrhagic blood products.
    - The mushroom cap sign refers to the appearance of rectosigmoid lesions on T2 weighted images as a hypointense fibrotic mass in the muscularity slayer that

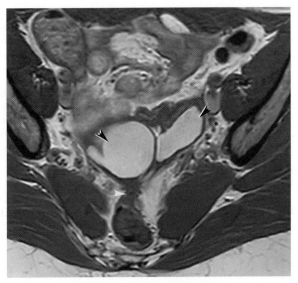

Fig. 138.2 Axial T1 weighted magnetic resonance imaging (MRI) of the pelvis shows two hyperintense cystic masses *(red arrows)* suggesting presence of blood within them and consistent with endometriomas. Note the T1 hypointense area *(yellow arrow)* seen posterior to the endometriomas anterior to the rectum consistent with fibrotic tissue from rectal endometriosis.

protrudes into the intestinal lumen with hyperintense submucosal and mucosa layers that cover the mass and create an outline similar to that of a mushroom cap.
- Other findings include bowel wall thickening, loss of fat planes between bowel segments and adjacent organs, and abnormal angulation of the bowel loops.
- The posterior compartment may be significantly involved by DIE, which includes the rectum, pouch of Douglas, torus uterinus, uterosacral ligaments, posterior vaginal fornix, and rectovaginal septum.
- Fibrotic changes are commonly seen in this area, which manifest as predominantly T2 dark bands.

REFERENCES

Darvishzadeh, A., McEachern, W., Lee, T. K., Bhosale, P., Shirkhoda, A., … Menias, C. (2016). Deep pelvic endometriosis: A radiologist's guide to key imaging features with clinical and histopathologic review. *Abdominal Radiology (New York)*, *41*(12), 2380–2400. doi:10.1007/s00261-016-0956-8.

Sourial, S., Tempest, N., & Hapangama, D. K. (2014). Theories on the pathogenesis of endometriosis. *International Journal of Reproductive Medicine*, *2014*, 179515. doi:10.1155/2014/179515.

CASE 139
Cervical Carcinoma Staging

1. A, B, C, D. The FIGO staging system stages malignancies of the cervix, endometrium, vulva, ovary, fallopian tube, peritoneum, and uterine sarcomas. The purpose of the staging system is to provide uniform terminology for better communication among health professionals, to allow comparison of patients between centers and to assign patients and their tumors to prognostic groups requiring specific treatments.
2. C. Stage III cervical carcinomas extend to the pelvic wall, involve the lower one-third of the vagina, or cause hydronephrosis or a nonfunctioning kidney.
3. D. Stage IV cervical cancer extends beyond the true pelvis or involves the bladder or rectal mucosa (biopsy proven). In

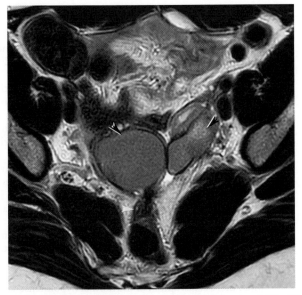

Fig. 138.1 Axial T2 weighted magnetic resonance imaging (MRI) of the pelvis shows two cystic masses *(red arrows)* with "shading artifact" within them consistent with endometriomas. Note the T2 hypointense area *(yellow arrow)* with small hyperintense areas within it seen posterior to the endometriomas anterior to the rectum consistent with fibrotic tissue from rectal endometriosis.

stage IVA there is spread to adjacent organs, and in stage IVB there is spread to distant organs. Distant metastases include peritoneal spread; involvement of supraclavicular, mediastinal, or paraaortic lymph nodes; and lung, liver, or bone metastasis.

4. D. Stage IV cervical cancer extends beyond the true pelvis or involves the bladder or rectal mucosa (biopsy proven). In stage IVA there is spread to adjacent organs and in stage IVB there is spread to distant organs. Distant metastases include peritoneal spread; involvement of supraclavicular, mediastinal, or paraaortic lymph nodes; and lung, liver, or bone metastasis.

Stage I

IA Invasive carcinoma that can be diagnosed only by microscopy, with maximum depth of invasion <5 mm

IB Invasive carcinoma with measured deepest invasion ≥5 mm (greater than stage IA), lesion limited to the cervix uteri

Stage II

IIA Involvement limited to the upper two-thirds of the vagina without parametrial involvement

IIB With parametrial involvement but not up to the pelvic wall

Stage III

IIIA Carcinoma involves the lower third of the vagina, with no extension to the pelvic wall

IIIB Extension to the pelvic wall and/or hydronephrosis or nonfunctioning kidney (unless known to be due to another cause)

IIIC Involvement of pelvic and/or paraaortic lymph nodes, irrespective of tumor size and extent (with r and p notations)

Stage IV

IVA Spread of the growth to adjacent organs

IVB Spread to distant organs

Comment

- Introduction: Although similar systems exist for staging cervical cancer, the American Joint Committee on Cancer (AJCC) tumor node metastasis (TNM) staging system and the FIGO system, gynecologists and gynecologic oncologists use the FIGO system.
- New FIGO Classification for Cervical Carcinoma (revised in 2018): The new revised FIGO classification of cervical carcinoma was reached by consensus at the FIGO regional meeting in April 2018 and is as follows:

IA1 Measured stromal invasion <3 mm in depth

IA2 Measured stromal invasion ≥3 mm and <5 mm in depth

IB1 Invasive carcinoma ≥5 mm depth of stromal invasion and <2 cm in greatest dimension

IB2 Invasive carcinoma ≥2 cm and <4 cm in greatest dimension

IB3 Invasive carcinoma ≥4 cm in greatest dimension

The carcinoma invades beyond the uterus, but has not extended onto the lower third of the vagina or to the pelvic wall

IIA1 Invasive carcinoma <4 cm in greatest dimension

IIA2 Invasive carcinoma ≥4 cm in greatest dimension

The carcinoma involves the lower third of the vagina and/or extends to the pelvic wall and/or causes hydronephrosis or nonfunctioning kidney and/or involves pelvic and/or paraaortic lymph nodes

IIIC1 Pelvic lymph node metastasis only

IIIC2 Paraaortic lymph node metastasis

The carcinoma has extended beyond the true pelvis or has involved (biopsy proven) the mucosa of the bladder or rectum. A bullous edema, as such, does not permit a case to be allotted to stage IV

- Imaging:
  - MRI: obviates the use of invasive procedures such as cystoscopy and proctoscopy, especially when there are no signs of local invasion
    - Can also be used to identify important prognostic factors such as lesion volume and metastatic lymph node involvement that help determine whether treatment will be palliative a curative
    - Tumor: Cervical carcinoma has intermediate signal intensity on T2 weighted imaging and disrupts the low signal intensity fibrous stroma of the normal cervix
      - Tumor can be exophytic, infiltrating, or endocervical with a barrel shape
      - Bulk of the lesion is centered at the level of the cervix with either protrusion into the vagina or invasion of the lower myometrium. This helps in differentiating from an endometrial mass (polyp or adenocarcinoma), which is centered in the endometrial cavity.
      - Smaller tumors may be more easily identified on dynamic contrast enhanced imaging due to the early enhancement
    - Vagina: disruption of the hypointense vaginal wall with hyperintense thickening at T2 weighted imaging and contrast material enhancement at T1 weighted imaging are signs of vaginal invasion. Invasion of the lower one-third of the vagina increases the stage and will modify the strategy for radiation therapy.
  - Parametria: In presence of parametrial invasion, the hypointense fibrous stromal ring seen at T2 weighted MRI is interrupted
    - Preservation of this hypointense fibrous stromal ring has a high negative predictive value for parametrial invasion
    - With disruption of the stromal ring but no definite parametrial mass, there may be microscopic invasion
    - Complete disruption of the ring with nodular or irregular tumor extending into the parametrium are reliable signs of invasion
  - Pelvic wall: Tumor extending to involve the internal obturator, piriform, or levator ani muscles with or without dilated ureter indicates pelvic wall invasion
  - Bladder and rectum: Bladder or rectal invasion is present when there is disruption of the normal hypointense walls seen on T2 weighted imaging with or without the mass protruding into the lumen. Dynamic gadolinium-enhanced T1 weighted sequences are helpful for confirming invasion and identifying fistulous tracks.
  - Lymph nodes: Lymph node disease detection is based on size criteria with >10 mm considered to be suspicious

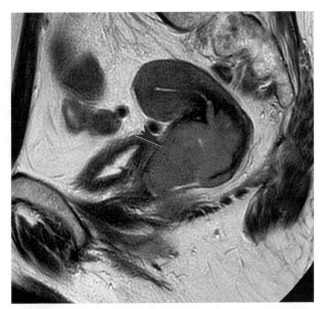

Fig. 139.1 Sagittal T2 weighted magnetic resonance image (MRI) of the uterus shows intermediate signal intensity cervical mass *(red arrow)* replacing the expected T2 dark cervical fibrous stroma with a large mass seen bulging into the vagina. Note the involvement of the lower one-third of the vagina suggesting Stage III cancer as per the FIGO guidelines

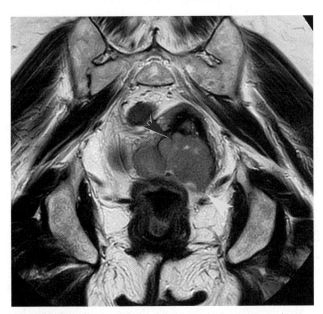

Fig. 139.2 Coronal oblique T2 weighted magnetic resonance image shows large cervical mass *(red arrow)* proven to be squamous cell carcinoma with parametrial tumor invasion *(yellow arrow)* suggesting Stage III cancer as per the FIGO guidelines

REFERENCES

Bhatla, N., Berek, J. S., Cuello Fredes, M., Denny, L. A., Grenman, S., … Karunaratne, K. (2019). Revised FIGO staging for carcinoma of the cervix uteri. *International Journal of Gynaecology and Obstetrics*, *145*(1), 129–135. doi:10.1002/ijgo.12749.

Nicolet, V., Carignan, L., Bourdon, F., & Prosmanne, O. (2000). MR imaging of cervical carcinoma: A practical staging approach. *Radiographics*, *20*(6), 1539–1549. doi:10.1148/radiographics.20.6.g00nv111539.

Raithatha, A., Papadopoulou, I., Stewart, V., Barwick, T. D., Rockall, A. G., & Bharwani, N. (2016). Cervical cancer staging: A resident's primer: Women's imaging. *Radiographics*, *36*(3), 933–934. doi:10.1148/rg.2016150173.

CASE 140
Endometrial Carcinoma Staging

1. A, B, C, D. Staging of endometrial cancer is always surgical and consists of hysterectomy, BSO, node dissection, peritoneal washing, and omental biopsy.
2. D. MRI has been shown to be superior to CT in local staging of endometrial carcinoma; however, for detection of metastasis to pelvic or paraaortic lymph nodes and detection of tumor invasion to the bladder bowel or distant metastasis, both MRI and CT have similar accuracy.
3. C. Stage III endometrial carcinoma is local or regional spread of tumor outside the uterus, to include tumor invasion of the serosa of the corpus uteri or adnexae, vaginal or parametrial involvement, and metastasis to pelvic or paraaortic lymph nodes.
4. D. Stage II endometrial carcinoma involves the connective tissue of the cervical stroma but has not invaded outside of the uterus. Treatment options at this stage include surgery first (a radical hysterectomy, BSO, and pelvic and priority lymph node dissection [LND] or sampling) followed by radiation (both vaginal brachytherapy and external pelvic radiation). An alternative approach is radiation therapy first followed by simple hysterectomy, BSO, and possible LND or lymph node sampling. Hysterectomy and BSO are the standard components of treatment for endometrial cancer.

Comment

- Staging: Endometrial cancer is staged with the International Federation of Gynecology and Obstetrics (FIGO) system, which is as follows:
  - Stage 0: carcinoma in situ
  - Stage I: limited to the body of the uterus
    - Ia: no or less than half ($\leq 50\%$) myometrial invasion
    - Ib: invasion equal to or more than half ($\geq 50\%$) of the myometrium
  - Stage II: cervical stromal involvement
    - Endocervical glandular involvement only is stage I
  - Stage III: local or regional spread of the tumor
  - IIIa: tumor invades the serosa of the body of the uterus and/or adnexa
  - IIIb: vaginal or parametrial involvement
  - IIIc: pelvic or paraaortic lymphadenopathy
    - IIIc1: positive pelvic nodes
    - IIIc2: positive paraaortic nodes with or without pelvic nodes
  - Stage IV: involvement of rectum and or bladder mucosa and or distant metastasis
    - IVa: bladder or rectal mucosal involvement
    - IVb: distant metastases, malignant ascites, peritoneal involvement
- Prognosis in endometrial carcinoma depends on a number of factors, including stage, depth of myometrial invasion, lymphovascular invasion, histologic grading, and nodal status. Most women (80% of cases) with endometrial carcinoma present in the early stage of the disease (Stage I, cancer confined to the corpus uteri).
- Imaging findings: MRI provides the best assessment of the depth of the tumor invasion.
  - Both MRI and CT have similar accuracy in detection of metastasis to pelvic or paraaortic lymph nodes and detection of tumor extension to the bladder or bowel or distant metastasis
  - Prevalence of malignant lymphadenopathy is low if the tumor is confined to the endometrium or superficial

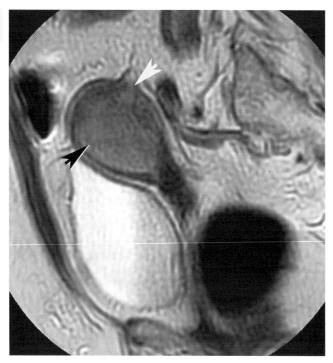

Fig. 140.1 Sagittal T2 weighted magnetic resonance imaging (MRI) of the pelvis shows expanded endometrial cavity filled with a mass with intermediate T2 signal *(red arrow)*. This was consistent with endometrial carcinoma and showed an area of extension into the myometrium posteriorly *(yellow arrow)* suggesting tumor invasion.

myometrium and increases to 46% when endometrial cancer invades the outer myometrium
- Tumor can be differentiated from the underlying myometrium based on T2 weighted images and on the late phase postcontrast imaging (3–4 minutes after contrast injection) where the tumor appears hypointense in comparison to the underlying myometrium allowing for assessment of tumor to myometrium interface and the depth of myometrial invasion as well as the cervical stromal invasion
- 18F-FDG PET/CT (18 fluorodeoxyglucose positron emission computed tomography) is a highly sensitive and specific modality for detecting recurrence and posttherapy patients with endometrial carcinoma. It is also helpful for detecting distant metastasis in the abdomen and extraabdominal regions in high-risk patients with endometrial carcinoma.

REFERENCES

Freeman, S. J., Aly, A. M., Kataoka, M. Y., Addley, H. C., Reinhold, C., & Sala E. (2012). The revised FIGO staging system for uterine malignancies: Implications for MR imaging. *Radiographics, 32*(6), 1805–1827. doi:10.1148/rg.326125519.

Kinkel, K., Forstner, R., Danza, F. M., Oleaga, L., Cunha, T. M., ... Bergman, A. (2009). Staging of endometrial cancer with MRI: Guidelines of the European Society of Urogenital Imaging. *European Radiology, 19*(7), 1565–1574. doi:10.1007/s00330-009-1309-6.

Manfredi, R., Mirk, P., Maresca, G., Margariti, P. A., Testa, A., ... Zannoni, G. F. (2004). Local-regional staging of endometrial carcinoma: Role of MR imaging in surgical planning. *Radiology, 231*(2), 372–378. doi:10.1148/radiol.2312021184.

CASE 141

Ovarian Metastasis

1. A, B, C. Primary ovarian tumors, ovarian metastases, and lymph nodal masses can present as bilateral solid pelvic masses.
2. A, B, C, D. All of these can result in ovarian metastasis.
3. D. Radiologic feature that suggests metastatic carcinoma is bilaterality.
4. A, B, C, D. All of the mentioned features can be seen in Krukenberg tumors on CT scan.

Comment

- Ovary is one preferential site for metastatic disease.
- Common primary sites for metastatic disease to the ovaries include the colon, stomach, breast, and the genitourinary tract; hematologic malignancies include lymphoma and leukemia.
- May metastasize to the ovary through hematogenous, lymphatic, or transperitoneal spreads, as well as by direct extension
- Radiologic feature that suggests metastatic carcinoma is bilaterality, seen in 60% to 80% of cases
  - Bilaterality can be seen in some primary ovarian carcinomas as well: serous papillary adenocarcinomas and endometrioid carcinomas
- Krukenberg tumor (metastatic gastric cancer)
  - Grossly characterized by moderate solid multinodular enlargement
  - Microscopic evaluation reveals diffuse infiltration by signet ring cells
  - Commonly bilateral and are associated with marked stromal proliferation and variable degrees of luteinization
  - Imaging:
    - Commonly bilateral, lobulated, and solid tumors

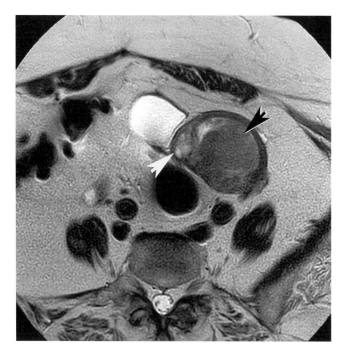

Fig. 140.2 Axial T2 weighted magnetic resonance imaging (MRI) of the pelvis shows expanded endometrial cavity filled with a mass with intermediate T2 signal *(red arrow)*. This was consistent with endometrial carcinoma and showed an area of extension into the myometrium posteriorly and along the right lateral myometrium *(yellow arrow)* suggesting tumor invasion.

- CT
  - Oval or kidney-shaped masses, which tend to preserve the ovary contour
  - Solid or predominantly solid with central necrosis or cysts
  - May attain a large size
  - Strong enhancement of solid components or septations is usually seen after contrast media administration.
- MRI
  - T2 weighted MRI, the solid tumor components typically show heterogeneously low to high signal intensity
  - On postcontrast images solid components usually demonstrate homogeneous enhancement
- Metastases from colorectal carcinoma
  - More frequently in women <40 years of age
  - Imaging on CT and MR:
    - Unilocular or multilocular cystic masses with a stained-glass appearance, associated with variable degrees of solid components
    - Enhancement of the septations and solid components within the predominantly cystic tumors
- Metastases from appendiceal tumors
  - Often associated with pseudomyxoma peritonei
  - Frequently bilateral
  - Unilateral involvement, the right ovary is more commonly involved
  - Imaging:
    - Cystic ovarian tumors and irregularly localized fluid within the peritoneal cavity
    - Mucinous tumor implantation on the peritoneum or omentum
- Metastases from breast carcinoma
  - Rarely produces symptoms related to ovarian tumors
  - Bilaterality and a relatively small lesion size (i.e., usually <5 cm)
  - Imaging:
    - Solid masses with a multinodular appearance, occasionally containing cysts

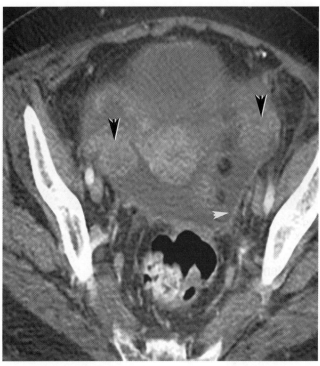

Fig. 141.2 Axial postcontrast computed tomography (CT) image through the lower abdomen shows enlarged ovaries *(red arrow)* with free fluid in the abdomen with peritoneal enhancement and nodularity *(yellow arrow)*. These were new from the prior exam performed 6 months ago and arose from the ovaries bilaterally and were consistent with Krukenberg tumors.

- Secondary ovarian involvement by hematologic malignancies
  - Usually non-Hodgkin lymphoma of B-cell lineage, in particular diffuse large cell lymphoma and follicular lymphoma
  - Commonly bilateral
  - Imaging:
    - Predominantly solid tumors of diffusely intermediate signal intensity, structures resembling septations of increased intensity on T2 weighted images
    - Enlarged lymph nodes

REFERENCE
Koyama, T., Mikami, Y., Saga, T., Tamai, K., & Togashi, K. (2007). Secondary ovarian tumors: Spectrum of CT and MR features with pathologic correlation. *Abdominal Imaging, 32*(6), 784–795. doi:10.1007/s00261-007-9186-4.

CASE 142

Ovarian Carcinoma Staging

1. A, B, C. All epithelial ovarian cancers can present as solid and cystic masses in the ovaries with peritoneal metastasis. Mature teratoma is a benign tumor and does not have peritoneal metastasis.
2. C. Extrapelvic metastasis from ovarian carcinoma most frequently occur by intraperitoneal seeding with ~70% of patients having peritoneal metastasis at staging laparotomy.
3. C. Ovarian cancer with peritoneal implants outside the pelvis is considered FIGO stage III.
4. C. Ovarian cancer with retroperitoneal lymph nodes outside the pelvis is considered FIGO stage III.

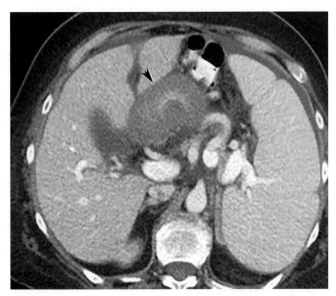

Fig. 141.1 Axial postcontrast computed tomography (CT) image through the upper abdomen shows a thickening in the gastric antrum *(red arrows)*. This was consistent with gastric adenocarcinoma.

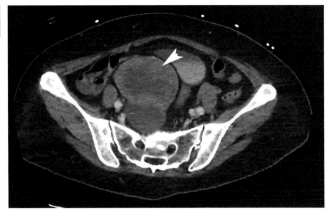

Fig. 142.1 Axial postcontrast computed tomography image of the pelvis demonstrates a complex cystic and solid right adnexal mass *(arrow)*.

Comment

- Ovarian carcinoma stage is determined surgically and pathologically.
- Five-year survival rate is 80% for stage I disease and declines to 8% for stage IV disease. Patients typically present late as stage III or IV disease after the disease has spread out of the pelvis.
- Two staging systems exist: the TNM (tumor, node, metastasis) system and the more commonly used FIGO (International Federation of Gynecology and Obstetrics) system.
  - FIGO staging system is the most commonly adopted ovarian carcinoma staging system.
- Role of imaging: currently no imaging modality allows microscopic spread of disease to be ruled out, and the full staging laparotomy is always required. Diagnostic imaging serves as an adjunctive surgical staging by helping characterize ovarian masses, predict tumor resectability, determine the extent of preoperative disease, and evaluate lymph node metastasis.
  - US: important role in the initial evaluation of adnexa mass as well as in screening of high-risk patients. Not the imaging modality to stage of ovarian cancer.
  - CT: recommended imaging modality for staging ovarian cancer
    - Provides clinically relevant information, including size of the primary tumor, size and location of any peritoneal implants, and lymph nodes
    - Particularly useful in patients with large amount of ascites, small peritoneal metastasis may be missed
  - MRI: provides excellent tissue differentiation and can be used as a problem-solving tool for characterization of indeterminate lesions seen on CT and US
    - Staging accuracy similar to CT scan
  - PET/CT: limited and characterizing ovarian masses but is helpful in staging ovarian cancer and for detecting recurrent disease
- FIGO staging system

Stage I	Tumor limited to the ovaries or fallopian tubes
IA	Tumor limited to one ovary (capsule intact) or fallopian tube
	No tumor on the external surface of the ovary or fallopian tube
	No malignant cells in the ascites or peritoneal washings
IB	Tumor limited to both ovaries (capsule intact) or fallopian tubes
	No tumor on the external surface of the ovaries or fallopian tubes
	No malignant cells in the ascites or peritoneal washings
IC	Tumor limited to one or both ovaries or fallopian tubes, but any of the following:
	Stage 1C1: surgical spill
	Stage IC2: capsule ruptured before surgery or tumor on ovarian or fallopian tube surface
	Stage IC3: malignant cells in the ascites or peritoneal washings
Stage II	Tumor involves one or both ovaries or fallopian tubes with pelvic extension (below the pelvic brim) or primary peritoneal cancer
IIA	Extension and/or implants on the uterus and/or ovaries and/or fallopian tubes
IIB	Extension to other pelvic intraperitoneal tissues
Stage III	Tumor involves one or both ovaries or fallopian tubes or primary peritoneal cancer with cytologically or histologically confirmed spread to the peritoneum outside the pelvis and/or metastasis to the retroperitoneal lymph nodes
IIIA1	Positive (cytologically or histologically proven) retroperitoneal lymph nodes only
	IIIA1(i): metastasis up to 10 mm in greatest dimension
	IIIA1(ii): metastasis >10 mm in greatest dimension
IIIA2	Microscopic extrapelvic (about the pelvic brim) peritoneal involvement with or without positive retroperitoneal lymph nodes
III B	Macroscopic peritoneal metastasis beyond the pelvis up to 2 cm in greatest dimension with or without metastasis to the retroperitoneal lymph nodes
III C	Macroscopic peritoneal metastasis beyond the pelvis >2 cm in greatest dimension with or without metastasis to the retroperitoneal lymph nodes
Stage IV	Distant metastasis excluding peritoneal metastasis
IV A	Pleural effusion with positive psychology
IV B	Parenchyma metastasis and metastasis to extraabdominal organs (including inguinal lymph nodes and lymph nodes outside of the abdominal cavity)

REFERENCE
Javadi, S., Ganeshan, D. M., Qayyum, A., Iyer, R. B., & Bhosale, P. (2016). Ovarian cancer, the revised FIGO staging system, and the role of imaging. *American Journal of Roentgenology, 206*(6), 1351–1360. doi:10.2214/AJR.15.15199.

CASE 143

Ovarian Serous Low-Grade Tumor

1. A, C, D. Serous cystadenoma, granulosa cell tumor, and cystadenocarcinoma could be included in the differential diagnosis of the imaging finding shown. The complexity of the lesion with amount of solid area within it makes cystadenocarcinoma most likely. Granulosa cell tumor is usually seen in postmenopausal patients and hence is unlikely in this patient. Serous cystadenoma usually appear as unilocular or multilocular cystic mass with thin regular wall or septum and no solid areas within it.
2. A, B, C, D. All features listed increase the likelihood of an ovarian mass being malignant.
3. B. Peritoneal carcinomatosis is more frequently seen in serous cystadenocarcinoma compared to mucinous cystadenocarcinoma.
4. A, B. Serous and mucinous tumors are the two most common types of epithelial tumors.

Comment

- Ovarian tumors are classified on the basis of tumor origin as the following:
  - Epithelial tumors: serous and mucinous tumors, endometrioid and clear cell carcinomas, Brenner tumor
  - Germ cell tumors: mature and immature teratomas, dysgerminoma, endodermal sinus tumor, embryonal carcinoma
  - Sex cord stromal tumors: fibrothecoma, granulosa cell tumor, sclerosing stromal, and Sertoli-Leydig cell tumors
  - Metastatic tumors
- Epithelial tumors represent 60% of all the ovarian neoplasms and 85% of malignant ovarian neoplasms.
- Rare in prepubescent patients, prevalence increases with age and peaks in the sixth or seventh decade of life.
- Can also be classified as benign (60% of cases), malignant (35%), or borderline (low malignant potential: 5%)
- Two most common types of epithelial neoplasms are serous and mucinous tumors.
- Serous epithelial tumors: 60% of all the serous ovarian neoplasms are smooth-walled benign cystadenomas, 15% are of low malignant potential, and 25% are malignant. They appear as unilocular or multilocular cystic mass with homogeneous CT attenuation or MRI signal intensity of the locules, a thin regular wall or septum, and no endocystic or exocystic vegetation is considered to be a benign serous cystadenoma.
- Mucinous cystadenomas tend to be larger than serous cystadenomas at presentation: 80% of all mucinous ovarian neoplasms are smooth-walled benign cystadenomas, 10% to 15% are of low malignant potential, and 5% to 10% are malignant. They appear as multilocular cystic mass that has a thin regular wall and septa or that contains liquids of different attenuation or signal intensity, but no endocystic or exocystic vegetation is considered to be a benign mucinous cystadenoma.
- Bilaterality and peritoneal carcinomatosis are seen more frequently in serous than in mucinous cystadenocarcinomas.
- Mucinous adenocarcinoma can rupture and is associated with pseudomyxoma peritonei.

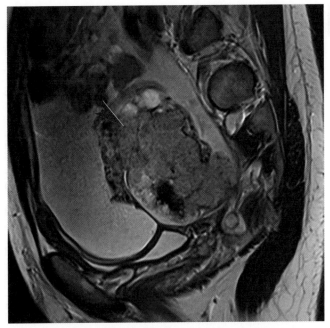

Fig. 143.2 Sagittal T2 weighted magnetic resonance imaging (MRI) shows solid mass *(red arrow)* arising from the right ovary with intermediate signal intensity seen within it. Note presence of ascites.

- Features that are more suggestive of benign epithelial tumors include a diameter <4 cm, entirely cystic components, a wall thickness <3 mm, lack of internal structure, and the absence of both ascites and invasive characteristics such as peritoneal disease or adenopathy.
- Imaging findings that are suggestive of malignant tumors include a thick, irregular wall; thick septa; papillary projections; and a large soft tissue component with necrosis. Ancillary findings of pelvic organ invasion, implants (peritoneal, omental, mesenteric), ascites, and adenopathy increase diagnostic confidence for malignancy.

REFERENCE

Jung, S. E., Lee, J. M., Rha, S. E., Byun, J. Y., Jung, J. I., & Hahn, S. T. (2002). CT and MR imaging of ovarian tumors with emphasis on differential diagnosis. *Radiographics*, 22(6), 1305–1325. doi:10.1148/rg.226025033.

CASE 144

Granulosa Cell Tumor

1. A, B, C, D. All the various ovarian tumors mentioned can be included in the differential diagnosis of imaging findings presented. These tumors can present as large cystic masses with heterogenous components in it; however, steroid cell tumors are usually small solid masses.
2. A. Granulosa cell tumors arise from granulosa cells, which are a type of primitive sex cord cells.
3. C. Fibromas show delayed enhancement on contrast administration due to abundant collagen and fibrous content.
4. A, B. Fibromas can be associated with Meigs syndrome (ascites, an ovarian tumor, and right pleural effusion), and metastatic ovarian adenocarcinoma can present with metastatic pleural effusion.

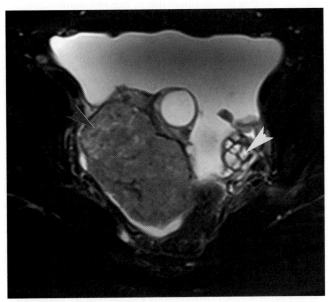

Fig. 143.1 Axial T2 weighted magnetic resonance imaging (MRI) shows solid mass *(red arrow)* arising from the right ovary with intermediate signal intensity seen within it. Left ovary appears normal *(yellow arrow)*. Note presence of ascites.

Comment

- Sex cord stromal tumors of the ovary are rare and make up about 8% of all ovarian neoplasms.

- Affect all age groups and are hormonally active tumors
- 70% of patients with these tumors are usually Stage I at presentation.
- Type of sex cord stromal tumors: arise from two groups of cells
  - Stromal cells: contain fibroblasts, theca cells, Leydig cells
  - Primitive sex cord cells: include granulosa cells and Sertoli cells
- Imaging: tumors have characteristic imaging features
  - Granulosa cell tumors: <5% of all malignant ovarian tumors, adult types are more common (usually in postmenopausal patients) than juvenile types
    - Present with abnormal vaginal bleeding due to endometrial hyperplasia, polyps, and carcinoma from estrogen secretion
    - Show a spectrum of imaging manifestations from solid masses with hemorrhagic or fibrotic changes, multilocular cystic lesions, or completely cystic tumors
    - Heterogeneity in these tumors is due to intratumoral bleeding, infarct, fibrous degeneration, and irregular arrangement of cells.
    - Can rupture and lead to hemoperitoneum
  - Fibroma, fibrothecoma, and thecoma: spectrum of benign tumors occurs in premenopausal and postmenopausal women
    - Fibromas are nonfunctioning; however, thecomas can show estrogenic activity
    - Fibromas can be associated with Meigs syndrome (ascites, an ovarian tumor, and right pleural effusion)
    - Due to abundant collagen and fibrous content, appear homogenous solid masses with delayed enhancement on CT and as hypointense mass on T1 weighted MRI with a very low signal intensity on T2 weighted imaging.
    - Dense calcification and high-signal-intensity areas due to cystic degeneration and edema can be seen
  - Sclerosing stromal tumor of the ovary: occur in young women, cause menstrual irregularity
    - Imaging findings include a large mass with hyperintense cystic components or a heterogenous solid mass of intermediate high signal intensity on T2 weighted MRI
    - Striking enhancement on postcontrast images with early peripheral enhancement and centripetal progression

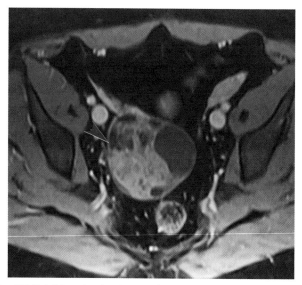

Fig. 144.2 Axial postcontrast magnetic resonance imaging (MRI) shows a large mixed solid and cystic mass *(red arrow)* arising from the right ovary with significant enhancement seen in the solid components in the mass. This was shown to be a granulosa cell tumor on histopathology.

- Sertoli-Leydig cell tumor: most common virilizing ovarian tumor, very rare, and occur in young women
  - Clinical features are usually due to androgenic activity
  - Usually unilateral tumors that can be solid, solid and cystic, and cystic or even papillary
  - Well-defined solid enhancing mass with intratumoral cysts on CT and as hypointense with multiple variable-sized cystic areas on MRI
- Steroid cell tumor: rare and affect patients of all ages but usually fifth and sixth decades
  - Usually virilizing and small (<3 cm) nodules and always unilateral
  - Seen as a small mass with hyperintense areas on T1 weighted images due to abundant intracellular lipid and intense enhancement due to rich vascularity

REFERENCES

Bekiesińska-Figatowska, M., Jurkiewicz, E., Iwanowska, B., Uliasz, M., Romaniuk-Doroszewska, A., … Bragoszewska, H. (2007). Magnetic resonance imaging as a diagnostic tool in case of ovarian masses in girls and young women. *Medical Science Monitor, 13*(Suppl. 1), 116–120.

Jung, S. E., Rha, S. E., Lee, J. M., Park, S. Y., Oh, S. N., … Cho, K. S. (2005). CT and MRI findings of sex cord-stromal tumor of the ovary. *American Journal of Roentgenology, 185*(1), 207–215. doi:10.2214/ajr.185.1.01850207.

CASE 146

Cesarean Section Scar Implantation of Pregnancy

1. B. The earliest time at which a gestational sac in a normal intrauterine pregnancy is shown by transvaginal ultrasound is 4.5 weeks after last menstrual period.
2. D. In a patient with a positive serum β-HCG test, nonvisualization of an intrauterine pregnancy may represent very early intrauterine pregnancy, failed pregnancy, or ectopic pregnancy.
3. C. The classic triad of symptoms of ectopic pregnancy are pelvic pain, vaginal bleeding, and tender adnexal mass.
4. B. Provided images demonstrate a gestational sac implanted in the lower uterine segment, at the site of prior cesarean section.

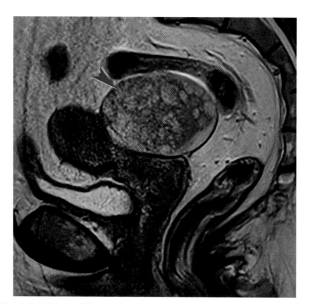

Fig. 144.1 Sagittal T2 weighted magnetic resonance image (MRI) that shows a large mixed solid and cystic mass *(red arrow)* posterior to the uterus.

Case 145 is online only and accessible at www.expertconsult.com.

Comment

Abnormal Implantation of Pregnancy

- Accounts for 2% of all pregnancies
  - In the first trimester, represents leading cause of death (9%–14% mortality)
  - Typically presents 6 to 8 weeks after last menstrual period
  - Classic symptom triad of ectopic (extrauterine) pregnancy: abdominal/pelvic pain, vaginal bleeding, tender adnexal mass
  - As ectopic pregnancy enlarges in size, risk for hemorrhagic rupture increases, with associated morbidity/mortality
  - Biochemical correlation with serum β-HCG
    - Increases during the first trimester to plateau at 9 to 11 weeks
    - Transvaginal US should show gestational sac at β-HCG ≥2000 mIU/mL
    - Average doubling time in a normal intrauterine pregnancy is ~48 hours
    - In ectopic pregnancy, serum β-HCG rises at a slower rate, typically <50% increase in 48 hours
- Extrauterine (ectopic pregnancy):
  - Fallopian tube: most common location of ectopic pregnancy (95%)
    - Adnexal mass separate from the ovary
    - Tubal ring sign: hyperechoic ring surrounding extrauterine gestational sac
  - Interstitial (2%–4%)
    - Intramyometrial segment of fallopian tube
    - Rupture may lead to life-threatening bleeding due to proximity to uterine artery
    - Eccentrically located gestational sac, surrounded by thin layer of myometrium measuring <5 mm thickness
  - Ovarian (3%)
    - Ovum is fertilized and retained in the ovary
  - Intraabdominal (1%)
    - Implantation at intraperitoneal location
- Intrauterine (abnormal implantation):
  - Cesarean section scar (<1%)
    - Within scar of prior cesarean section, within the anterior wall of the lower uterine segment, distinct from the endometrial cavity

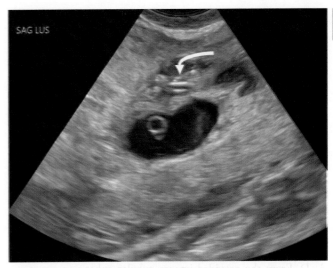

Fig. 146.2 Grayscale transvaginal ultrasound with smaller field of view demonstrates the gestational sac in close proximity to prior cesarean section scar with associated thinning of the overlying myometrium *(curved arrow)*. Findings are consistent with cesarean section implantation.

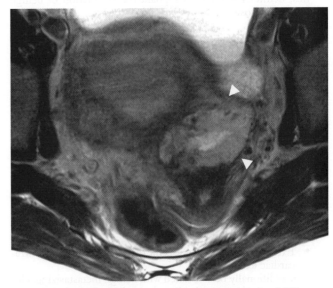

Fig. 146.3 Axial T2 weighted magnetic resonance imaging (MRI) confirms eccentric position of the gestational sac within the lower uterine segment with thinning of the overlying myometrium and bulging of the lower uterine segment contour *(arrowheads)*.

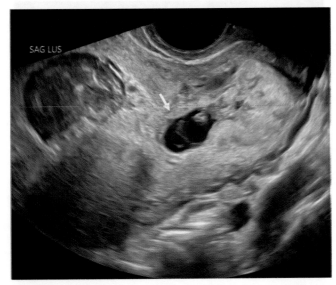

Fig. 146.1 Grayscale transvaginal ultrasound image demonstrating a gestational sac *(arrow)* with amnion and small embryo at the anterior lower uterine segment.

- Myometrium may be focally thinned, adding to the risk of rupture
- Cervical (<1%)
  - Implantation in cervical canal
- Cornual (<1%)
  - Cornual implantation in a bicornuate or septate uterus
- Heterotopic (1%)
  - Simultaneous intrauterine and extrauterine pregnancy

REFERENCES

Chukus, A., Tirada, N., Restrepo, R., & Reddy, N. I. (2015). Uncommon implantation sites of ectopic pregnancy: Thinking beyond the complex adnexal mass. *Radiographics, 35*, 946–959.

Kao, L. Y., Scheinfled, M. H., Chernyak, V., Rozenblit, A. M., Oh, S., & Dym, R. J. (2014). Beyond ultrasound: CT and MRI of ectopic pregnancy. *American Journal of Roentgenology, 202,* 904–911.

Lin, E. P., Bhatt, S., & Dogra, V. S. (2008). Diagnostic clues to ectopic pregnancy. *Radiographics, 28,* 1661–1671.

Rodgers, S. K., Chang, C., DeBardeleben, J. T., & Horrow, M. M. (2015). Normal and abnormal US findings in early first-trimester pregnancy: Review of the Society of Radiologists in Ultrasound 2012 Consensus Panel Recommendations. *Radiographics, 35,* 2135–2148.

CASE 147

Intravascular Leiomyomatosis

1. D. On MRI, flow voids result from the motion of protons out of the plane of spatially selective radiofrequency pulses and thus are an indicator of vascular patency.
2. D. Flow voids are most apparent on MR sequences with long TE, such as T2 weighted and proton density weighted image sequences.
3. D. From the provided images, tubular enhancing structures are shown in adnexal vessels, and may represent malignant pelvic vascular invasion or intravascular leiomyomatosis. Bland pelvic vein thrombosis would not be expected to enhance at postcontrast imaging.
4. D. Both metastasizing leiomyomatosis and intravascular leiomyomatosis represent benign yet clinically aggressive entities; neither represents malignant transformation of benign leiomyomatosis.

Comment

Intravascular Leiomyomatosis

- Rare condition, first described at autopsy in 1896
- Typically found among premenopausal women with history of hysterectomy or myomectomy for uterine leiomyoma
- Theorized to arise from either local extension of uterine leiomyoma into pelvic veins or to develop within pelvic veins from intimal smooth muscle proliferation
- Pathways of venous spread:
  - Veins in the myometrium and broad ligament
  - Subsequently may access systemic venous circulation via:
    - Uterine vein (more common), then pelvic veins
    - Ovarian vein (less common), then IVC or left renal vein
  - Extensive disease may ascend the IVC, resulting in intracardiac extension
- Can additionally be associated with benign metastasizing leiomyomatosis (e.g., to the lungs), or disseminated peritoneal leiomyomatosis after surgery

Imaging Features

- Coiled or nodular soft tissue mass, with tubular extension into veins
- On US, presents as hypoechoic tubular signal in pelvic vessels; flow around tubular filling defects in affected vessels can be seen on color Doppler US
- On CT, typically hypoenhancing serpiginous structures within contrast enhanced vessels
- On MRI, predominantly heterogeneous hyperintensity on T2 weighted images, with variable enhancement on postcontrast imaging
- Mimics:
  - Leiomyosarcoma: either arising from uterus or IVC
  - Bland thrombus: bland venous thrombus does not enhance following contrast administration
  - Malignant thrombus: such as arising from renal cell carcinoma

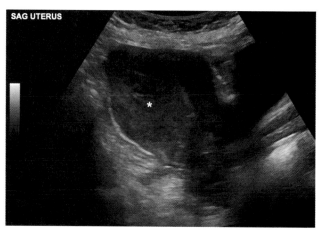

Fig. 147.1 Sagittal transabdominal grayscale ultrasound image of the uterus demonstrates an enlarged uterus with heterogeneous mass *(asterisk),* representing fibroid uterus.

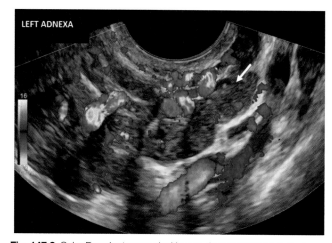

Fig. 147.2 Color Doppler transvaginal image demonstrating tubular hypoechoic material within the left adnexa *(arrow),* with internal Doppler flow.

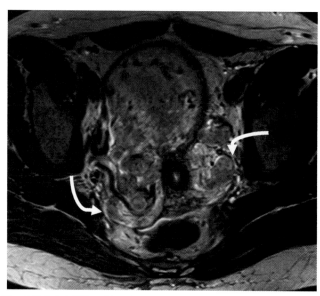

Fig. 147.3 Axial T2 weighted magnetic resonance imaging (MRI) shows T2 hyperintense tubular signal at left and right adnexa *(curved arrows)* suggesting intravascular mass.

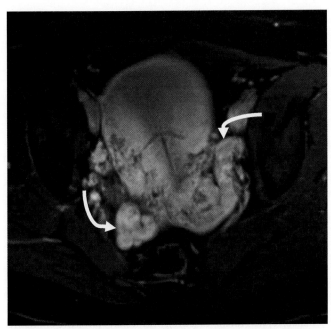

Fig. 147.4 Axial postcontrast magnetic resonance imaging (MRI) shows enhancement in the tubular signal in both adnexae *(curved arrows)*, likely representing intravascular leiomyomatosis. IUD is located in the lower uterine segment with arms imbedded in the adjacent myometrium.

Treatment

- Surgical management is preferred, including total hysterectomy, bilateral salpingo-oophorectomy, and removal of intravenous tumor.
- Staged surgical interventions may be necessary, depending on extent of disease.
- 30% risk of recurrence is reported, for which serial imaging follow-up is indicated after therapy.

REFERENCES

Bender, L. C., Mitsumori, L. M., Lloyd, K. A., & Stambaugh III, L. E. (2011). Intravenous leiomyomatosis. *Radiographics, 31*, 1053–1058.

Low, G., Rouget, A. C., & Crawley, C. (2012). Intravenous leiomyomatosis with intracaval and intracardiac involvement. *Radiology, 265*, 971–975.

CASE 148

Placenta Accreta Spectrum

1. D. The provided images demonstrate features typical of invasive placentation (placenta accreta spectrum). The US image shows bulging uterine contour, vascular lacunae, and the MR images additionally show intraplacental T2 hypointense bands and increased vascular channels. While preeclampsia and HELLP syndrome are related to abnormalities of placentation, no specific imaging features of the placenta are known to be associated.
2. E. Major risk factors for placenta accreta are prior cesarean section and placenta previa. The other risk factors are considered minor in comparison.
3. B. Placenta increta refers to chorionic villi partially invading myometrium; placenta increta is not readily distinguished from placenta accreta by conventional imaging.
4. D. Typical MR features of invasive placentation include rounded or lumpy placental contour, uterine bulging, and T2 hypointense bands (not T2 hyperintense bands).

Comment

Placenta Accreta Spectrum

- Normally, decidua basalis separates placental chorionic villi from myometrium
  - At birth, allows for complete separation of placenta from contracting myometrium
- Abnormality of decidua basalis results in invasive placentation of chorionic villi invading myometrium
- If undiagnosed before delivery, can lead to potentially life-threatening perinatal hemorrhage
- Spectrum of abnormality, defined by depth of myometrial invasion
  - Accreta: villi attached to myometrium, do not invade muscle
  - Increta: partial invasion of myometrium
  - Percreta: invasion of myometrium, and potentially beyond into adjacent organs
- Risk factors:
  - Placenta previa
  - Prior cesarean section: risk increases with increasing cesarean section deliveries
  - Minor risk factors: advanced maternal age, uterine anomaly, prior uterine surgery including myomectomy

Imaging Findings

- Ultrasound
  - Sensitivity 91%, specificity 97%
  - Placenta typically assessed at the 18- to 20-week fetal screening examination
  - Imaging features associated with accreta:
    - Placenta previa
    - Vascular lacunae, result in "Swiss cheese" appearance
    - Abnormal color Doppler; turbulent flow in placental lacunae
    - Loss of retroplacental hypoechoic zone/clear space
    - Reduced myometrial thickness
- MRI
  - For equivocal US findings, high clinical risk factors, or surgical planning, such as for extrauterine organ involvement in percreta

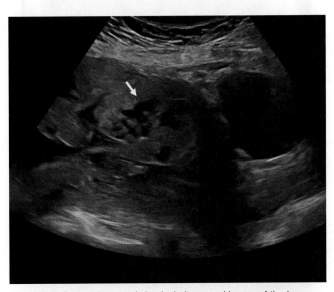

Fig. 148.1 Grayscale transabdominal ultrasound image of the lower uterine segment demonstrates anterior placenta with multiple irregularly shaped lacuna *(arrow)*, loss of the retroplacental hypoechoic zone, and bulging uterine contour, representing placenta accreta spectrum.

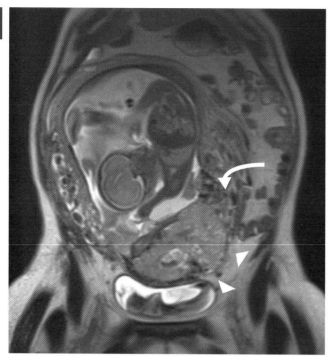

Fig. 148.2 Coronal T2 weighted magnetic resonance imaging (MRI) demonstrates heterogeneous signal of the placenta and prominent intraplacental vessels *(curved arrow),* with lumpy rounded contours *(arrowheads).*

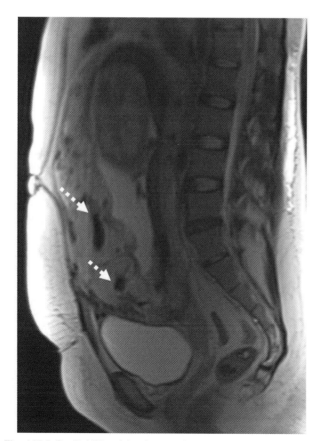

Fig. 148.3 Sagittal T2 weighted magnetic resonance imaging (MRI) demonstrates T2 hypointense intraplacental bands *(dashed arrows).* Off-axis image partially images placenta previa *(not shown).*

- Optimal time for MR assessment of accreta reported at 24 to 30 weeks
  - Before 24 weeks, immature placenta remains subject to physiologic changes
  - After 30 weeks, placental appearance becomes more heterogeneous, may confound interpretation
- At this time, placenta is typically of homogeneous intermediate signal
- Imaging features associated with accreta:
  - Placenta previa
  - Lumpy, rounded placental contour
  - Uterine bulging
  - Heterogeneous placenta signal intensity
  - T2 hypointense intraplacental bands
  - Percreta may be indicated by loss of fat plane to adjacent organs, or intermediate placental signal involving bladder, bowel, or abdominopelvic musculature

REFERENCES

Baughman, W. C., Corteville, J. E., & Shah, R. R. (2008). Placenta accreta: Spectrum of US and MR imaging findings. *Radiographics, 28,* 1905–1916.

Bourgioti, C., Zafeiropoulou, K., Fotopoulos, S., Nikolaidou, M. E., Antoniou, A., … Tzavara, C. (2018). MRI features predictive of invasive placenta with extrauterine spread in high-risk gravid patients: A prospective evaluation. *American Journal of Roentgenology, 211,* 701–711.

Kilcoyne, A., Shenoy-Bhangle, A. S., Roberts, D. J., Sisodia, R. C., Gervais, D. A., & Lee, S. I. (2017). MRI of placenta accreta, placenta increta, and placenta percreta: Pearls and pitfalls. *American Journal of Roentgenology, 208,* 214–221.

CASE 149

Penile Fracture

1. C, D. Images show hematoma in the right corpus cavernosum with air within it, which can be seen with penile fracture and/or urethral rupture.
2. D. Penile fracture result of traumatic coitus usually from thrusting the erect penis against the symphysis pubis or perineum.
3. B. Nonoperative treatment can be tried in penile fracture; however, these can lead to long-term complications, and surgery is the preferred treatment for penile fracture.
4. A, B, D. Rupture of the Buck fascia can lead to extension of the hematoma into the scrotum. Urethral injury is rare; however, it can be seen in approximately 1% to 3% of cases. Long-term complications after penile fracture include penile deviation, painful intercourse, painful erection, erectile dysfunction, priapism, skin necrosis, arteriovenous fistula, urtherocavernous fistula, and urethral stricture. Penile fracture leads to detumescence and loss of erection.

Comment

- Normal penile anatomy:
  - Penis is divided into two parts: the body (corpus) and the root (radix)
  - Corpus is composed of three parallel cylindrical masses of erectile tissue: two lateral corpora cavernosum and the ventromedial corpus spongiosum
  - At the distal end of the penis, the corpus spongiosum expands to form the glans penis
  - Each of these three erectile bodies are enveloped by a fibrous sheet called the tunica albuginea
  - Buck fascia (deep fascia of the penis) is a fibrous sheet that surrounds the tunica albuginea and is divided into dorsal and ventral compartments. Dorsal compartment encloses the two corpora cavernosa and the ventral compartment encloses the corpus spongiosum.

- Penile artery arises from the internal predental artery and divides into two main branches, the cavernous artery and the dorsal artery
  - Cavernous artery courses through the center of the corpus cavernosum and gives off many helicine arteries, which supply the sinusoids in the corpus cavernosum
  - Dorsal artery courses in the dorsum of the penis
  - Blood from the sinusoids drains via the subalbugineal venous plexus into the deep dorsal vein in the dorsum of the penis and then via the periprostatic venous plexus into the internal predental vein
- Penile fracture refers to a rupture of the corpus cavernosum induced by blunt trauma to the erect penis.
- Majority of the cases are the result of traumatic coitus usually from thrusting the erect penis against the symphysis pubis or perineum.
- Diagnosis is from typical clinical presentation of patients commonly hearing a "pop" or cracking sound from the erect penis at the moment of injury. This is followed by detumescence and acute swelling, pain, and deformity of the penis.
- Urethral injury from penile fracture is rare and the incidence ranges from 0% to 3%.
- Imaging:
  - Ultrasound imaging may demonstrate the break in the tunica of the penis with a hematoma. In presence of urethral injury, fluid collection may be seen adjacent to the urethra.
  - Magnetic resonance imaging can detect the presence, location, and extent of the tunical tear. Penile or scrotal hematomas are best demonstrated at T2 weighted MRI than postcontrast T1 weighted images.
  - Rupture of the Buck fascia can lead to extension of the hematoma into the scrotum
- Treatment:
  - Nonoperative treatment of penile fracture includes use of compression bandages, erection-inhibiting estrogens, penis splints, antibiotics, and fibrinolytic agents
  - Surgical treatment includes evacuation of the hematoma, identification of the tunica injury, local corpora debridement, closure of the tunica laceration, and ligation of any destructive vasculature

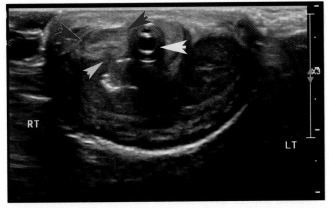

Fig. 149.1 Transverse image of the penis showing the two corpora cavernosa *(C)* with the Foley catheter *(yellow arrow)* seen in the urethra in the corpus spongiosum. Note the discontinuity in the tunica along the right corpus cavernosa *(green arrow)* with hematoma seen superficial to the right corpus cavernosa suggesting a penile fracture.

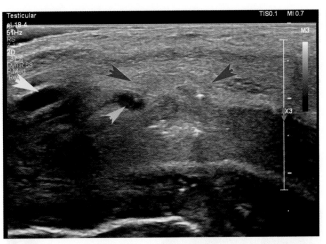

Fig. 149.2 Longitudinal image of the penile shaft in right corpus cavernosa showing a hypoechoic collection with echogenic areas *(red arrow)* within it suggestive of air. Note small fluid collection *(green arrow)* seen in between the urethra with the Foley catheter within it *(yellow arrow)* and the hematoma in the corpus cavernosum. This was suspicious for urethral injury, which is confirmed during surgery.

REFERENCES

Choi, M. H., Kim, B., Ryu, J. A., Lee, S. W., & Lee, K. S. (2000). MR imaging of acute penile fracture. *Radiographics, 20*(5), 1397–1405. doi:10.1148/radiographics.20.5.g00se051397.

Kachewar, S., & Kulkarni, D. (2011). Ultrasound evaluation of penile fractures. *Biomedical Imaging and Intervention Journal, 7*(4), e27. doi:10.2349/biij.7.4.e27.

CASE 150
Penile Mass

1. A, B. Multiple penile masses seen in the images suggest a penile neoplasm like metastasis (more likely) or a primary penile carcinoma.
2. D. Secondary metastatic tumors of the penis are most commonly seen in patients who have primary malignancy located in the urogenital tract, for example bladder carcinoma.
3. B, C. Main prognostic factor for carcinoma of the penis of the degree of invasion by the primary tumor and the status of draining lymph nodes.
4. A. Primary penile cancers are most often solitary, ill-defined infiltrating tumors that are hypointense relative to the corpora on both T1 and T2 weighted images.

Comment

- Penile cancer is relatively rare and accounts for 10% to 20% of all malignancies worldwide and only 0.4% of all male malignancies in the United States.
- Most important factor in penile cancer is the presence of foreskin with the resultant accumulation of smegma. Other risk factors include chronic inflammatory conditions, smoking, treatment with psoralen or ultraviolet A photo chemotherapy, and human papillomavirus 16 and 18.
- Primary neoplasms of the penis are commonly squamous cell carcinomas with a smaller number of sarcomas, melanomas, and lymphomas.
- Secondary metastatic tumors of the penis are most commonly seen in patients with primary tumor located in the urogenital tract. Metastasis from other primary cancers include rectum, stomach, bronchus, and thyroid gland.

- Primary squamous cell carcinoma of the penis is most commonly located in the glans penis.
- Main prognostic factor for carcinoma of the penis is the degree of invasion by the primary tumor and the status of draining lymph nodes.
- Imaging:
  - MRI is superior to CT in evaluation of tumors in the penis.
  - T2 weighted and gadolinium-enhanced T1 weighted MRI are the most useful in defining local extent of a penile neoplasm.
  - Primary penile cancers are most often solitary, ill-defined infiltrating tumors that are hypointense relative to the corpora on both T1 and T2 weighted images. Enhancement is

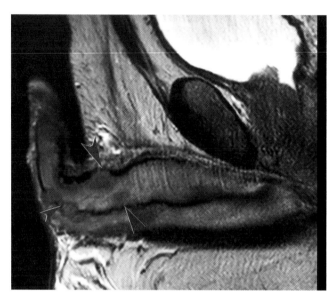

Fig. 150.1 Sagittal T2 weighted magnetic resonance imaging (MRI) shows multiple hypointense masses *(red arrowheads)* in the corpora cavernosa and corpus spongiosum. This patient had history of urinary bladder carcinoma, and hence these are suspicious for metastasis.

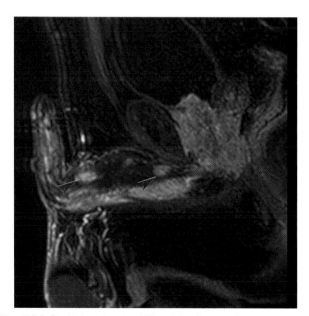

Fig. 150.2 Sagittal postcontrast T1 weighted magnetic resonance imaging (MRI) shows multiple enhancing masses *(red arrowheads)* in the corpora cavernosa. This patient had history of urinary bladder carcinoma and hence these are suspicious for metastasis.

seen on postgadolinium images, although to a lesser extent than the corpora cavernosa.
- Metastasis typically manifests as multiple discrete masses in the corpora cavernosa and corpus spongiosum. These are seen as low-signal-intensity areas within the corporal bodies compared to normal corporal tissue on both T1 and T2 weighted sequences.
- Treatment: varies depending on the site and extent of the primary cancer and the presence of metastatic groin lymph nodes. Surgical resection, radiation therapy with external beam irradiation, and brachytherapy have been used.

REFERENCES

Singh, A. K., Saokar, A., Hahn, P. F., & Harisinghani, M. G. (2005). Imaging of penile neoplasms. *Radiographics*, 25(6), 1629–1638. doi:10.1148/rg.256055069.

Suh, C. H., Baheti, A. D., Tirumani, S. H., Rosenthal, M. H., Kim, K. W., … Ramaiya, N. H. (2015). Multimodality imaging of penile cancer: What radiologists need to know. *Abdominal Imaging*, 40(2), 424–435. doi:10.1007/s00261-014-0218-6.

CASE 152
Prostate Cancer With Extraprostatic Extension

1. C. Fig. 152.1 depicts prostate cancer on multiparametric MRI with extraprostatic extension of tumor into the left seminal vesicle, compatible with T3b disease. The tumor is not T2 because there is extraprostatic disease. It is not T3a because it involves the seminal vesicle. It is not T4 because it does not involve another nearby organ such as the bladder or rectum.
2. B. Tumor is seen on T2 weighted imaging and the ADC map in the left posterior peripheral zone, extending beyond the margins of the prostate at the level of the left neurovascular bundle. The tumor does not invade the rectum, bladder, or levator sling.
3. A. Loss of the normally acute rectoprostate angle is useful for detecting extraprostatic extension of posteriorly oriented peripheral zone tumors. Transition zone, central zone, or anterior tumors with extraprostatic extension will not invade the rectoprostate angle unless very large.
4. D. Broad capsular contact (>10 mm contact between the prostate tumor and capsule) is the least specific sign for predicting extraprostatic extension of tumor. Neurovascular bundle invasion, loss of the rectoprostatic angle, and capsular bulge are all more specific (in descending order).

Comment

- Prostate cancer is the most common malignant tumor in men and the second leading cause of cancer deaths in men.
- The traditional role of imaging in prostate cancer is to stage disease. MRI has emerged as a tool for local staging and continues to increase in importance as a guide for targeted biopsy in men with suspected prostate carcinoma.
- A critical finding at multiparametric MRI is determination of extraprostatic (commonly referred to as extracapsular) extension of tumor, in which tumor grows beyond the fibromuscular band surrounding the prostate and into the periprostatic fat.
- Extraprostatic extension of tumor classifies a prostate carcinoma as T3, with T3a disease referring to extraprostatic extension without seminal vesicle invasion and T3b disease referring to seminal vesicle invasion.
- Identification of extraprostatic extension on imaging is important for surgical planning to guide expectations for postoperative

Case 151 is online only and accessible at www.expertconsult.com.

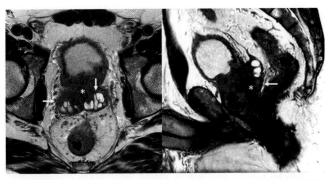

Fig. 152.1 Axial and sagittal T2 weighted magnetic resonance imaging (MRI) demonstrates ill-defined T2 hypointense signal abnormality representing prostate cancer (*), with extension to the bilateral seminal vesicles *(arrows)*.

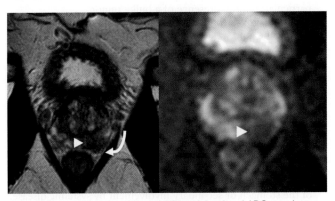

Fig. 152.2 In a different patient, axial T2 weighted and ADC map images demonstrate left midgland peripheral zone signal abnormality *(arrowhead)* involving the left neurovascular bundle *(curved arrow)*.

morbidity, particularly if the neurovascular bundle is involved. Extraprostatic extension also confers a higher risk of recurrence and metastatic disease after prostatectomy.

- Multiparametric MRI findings of prostate cancer with extra-prostatic extension:
  - Invasion of the seminal vesicle (asymmetric loss of T2 hyper-intensity) or neurovascular bundle (asymmetric nodularity/thickening)
  - Macroscopic tumor signal beyond the prostate in the peri-prostatic fat or adjacent organs
  - Loss of the rectoprostatic angle
  - Capsular bulge
  - Broad capsular contact (>10 mm contact between tumor and capsule)

REFERENCES

Mehralivand, S., Shih, J. H., Harmon, S., Smith, C., Bloom, J., ... Czarniecki, M. (2019). A grading system for the assessment of risk of extraprostatic extension of prostate cancer at multiparametric MRI. *Radiology, 290*(3), 709–719.

Wibmer, A., Vargas, H. A., Donahue, T. F., et al. (2015). Diagnosis of extracapsular extension of prostate cancer on prostate MRI: Impact of second-opinion readings by subspecialized genitourinary oncologic radiologists. *American Journal of Roentgenology, 205*(1), W73–W78.

Woo, S., Cho, J. Y., Kim, S. Y., & Kim, S. H. (2015). Extracapsular extension in prostate cancer: Added value of diffusion-weighted MRI in patients with equivocal findings on T2-weighted imaging. *American Journal of Roentgenology, 204*(2), W168–W175.

CASE 153

Postprostatectomy Prostate Cancer Recurrence

1. A. Following radical prostatectomy, the most common site of local recurrence is at the vesicourethral anastomosis.
2. B. Images demonstrate, at the level of the vesicourethral anastomosis, a T2 intermediate/hypointense focus with intense postcontrast enhancement, most likely representing recurrent prostate cancer.
3. D. Whereas T2 weighted and diffusion weighted imaging are of primary importance in the PI-RADS assessment of the transitional and peripheral zones in the treatment-naïve prostate, dynamic contrast-enhanced imaging is of increased importance in the posttreatment assessment of prostate cancer.
4. D. Compared to its pretreatment appearance, the MRI appearance of the postradiation prostate is typically atrophic and with decreased T2 signal intensity.

Comment

Biochemical Recurrence of Prostate Cancer

- Following radical prostatectomy for organ-confined prostate cancer, serum PSA level should be undetectable, <0.10 ng/mL.
- Biochemical recurrence is defined as:
  - Undetectable PSA level after radical prostatectomy, with two or more subsequent PSA level increases
  - Two PSA level measurements >0.2 ng/mL after radical prostatectomy
- PSA recurrence after prostatectomy occurs in 20% to 35% of cases, with median time to biochemical recurrence of 2 to 3 years after surgery.
- Following radiation therapy, some residual serum PSA level is expected; biochemical recurrence is defined as PSA rise of >2.0 ng/mL above the postradiation nadir.

Postprostatectomy MR Appearance

- Bladder and levator sling descend in the low pelvis to occupy the prostatectomy bed.
- Retained seminal vesicles are shown in up to 20% of patients.
- Lymphocele may be present if lymphadenectomy was performed.
- Less common: hematoma, abscess, urinoma
- Local recurrence:
  - The most common site of local recurrence after prostatectomy is at the vesicourethral anastomosis
  - The normal appearance of the vesicourethral anastomosis is isointense to muscle on T1 weighted imaging, and slightly hyperintense to muscle on T2 weighted imaging
  - Recurrent tumor typically is slightly hypointense to muscle on T2 weighted imaging, and with early dynamic contrast enhancement and restricted diffusion

Postradiation MR Appearance

- Two main types of radiation therapy for prostate cancer
  - Interstitial brachytherapy
  - External-beam radiation therapy (EBRT)
- Radiation therapy results in decreased size/relative atrophy of the prostate gland, with diffusely decreased T2 signal
- Local recurrence:
  - Recurrent disease is most commonly seen at the site of prior tumor
  - Postradiation appearance reduces conspicuity of disease recurrence on T2 weighted imaging; early dynamic contrast enhancement and restricted diffusion increase sensitivity of detection

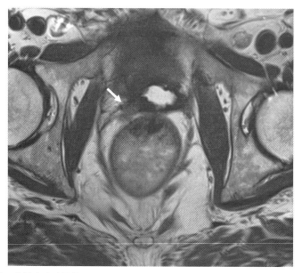

Fig. 153.1 Axial T2 weighted image of the prostatectomy bed, at a level superior to the vesicourethral anastomosis, demonstrates focal T2 intermediate/hypointense signal rightward adjacent *(arrow)*.

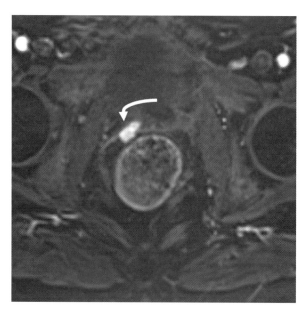

Fig. 153.2 Dynamic contrast-enhanced image shows intense early enhancement at the focal area *(curved arrow)*.

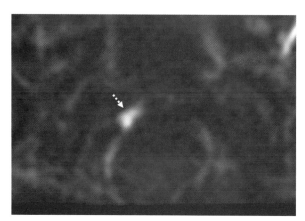

Fig. 153.3 Diffusion weighted image shows restricted diffusion *(dashed arrow)*. Together, these imaging findings are characteristic of locally recurrent prostate cancer.

REFERENCES

Patel, P., Mathew, M. S., Trilisky, I., & Oto, A. (2018). Multiparametric MR imaging of the prostate after treatment of prostate cancer. *Radiographics, 38*, 437–449.

Tanaka, T., Yang, M., Froemming, A. T., Bryce, A. H., Inai, R., ... Kanazawa, S. (2020). Current imaging techniques for and imaging spectrum of prostate cancer recurrence and metastasis: A pictorial review. *Radiographics, 40*, 709–726.

CASE 154

Gastric Lymphoma

1. A, B, D. Gastric carcinoma, gastric lymphoma, and gastrointestinal stromal tumor can present with diffuse thickening of the stomach wall.
2. B. Stomach is the most commonly affected site in the bowel followed by small intestine and colon.
3. C. Preservation of the perigastric fat planes at CT is more likely to be seen in lymphoma than in adenocarcinoma, particularly in the presence of a bulky tumor.
4. A. Esophagogastroduodenoscopy (EGD) with biopsy sampling is the gold standard for diagnosis of PGL. CT, MRI, and PET exams are most helpful for staging and follow-up of patients with gastric lymphoma.

Comment

- Gastrointestinal (GI) lymphoma accounts for 5% to 20% of extranodal lymphomas: the stomach is the most common site, followed by small intestine (ileum, 60%–65%; jejunum, 20%−25%; duodenum, 6%–8%; and then colorectal lymphomas, 6%–12%).
- Gastric lymphoma may either be due to primary involvement of the stomach or secondary involvement by systemic disease.
- Primary gastrointestinal lymphoma is the most common extranodal manifestation of non-Hodgkin lymphoma, accounting for up to 20% of all cases.
- Most commonly accepted hypothesis for gastric lymphoma is that a chronic infection of the stomach by *Helicobacter pylori* causes lymphoid proliferation in the gastric mucosa, with subsequent development of gastric mucosa associated lymphoid tissue (MALT) lymphoma.
- The most common CT pattern of gastric lymphoma is the presence of diffuse or segmental wall thickening of 2 to 5 cm with low contrast enhancement and extensive lateral extension of the tumour due to submucosal spread.
  - CT can also evaluate the presence of lymph node enlargement.
  - It may also present less commonly as a polypoidal mass, an ulcerative lesion, or a mucosal nodularity.

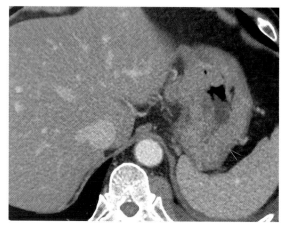

Fig. 154.1 Axial postcontrast computed tomography (CT) image through the upper abdomen shows diffuse thickening of the stomach wall *(red arrow)*.

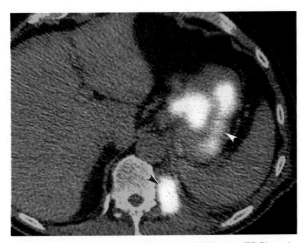

Fig. 154.2 Axial image from an 18-fluorodeoxyglucose (FDG) positron emission tomography (PET) scan shows uptake in the stomach wall *(white arrow)* in addition to a large lymph nodal mass in the paraspinous region in the lower thorax *(black arrow)*. This was consistent with non-Hodgkin lymphoma with involvement of the stomach.

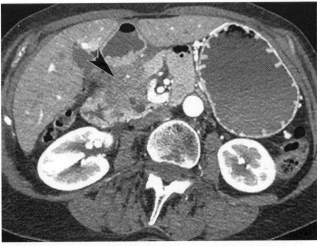

Fig. 155.1 Axial postcontrast computed tomography (CT) image through the upper abdomen shows a large hypointense mass in the pancreatic head *(red arrows)* with small area of calcification within it. This is consistent with pancreatic adenocarcinoma.

REFERENCES
Ghai, S., Pattison, J., O'Malley, M. E., Khalili, K., & Stephens, M. (2007). Primary gastrointestinal lymphoma: Spectrum of imaging findings with pathologic correlation. *Radiographics*, 27(5), 1371–1388. doi:10.1148/rg.275065151.
Lo Re, G., Federica, V., Midiri, F., Picone, D., La Tona, G., … Galia, M. (2016). Radiological features of gastrointestinal lymphoma. *Gastroenterology Research and Practice*, 2016, 2498143. doi:10.1155/2016/2498143.

CASE 155

Krukenberg Tumor

1. A, B. Primary ovarian tumors and Krukenberg tumors can present as bilateral mixed solid and cystic ovarian masses.
2. A, B. Colon and stomach are the most common primary tumors that result in ovarian metastasis.
3. A. 10% of ovarian tumors represent metastatic tumors to the ovary.
4. D. CT appearance is indistinguishable from primary ovarian carcinoma. Features that favor a Krukenberg tumor include presence of primary neoplasm.

Comment

- Krukenberg tumor, also known as carcinoma mucocellulare, refers to the signet ring subtype of metastatic tumor to the ovary.
- Colon and stomach are the most common primary tumors that result in ovarian metastasis followed by breast, lung, contralateral ovary, pancreatic, and cholangiocarcinoma.
- Represent 5% to 10% of all the ovarian tumors and up to 50% of all metastatic tumors to the ovary.
- Time from diagnosis of primary neoplasm to the development of ovarian metastasis is variable and can range from several months to >10 years.
- Imaging:
  - Imaging features are nonspecific and often difficult to differentiate from other ovarian neoplasms
  - US: typically seen as bilateral solid ovarian masses with clear well-defined margins or irregular hypoechoic solid pattern or moth-eaten–like cyst formation
  - CT: appearance can be indistinguishable from primary ovarian carcinoma. Features that favor a Krukenberg tumor include presence of primary neoplasm.

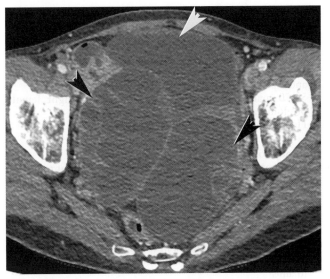

Fig. 155.2 Axial postcontrast computed tomography (CT) image through the lower abdomen shows two large cystic masses *(red arrows)* posterior to the bladder *(yellow arrow)* with septations and solid components within them. These were new from the prior exam performed 6 months ago and arose from the ovaries bilaterally and were consistent with Krukenberg tumors.

- MRI: typically seen as bilateral complex masses with hypointense solid components due to dense stromal reaction with internal hyperintensity due to mucin on T1 and T2 weighted MRI. Strong contrast enhancement is usually seen in the solid component or the wall of the intratumoral cyst.

REFERENCE
Koyama, T., Mikami, Y., Saga, T., Tamai, K., & Togashi, K. (2007). Secondary ovarian tumors: Spectrum of CT and MR features with pathologic correlation. *Abdominal Imaging*, 32(6), 784–795. doi:10.1007/s00261-007-9186-4.

CASE 156

Crohn's Disease: Active Inflammation

1. B. The images demonstrate typical MRI findings of active inflammatory Crohn's disease involving the distal ileum. There is no colonic wall thickening pictured that would strongly indicate ulcerative colitis. Small bowel adenocarcinoma does not typically present in a segmental distribution.
2. C. Crohn's disease most commonly involves the terminal ileum, although may involve any part of the gastrointestinal tract, from mouth to anus, sometimes multiple locations separated by normal bowel, called skip lesions.
3. E. Asymmetric wall abnormalities, worse on the mesenteric side, including hyperenhancement, are highly specific of Crohn's disease. All other listed findings may be seen in other infectious or inflammatory abnormalities of the small bowel and are not specific to Crohn's disease.
4. D. A classic imaging finding of ulcerative colitis is ahaustral colon, sometimes referred to as leadpipe colon. Unlike Crohn's disease, ulcerative colitis spares the anus and tends to involve the rectum and colon in a retrograde fashion, without skip lesions.

Comment

Crohn's Disease

Background
- Peak age of onset is bimodal (first peak 15–20 years old; second peak 50–80 years old)
- More common in Northern Europe, North America, Australia, and Japan
- 50:50 male to female ratio, with possible slight female predominance
- Has familial predisposition

Pathophysiology
- Pathogenesis is incompletely understood; thought to be due to an environmental or triggering event in a genetically susceptible patient.
- Chronic granulomatous inflammatory disease of the gastrointestinal tract
- Often has a relapsing and remitting course
- Involves the entire bowel wall (transmural)
- May involve any part of the gastrointestinal tract from mouth to anus
  - Small bowel is involved in ~80% of cases, most commonly the terminal ileum
  - More than one area may be involved with intervening normal bowel (skip lesions)
- Three phenotypes that may exist independently or coexist
  - Active inflammation
  - Stricturing disease
  - Penetrating disease
- Perianal disease (e.g., skin tags, sinus tracts, fistula, abscesses) may be seen with any phenotype

Imaging Appearance: Active Inflammation
- On CT and MRI: single or multiple segments of bowel demonstrating:
  - Mural hyperenhancement
    - Asymmetric wall involvement, worse on the mesenteric side (most specific finding of Crohn's disease)
    - May also have diffuse hyperenhancement or mural stratification (target sign)

- Intramural edema (only seen by MRI on T2 fat-saturated images)
- Mural ulcerations (finding most indicative of severe disease)
- Restricted diffusion
  - Nonspecific sign in the absence of other signs of active inflammation
  - If seen with other signs of active inflammation, indicates more severe disease
- Vasa recta hyperemia
  - Nonspecific sign, may be seen with current or previous bowel inflammation
- Fibrofatty proliferation

Mimics
- Ulcerative colitis
  - Usually spares anus, starts in rectum and involves colon in a sequential retrograde fashion
  - May see backwash ileitis
  - Involves only the mucosal layer of the colon
  - Classic finding is ahaustral colon (leadpipe colon)
- Infectious enteritis
  - Several infections are known to cause ileitis, including *Yersinia*, *Salmonella*, *Cytomegalovirus*, and *Mycobacterium tuberculosis*, among others
  - Tuberculosis may mimic Crohn's disease with associated penetrating features (fistulae, abscesses)
- Vasculitis
  - Most commonly due to small and midsize vessel vasculitides, including systemic lupus erythematosus, polyarteritis nodosa, Henoch-Schönlein purpura, and Behçet disease

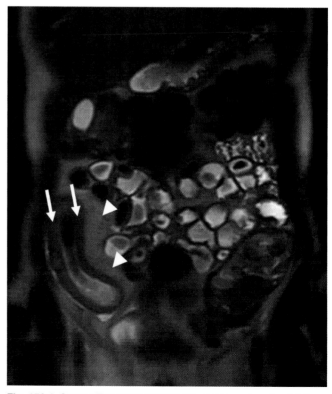

Fig. 156.1 Coronal T2 weighted magnetic resonance imaging (MRI) demonstrates segmental wall thickening of the distal ileum *(arrows)*, with fibrofatty proliferation *(arrowheads)*.

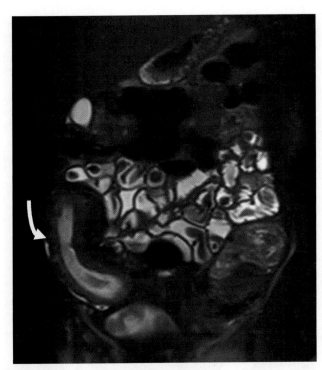

Fig. 156.2 Coronal T2 weighted fat-saturated image shows corresponding mural edema *(curved arrow).*

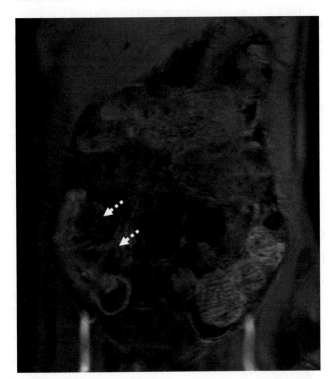

Fig. 156.3 Coronal T1 early postcontrast image demonstrates vasa recta hyperemia *(dashed arrows).*

- Tends to be diffuse and may involve mucosa only or transmural involvement
- Often have evidence of generalized disease activity elsewhere
- Small bowel angioedema
  - May be congenital or acquired (most commonly associated with use of angiotensin-converting enzyme inhibitors)

- Due to increased capillary permeability in the mucosa resulting in submucosal edema
- Imaging features of segmental small bowel dilatation, thickening, straightening, and ascites
- Radiation enteritis
  - Usually a geographic distribution that corresponds to the radiation field
- Malignancy
  - Lymphoma: typically homogeneous wall thickening, often with aneurysmal dilatation
  - Adenocarcinoma: heterogeneous, irregular, and often focal eccentric bowel wall thickening
  - Metastases: usually presents as serosal mass

REFERENCES

Bruining, D. H., Zimmerman, E. M., Loftus, E. V., Sandbom, W. J., Sauer, C. G., ... Strong, S. A. (2018). Consensus recommendations for evaluation, interpretation, and utilization of computed tomography and magnetic resonance enterography in patients with small bowel Crohn's disease. *Radiology, 286,* 776–799.

DiLauro, S., & Crum-Cianflone, N. F. (2010). Ileitis: When is it not Crohn's disease. *Current Gastroenterology Reports, 12,* 249–258.

Guglielmo, F. F., Anupindi, S. A., Fletcher, J. G., Al-Hawary, M. M., Dillman, J. R., ... Grand, D. J. (2020). Small bowel Crohn's disease at CT and MR enterography: Imaging atlas and glossary of terms. *Radiographics, 40,* 354–375.

Macari, M., Megibow, A. J., & Balthazar, E. J. (2007). A pattern approach to the abnormal small bowel: Observations at MDCT and CT enterography. *American Journal of Roentgenology, 188,* 1344–1355.

CASE 158

Acute Graft-Versus-Host Disease (GVHD) Involving Small Bowel

1. D. The provided images demonstrate diffuse small bowel wall thickening and mucosal enhancement; differential considerations should include infectious enteritis and acute graft-versus-host disease. Pseudomembranous colitis commonly results in diffuse colonic wall thickening; small bowel abnormality is relatively uncommon.
2. E. Typical manifestations of acute graft-versus-host disease are dermatitis, enterocolitis, and cholestasis; meningitis is not a typical manifestation.
3. E. Typical abdominal imaging findings of acute graft-versus-host disease include diffuse, small bowel mucosal enhancement, fluid-filled small bowel, and vasa recta engorgement; small bowel obstruction is not a typical finding.
4. C. Clinical manifestations of acute and chronic forms have minimal overlap. While patients with acute GVHD often develop chronic GVHD, the history of acute GVHD is not necessary to develop chronic GVHD.

Comment

Graft-Versus-Host Disease (GVHD)

- Complication of hematopoietic stem cell transplant (HSCT)
  - Allogeneic and nonmyeloablative recipients at risk
  - Overall incidence of up to 59% after HSCT
- Results from interaction between donor T lymphocytes and the recipient's epithelial cells of the skin, gastrointestinal tract, and hepatobiliary system
  - Likelihood of developing GVHD and its resultant severity is related to the magnitude of differences between host and donor human leukocyte antigen (HLA) proteins

Case 157 is online only and accessible at www.expertconsult.com.

- US National Institutes of Health (NIH) classification:
  - Classic acute: presents <100 days of HSCT (typically 10–40 days); features rash, nausea, vomiting, anorexia, diarrhea, ileus, or cholestatic hepatitis
  - Late-onset acute: >100 days after HSCT
  - Classic chronic: any time after HSCT; without features of acute GVHD
  - Overlap syndrome: any time after HSCT; features of acute and chronic GVHD appear together

Imaging Findings in Acute GVHD

- Gastrointestinal
  - Bowel wall thickening: most commonly diffusely involving small bowel and colon, can be dilated and fluid filled
  - Mucosal enhancement: resulting appearance of target sign of bowel in cross section
  - Mesenteric edema
  - Vascular engorgement
  - Chronic GVHD: sequelae of chronic bowel wall thickening, including esophageal, small bowel, or colonic strictures
- Hepatobiliary
  - Generally less prevalent that gastrointestinal findings
  - When present, seen in conjunction with skin and gastrointestinal manifestations; isolated hepatic involvement is rare
  - Hepatosplenomegaly
  - Periportal edema
  - Gallbladder wall enhancement/thickening
  - Chronic GVHD: nonspecific; may developed extrahepatic bile duct stricture
- Mimics
  - Neutropenic enterocolitis (typhilitis): typically involves cecum/ascending colon and terminal ileum
  - Infectious enterocolitis
    - CMV colitis: viral enteritis is typically segmental, rather than diffuse
    - Pseudomembranous colitis: pancolitis; small bowel involvement is uncommon
  - Radiation enteritis

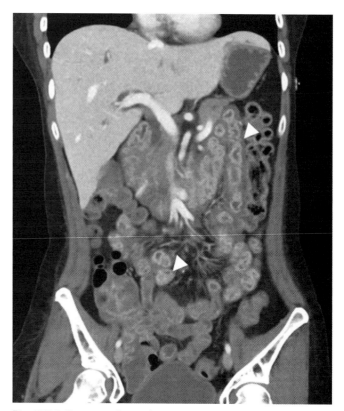

Fig. 158.2 Contrast-enhanced computed tomography (CT) of the abdomen and pelvis. Coronal image shows diffuse small bowel abnormality, involving jejunum and ileum *(arrowheads)*, representing small bowel involvement by acute graft-versus-host disease.

REFERENCES

Lubner, M. G., Menias, C. O., Agrons, M., Alhalabi, K., Katabathina, V. S., … Elsayes, K. M. (2017). Imaging of abdominal and pelvic manifestations of graft-versus-host disease after hematopoietic stem cell transplant. *American Journal of Roentgenology, 209,* 33–45.

Mahgerefteh, S. Y., Sosna, J., Bogot, N., Shapira, M. Y., Pappo, O., & Bloom, A. I. (2011). Radiologic imaging and intervention for gastrointestinal and hepatic complications of hematopoietic stem cell transplantation. *Radiology, 258,* 660–671.

CASE 159

Internal Hernia

1. A, B, D. Images show proximal bowel obstruction with collection of bowel loops in the right upper quadrant with convergence of the vessels and mesentery passing in the right upper quadrant likely at hernia orifice.
2. A. Paraduodenal hernia is the most common type of internal hernia.
3. A, B, C, D. CT features of internal hernia include all of the findings listed.
4. D. Complications of cholecystitis include gangrenous cholecystitis, gallbladder rupture with biliary peritonitis, and formation of abscesses and fistulas.

Comment

- Background: An internal hernia is defined as the protrusion of abdominal viscera, most commonly small bowel loops, through a peritoneal or mesenteric aperture into a compartment in the abdominal and pelvic cavity.

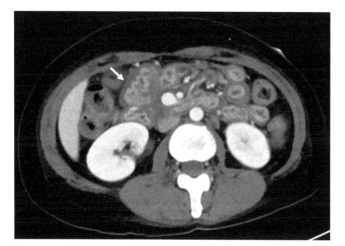

Fig. 158.1 Contrast-enhanced computed tomography (CT) of the abdomen and pelvis. Axial image demonstrates small bowel wall thickening and mucosal enhancement of the duodenum *(arrow).*

- Most common clinical symptoms are nausea, vomiting, abdominal pain, and abdominal distention.
- Can be congenital, including both normal foramina or recesses and unusual apertures resulting from anomalies of peritoneal attachment and internal rotation, or acquired if caused by inflammation, trauma, and previous surgery, like gastric bypass for bariatric treatment and liver transplantation.
- Classification:
  - On the basis of the topographic distribution of bowel loops related to the anatomic location of the orifice
    - Left paraduodenal hernia
    - Right paraduodenal hernia
    - Foramen of Winslow hernia
    - Pericecal hernia
    - Sigmoid mesocolon related hernia
    - Transmesenteric hernia
    - Transomental hernia
    - Supravesical and pelvic hernia
  - According to the type of hernia orifice
    - Normal foramen
      - Foramen of Winslow
    - Unusual peritoneal fossa or recess into retroperitoneum
      - Paradoudenal hernia
      - Pericecal hernia
      - Intersigmoid hernia
      - Pelvic internal hernia (except for broad ligament hernia)
    - Abnormal opening in a mesentery or peritoneal ligament
      - Small bowel mesentery related hernia
      - Greater omentum related hernia
      - Most types of lesser sac hernia (except foramen of Winslow)
      - Transverse mesocolon related hernia
      - Falciform ligament hernia
      - Broad ligament hernia
      - Roux-en-Y anastomosis related hernia
- Locations and relative frequencies of internal hernias are as follows:
  - Paraduodenal, 53%
  - Pericecal, 13%
  - Foramen of Winslow, 8%
  - Transmesenteric and transmesocolic, 8%

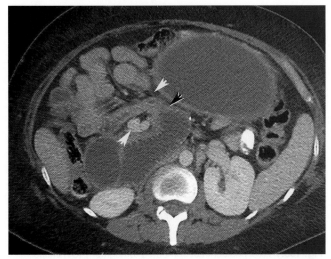

Fig. 159.1 Axial contrast-enhanced computed tomography (CT) shows dilatation of the stomach and proximal small bowel with transition point seen in the right upper abdomen *(red arrow)* with convergence of the mesentery and vessels *(yellow arrows)* in this region. This was consistent with a transmesenteric internal hernia.

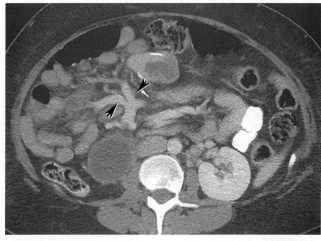

Fig. 159.2 Axial contrast-enhanced computed tomography (CT) at a lower level shows convergence of the mesentery and vessels *(red arrows)* in the region of internal hernia.

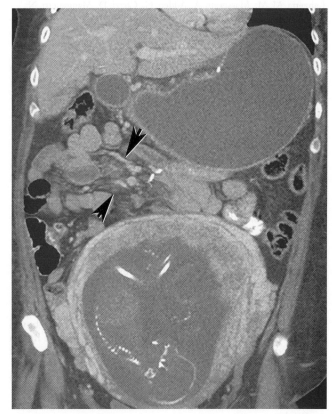

Fig. 159.3 Coronal reformat from a contrast-enhanced computed tomography (CT) shows dilatation of the stomach with convergence of the mesentery and vessels in the right upper quadrant *(red arrow)*. This was consistent with a transmesenteric internal hernia. Note fetus in the pregnant uterus.

- Pelvic and supravesical, 6%
- Sigmoid mesocolon, 6%
- Transomental, 1%–4%
- Imaging: CT is the imaging modality of choice
  - Protocol to be used:
    - Nonenhanced scan: to detect an increased bowel wall attenuation reflecting hemorrhagic congestion in cases of strangulation

- Contrast-enhanced scan: for depicting mesenteric vessels and for the assessment of bowel wall vascularity
- Key features of internal hernia on CT
  - Bowel configuration
    - Saclike mass or cluster of dilated small bowel loops within an abnormal anatomic location in the setting of small bowel obstruction
  - Mesenteric abnormalities
    - Convergence of vessels and mesenteric fat at the hernia orifice
    - Displacement of key mesenteric vessels
    - Engorgement, crowding, twisting, stretching of mesenteric vessels if strangulation is present
  - Position of surrounding viscera
    - Displacement of surrounding structures around the hernia sac

REFERENCES

Doishita, S., Takeshita, T., Uchima, Y., Kawasaki, M., Shimono, T., … Yamashita, A. (2016). Internal hernias in the era of multidetector CT: Correlation of imaging and surgical findings. *Radiographics, 36*(1), 88–106.

Lanzetta, M. M., Masserelli, A., Addeo, G., Cozzi, D., Maggialetti, N., … Danti, G. (2019). Internal hernias: A difficult diagnostic challenge. Review of CT signs and clinical findings. *Acta Biomedica, 90*(5-S), 20–37. doi:10.23750/abm.v90i5-S.8344.

Takeyama, N., Gokan, T., Ohgiya, Y., Satoh, S., Hashizume, T., … Hataya, K. (2005). CT of internal hernias. *Radiographics, 25*(4), 997–1015.

CASE 160

Intussusception

1. B. Images show a typical appearance of an intussusception in the left lateral abdomen with invagination of a small bowel loop into another small bowel loop.
2. B. Malignant tumors are less common in small bowel intussusceptions, and most intussusceptions in the small bowel are transient.
3. A, B, C. CT features of intussusception include bowel obstruction, target, and sausage-shaped appearance. Coiled-spring appearance is seen on barium exam.

Comment

- Background: Intussusception is the invagination of a bowel loop with its mesenteric fold (intussusceptum) into the lumen of a contiguous portion of bowel (intussuscipiens) as a result of peristalsis.
  - Intestinal intussusception in adults is uncommon: 5% of all intussusceptions
  - Most often secondary to an identifiable cause
- Etiology
  - Malignant or benign neoplasms
    - Malignant tumors more common in large bowel intussusception (60%–70% of cases)
    - Malignant tumors are less common in small bowel intussusceptions (30%–15%)
  - Polyps
  - Meckel diverticulum
  - Postoperative adhesions
- Can be classified based on location into three types
  - Enteroenteric, when confined to the small bowel
  - Colocolonic, when involving the large bowel
  - Enterocolonic, which can be ileocecal or ileocecocolonic
- Can be classified based on location into three types

- Can be classified on the basis of whether a lead point is present
  - Without a lead point tend to be transient, self-limiting, and nonobstructing
  - Intussusceptions with a lead point may manifest with atypical clinical findings.
- Ileocaecal intussusceptions are the most common of all the gastrointestinal intussusceptions, followed by enteroenteric intussusceptions, which can account for up to 40% of cases. Colocolonic intussusceptions are the less common type of intussusceptions.
- Imaging:
  - Plain radiographs: not sensitive or specific and usually have normal bowel gas pattern
  - Barium enema: "coiled spring" appearance with barium in the lumen of the intussusceptum and in the intraluminal space
  - Ultrasound (not pathognomonic)
    - Transverse: target or doughnut sign, with hypoechoic rim (edematous bowel wall) surrounding hyperechoic central area (intussusceptum and associated mesenteric fat)
    - Longitudinal: sandwich, trident or hayfork sign, with layering of hypoechoic bowel wall and hyperechoic mesentery
    - Oblique: pseudokidney sign, with hypoechoic bowel wall mimicking the renal cortex and hyperechoic mesentery mimicking the renal fat
    - Doppler may help determine viability of the tissue
    - Adults: may be less useful, as often cannot identify the pathologic lead point and is most useful when an abdominal mass is palpated
  - CT: imaging modality of choice for the detection and assessment of adult bowel intussusception
    - Three patterns:
      - Targetlike pattern: round mass with intraluminal soft tissue and eccentric fat density
      - Reniform pattern: bilobed mass with central low attenuation and peripheral higher density
      - Sausage-shaped pattern: alternating areas of low and high attenuation related to the bowel wall, mesenteric fat and fluid, intraluminal fluid, contrast material, or air

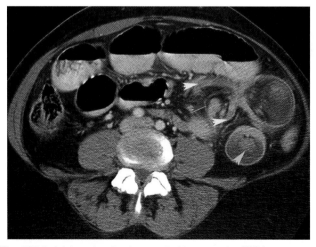

Fig. 160.1 Axial postcontrast computed tomography (CT) image showing invagination of a small bowel loop (intussusceptum; *red arrow*) into another small bowel loop (intussuscipiens; *yellow arrows*) in the left midabdomen suggesting an intussusception. Note the soft tissue mass (*green arrow*) seen at the tip of the intussusceptum.

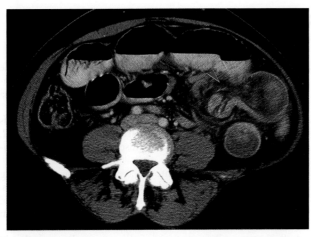

Fig. 160.2 Axial postcontrast computed tomography (CT) image showing invagination of a small bowel loop (intussusceptum) into another small bowel loop (intussuscipiens) in the left midabdomen suggesting an intussusception. Note the mesentery being pulled into the intussusception (*red arrow*).

- Composed of a central intussusceptum and outer intussuscipiens, separated by mesenteric fat, which appears as a low-attenuation layer. Enhanced vessels are often seen within the mesenteric fat.
- Intussusception with a lead point usually appears as an abnormal targetlike mass with a cross-sectional diameter greater than that of the normal bowel and may be associated with proximal bowel obstruction
- Treatment: depends on the type of intussusception
  - Colonic: surgical resection without reduction because of risk of venous embolization of tumor or seeding from a malignant tumor
  - Enteroenteric: depends on cause and symptoms; may require resection or manual reduction during surgery, may be treated with enema reduction, or may require no intervention

REFERENCES
Choi, S. H., Han, J. K., Kim, S. H., Lee, J. M., Lee, K. H., … Kim, Y. J. (2004). Intussusception in adults: From stomach to rectum. *American Journal of Roentgenology, 183*(3), 691–698. doi:10.2214/ajr.183.3.1830691.

Kim, Y. H., Blake, M. A., Harisinghani, M. G., Archer-Arroyo, K., Hahn, P. F., … Pitman, M. B. (2006). Adult intestinal intussusception: CT appearances and identification of a causative lead point. *Radiographics, 26*(3), 733–744. doi:10.1148/rg.263055100.

Valentini, V., Buquicchio, G. L., Galluzzo, M., Ianniello, S., Di Grezia, G., … Ambrosio, R. (2016). Intussusception in adults: The role of MDCT in the identification of the site and cause of obstruction. *Gastroenterology Research and Practice, 2016*, 5623718. doi:10.1155/2016/5623718.

CASE 161

Villous Adenoma of the Rectum

1. B. The most common location of villous adenomas is the rectum and rectosigmoid colon. The most common extracolonic location is the duodenum.
2. A. McKittrick-Wheelock syndrome is the name of the condition when a villous adenoma is associated with uncontrolled watery diarrhea leading to fluid, protein, and electrolyte imbalance.
3. C. The rate of malignant transformation is higher in villous adenomas (40%), compared with tubulovillous (22%) or tubular adenomas (5%).
4. A. In the images, the curved arrows represent vessels and desmoplastic response. It can sometimes be difficult to differentiate these two entities on MRI; vessels and desmoplastic response tend to appear T2 hypointense and linear, while extramural tumor is usually T2 intermediate signal (with MRI signal matching the primary tumor) and nodular.

Comment

Villous Adenoma
Background/Pathophysiology
- Adenomatous polyps are premalignant epithelial neoplasms
  - Three adenoma subtypes on a continuous spectrum: tubular adenomas are most common (>80%), followed by tubulovillous (10%–15%) and villous adenomas (<5%)
- Occur due to loss of the adenomatous polyposis coli (APC) gene, which is a tumor suppressor gene
- Most arise spontaneously (3%–7% prevalence in screening cohorts)
  - Individuals with hereditary polyposis syndromes, such as familial adenomatous polyposis (FAP), are at increased risk of developing adenomas
- Approximately 40% of villous adenomas demonstrate malignant degeneration to adenocarcinoma

Clinical Features
- Often asymptomatic
- May present as iron-deficiency anemia due to occult bleeding, obstruction, and/or prolapse/intussusception
- Rarely, associated with uncontrolled mucous secretion leading to watery diarrhea, dehydration, and electrolyte abnormalities known as McKittrick-Wheelock syndrome

Imaging Appearance
MRI
- Polypoidal, frondlike pedunculated masses; superficially spreading tumors are less common
- T2 intermediate signal, occasionally with T2 hyperintense layer along the periphery of the masses
- Most have a vascular stalk, demonstrating T2 hypointense and enhancing linear streak from the mesorectal fat
- In a small study of 23 villous adenomas, MRI staging was concordant with pathologic staging in 74% of cases; with 22% overstaged (pathologic T1 and T2 tumors were reported as T3 on MRI)

Transrectal Ultrasound (TRUS)/Endoscopic Ultrasound (EUS)
- Well-circumscribed, frondlike hypoechoic masses
- May show intratumoral cystic change
- Pedunculated masses may be difficult to assess due to mobility

MRI Versus TRUS/EUS for T-staging
- Similar to slightly improved accuracy for T-staging with TRUS/EUS
  - Studies have shown radiologic/pathologic T-staging concordance of MRI ranging from 45% to 74% versus 69% to 97% for TRUS/EUS

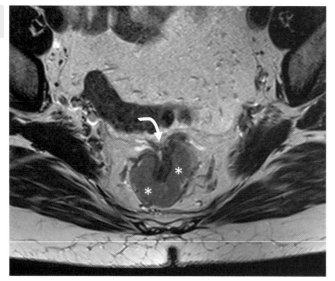

Fig. 161.1 Axial T2 weighted magnetic resonance imaging (MRI) demonstrates a polypoid, frondlike T2 intermediate signal mass *(asterisks)* within the midrectum, attached to the rectal wall by a stalk *(curved arrow)*.

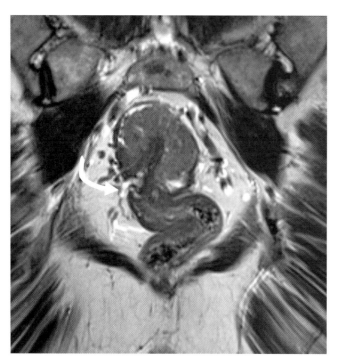

Fig. 161.2 Coronal T2 weighted image shows the site of the vascular stalk *(curved arrow)*, with mild tethering of the rectal wall. Endoscopic biopsy showed villous adenoma with associated rectal adenocarcinoma.

REFERENCES

De Vargas Macciucca, M., Casale, A., Manganaro, L., Floriani, I., Fabrizio, F., … Marchetti, L. (2010). Rectal villous tumours: MR features and correlation with TRUS in the preoperative evaluation. *European Journal of Radiology, 73,* 329–333.

Lubner, M. G., Menias, C. O., Johnson, R. J., Gaballah, A. H., Shaaban, A., & Elsayes, K. M. (2018). Villous gastrointestinal tumors: Multimodality imaging with histopathologic correlation. *Radiographics, 38,* 1370–1384.

Raynaud, L., Mege, D., Zappa, M., Guedj, N., Vilgrain, V., & Panis, Y. (2018). Is magnetic resonance imaging useful for the management of patients with rectal villous adenoma? A study of 45 consecutive patients treated by transanal endoscopic microsurgery. *International Journal of Colorectal Disease, 33,* 1695–1701.

CASE 162

T3 Rectal Adenocarcinoma

1. C. The layers of the rectal wall as visible on MRI from inside extending outward are the mucosa (T2 hypointense), the submucosa (mildly T2 hyperintense), and the muscularis propria (T2 hypointense).
2. B. A tumor that grows through the submucosa and extends into, but not beyond, the muscularis propria is staged as T2. Tumor that extends beyond the muscularis propria into mesorectal fat is staged as T3.
3. D. A tumor that grows into adjacent structures, including uterus, vagina, prostate gland, seminal vesicles, bone, muscles, pelvic fat beyond the mesorectum, nerves, ureters, and blood vessels, is staged as T4b. If the tumor invades the peritoneum but not any other structures, it is staged as T4a.
4. A. Squamous cell carcinomas of the anorectal region should be staged and treated as anal cancers regardless of where they are located. Anal/squamous cell carcinomas are staged differently than rectal/adenocarcinomas cancers.

Comment

Rectal Adenocarcinoma

Background/Pathophysiology
- Third most common cancer in men and second most common in women
- Third leading cause of cancer-related deaths in both men and women
- Approximately 44% of colorectal cancers occur in the rectum.
- Most colorectal adenocarcinomas arise from adenomatous polyps (see Case 161).

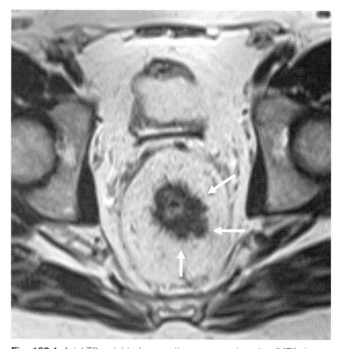

Fig. 162.1 Axial T2 weighted magnetic resonance imaging (MRI) demonstrates an ill-defined, annular midrectal mass with tumor extending beyond the muscularis propria from 3- to 6-o'clock *(arrows)*, consistent with T3 rectal adenocarcinoma.

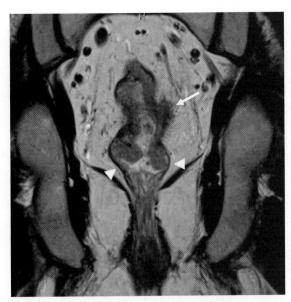

Fig. 162.2 Coronal T2 weighted image demonstrates an irregular mass arising from the left lateral wall of the rectum *(arrow)* consistent with rectal carcinoma with infiltration outside the rectal wall. For comparison, a segment of low rectum with linear T2 hypointense signal of muscularis propria, representing uninvolved intact muscularis propria *(arrowheads).*

Imaging Appearance

- MRI is essential for the staging and treatment planning for rectal adenocarcinoma
  - Tumors ≥ T3 AND/OR node positive are usually treated with neoadjuvant chemoradiation, while tumors ≤ T2 AND node negative usually go straight to surgery
- Layers of rectal wall on MRI (innermost to outermost)
  - Mucosa (T2 hypointense), the submucosa (mildly T2 hyperintense), and the muscularis propria (T2 hypointense)
- T stage:
  - T1 = invasion into submucosa
  - T2 = invasion through submucosa into muscularis propria
  - T3 = invasion through muscularis propria into mesorectal fat
  - T4a = invasion into visceral peritoneum
  - T4b = invasion into adjacent structures
- Tumors usually demonstrate T2 intermediate signal (exception: mucinous tumors that are T2 hyperintense) and may be annular, partially annular, or polypoidal.
- Tumors should be primarily staged on T2 weighted images (best anatomic distinction), oblique to the plane of the tumor, to reduce artifacts related to volume averaging.

REFERENCES
Gollub, M. J., Lall, C., Lalwani, N., & Rosenthal MH. (2019). Current controversy, confusion, and imprecision in the use and interpretation of rectal MRI. *Abdominal Radiology, 44*(11), 3549–3558.
Horvat, N., Tavares Rocha, C. C., Oliveira, B. C., Petkovska, I., & Gollub, M. J. (2019). MRI of rectal cancer: Tumor staging, imaging techniques, and management. *Radiographics, 39,* 367–387.
Matalon, S. A., Mamon, H. J., Fuchs, C. S., Doyle, L. A., Tirumani, S. H., ... Ramaiya, N. H. (2015). Anorectal cancer: Critical anatomic and staging distinctions that affect use of radiation therapy. *Radiographics, 35,* 2090–2107.

CASE 163

Cervical Cancer

1. B. The MRI for Patient B demonstrates loss of the T2 hypointense cervical stromal ring with nodular extension of soft tissue into the space lateral to the cervix, compatible with parametrial extension. Parametrial extension is not seen in the imaging for Patient A.

2. B. There is left-sided parametrial extension in Patient B, depicted as discontinuity of the T2 dark cervical ring and tumor extension into the tissues lateral to the left cervix. Contrast this appearance with the clean, intact T2 hypointense cervical ring seen in Patient A, who does not have parametrial extension. Also note the asymmetry of the cervix in Patient B due to the lack of right-sided parametrial extension.

3. A. Cervical carcinoma is staged clinically according to the FIGO staging system. Imaging is used to guide treatment. Ultrasound may detect some elements of local staging but is not first line. PET/CT is useful to evaluate for distant metastases or recurrence. MRI is the imaging gold standard for evaluating local extent of disease.

4. A, B, C, D. Tumor size, parametrial extension, vaginal invasion, and hydronephrosis are all critical elements of a staging cervical cancer MRI. Precise reporting of greatest dimension (more or less than 4 cm) and degree of vaginal invasion are important details to provide the gynecologic surgeon.

Comment

- Cervical cancer is the third most common gynecologic malignancy, typically presenting in young to middle-aged women.
- Squamous cell carcinoma in association with HPV exposure accounts for the majority of cervical cancer cases, with adenocarcinoma occurring less frequently.
- Patients may present with vaginal bleeding/discharge or an abnormal Pap smear.
- Tumor is staged clinically according to the FIGO staging system.
- Prognosis depends on size, stage, and histologic grade of the tumor.
- Although the tumor is staged clinically, imaging may be used for direct management and triage patients to primary surgery vs. neoadjuvant chemoradiotherapy.
- Imaging findings of cervical cancer:
  - US: heterogeneous hypoechoic cervical mass, which may show hypervascularity on color Doppler. US can be useful to determine certain local staging elements, such as size (smaller or larger than 4 cm), invasion into adjacent organs, and hydronephrosis.
  - CT: not utilized for local staging. Can be used to evaluate for adenopathy and distant metastases.
  - PET/CT: can be used for staging of disease and evaluation for recurrence
  - MRI: gold standard for imaging of local disease extent. Cervical cancer appears as hyperintense on T2 weighted and hyperenhancing on postcontrast T1 weighted imaging relative to the hypointense cervical stroma. The following should be described on reporting of cervical cancer on MRI:
    - Tumor size: a maximum size >4 cm is a tipping point for consideration of upfront surgery
    - Parametrial extension: presents as loss of the circumferential T2 hypointense cervical stromal ring with irregularity of the fat adjacent to the cervix. MRI has a high negative predictive value for evaluating parametrial extension (IIb or not IIb).
    - Vaginal invasion: if present, describe invasion of the upper two-thirds of the vagina (stage IIa) vs. lower one-third (stage IIIa)
    - Pelvic sidewall involvement
    - Hydronephrosis
    - Bladder or rectal invasion

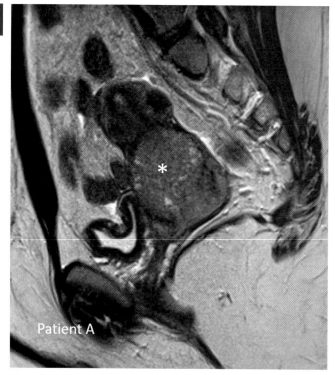

Fig. 163.1 Sagittal T2 weighted magnetic resonance imaging (MRI) of Patient A demonstrates a round cervical mass *(asterisk)* extending to the lower uterine segment.

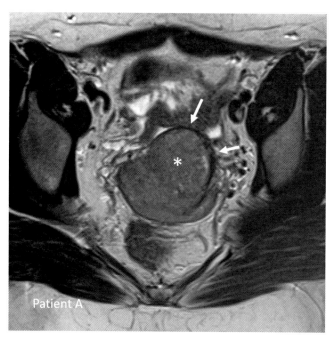

Fig. 163.2 Axial T2 weighted image of Patient A shows bulging contour of the mass *(asterisk)* leftward, with intact T2 hypointense band *(arrows),* indicating no parametrial extension.

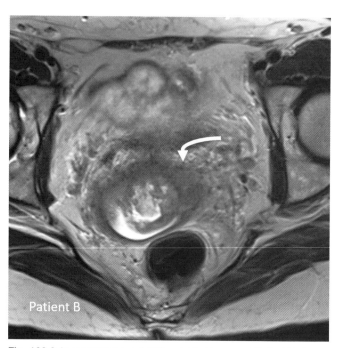

Fig. 163.3 In comparison, axial T2 weighted image of Patient B shows ill-defined T2 intermediate signal extending beyond the boundary of T2 hypointensity, indicating left parametrial extension *(curved arrow).*

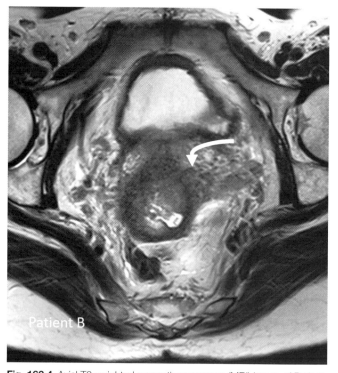

Fig. 163.4 Axial T2 weighted magnetic resonance (MRI) image of Patient B at a lower level in the pelvis showing ill-defined T2 intermediate signal extending beyond the boundary of T2 hypointensity of the wall, indicating left parametrial extension *(curved arrow).*

REFERENCES

Kaur, H., Silverman, P. M., Iyer, R. B., Verschraegen, C. F., Eifel, P. J., & Charnsangavej, C. (2003). Diagnosis, staging, and surveillance of cervical carcinoma. *American Journal of Roentgenology, 180*(6), 1621–1631.

Nicolet, V., Carignan, L., Bourdon, F., & Prosmanne, O. (2000). MR imaging of cervical carcinoma: A practical staging approach. *Radiographics, 20*(6), 1539–1549.

CASE 164

Fistula-in-Ano

1. B. Figs. 164.1 through 164.4 demonstrate MRI findings of fistula-in-ano (or perianal fistula) seen to the left of the anal canal on axial and coronal images. The rectum is not shown on the provided images. A diagnosis of rectocele requires dynamic observation with defecography. Hemorrhoids are not depicted.

2. A. The images depict a left-sided intersphincteric fistula with internal mucosal opening in the left lateral anal canal. This is the most common type of perianal fistula. It does not cross through (transphincteric) or above (suprasphincteric) the external anal sphincter, nor is it outside of the anal canal (extrasphincteric).

3. D. Extrasphincteric fistula is the least common fistula-in-ano, accounting for ~1% of cases. It originates outside of the anal canal and courses through the levator ani complex into the rectum. Intersphincteric is most common, followed by transphincteric. Suprasphincteric is also uncommon (~5%).

4. C. Active fistulous tracts are hyperintense on T2 weighted imaging and demonstrate enhancement on fat-saturated post-contrast T1 weighted images. T2 hypointense tracts that do not enhance are chronic fistulas without active inflammation.

Comment

- Fistula-in-ano (or perianal fistula) is an abnormal connection between the anal canal and the skin, coursing in between, through, or alongside the anal sphincters.
- The causes of fistula-in-ano may be inflammatory (i.e., Crohn's disease), infectious (viral, fungal, TB), iatrogenic (i.e., postsurgical), or malignant.
- Symptoms are variable and may include perianal pain, tenesmus, pruritis, and infection.
- The most widely used surgical classification system is the Parks classification, which categories perianal fistulas into four categories according to their anatomic relation to the internal and external anal sphincter in the coronal plane.
  - Intersphincteric: majority of perianal fistulas, accounting up to three-fourths of cases. The fistula traverses the internal anal sphincter and descends inferiorly through the intersphincteric fat without coursing through the external anal sphincter.
  - Transphincteric: second most common (20%–25%). The fistula courses through the intersphincteric space, through the external anal sphincter, and into the ischiorectal fossa.
  - Suprasphincteric: uncommon (~5%). The fistula courses superiorly into the intersphincteric space, above the puborectalis muscle and through the iliococcygeus muscle, then heads back inferiorly through the ischiorectal fossa to the skin.
  - Extrasphincteric: least common (1%). The fistula originates from the ischiorectal fossa and tracks superiorly through the levator sling into the rectum (external to the anal canal).
- Imaging findings of fistula-in-ano:
  - MRI: although fistulography and ultrasound are traditional imaging options, MRI is currently the modality of choice. Imaging report should describe:
    - Location of fistula with position of internal mucosal opening
    - Classification according to the Parks classification (intersphincteric, transphincteric, suprasphincteric, extrasphincteric)

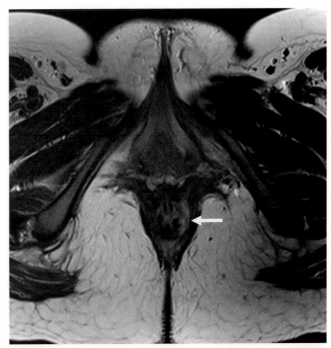

Fig. 164.1 Axial T2 weighted magnetic resonance imaging (MRI) of the anal canal demonstrates ill-defined signal of the leftward aspect of the internal anal sphincter *(arrow)* compared to the right.

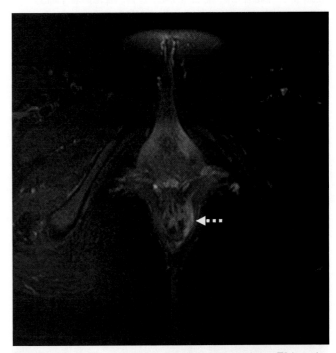

Fig. 164.2 Axial T2 weighted fat-suppressed image shows T2 hyperintense signal at the corresponding location *(dashed arrow)*, involving intersphincteric fat.

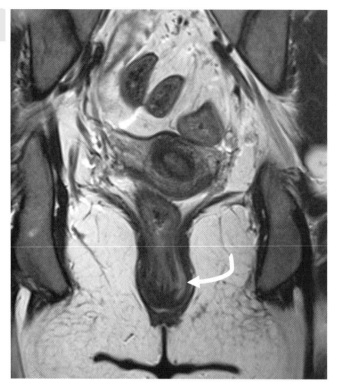

Fig. 164.3 Coronal T2 weighted image shows corresponding focal defect of the internal sphincter with adjacent crescentic signal abnormality at the intersphincteric fat *(curved arrow),* representing fistula-in-ano with intersphincteric focal fluid collection.

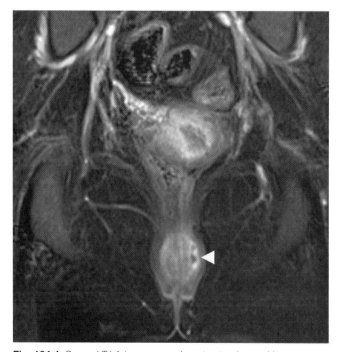

Fig. 164.4 Coronal T1 fat-suppressed contrast-enhanced image confirms rim-enhancing intersphincteric focal fluid collection *(arrowhead).*

- Fistula type (simple, branching, complex)
- Detection of fistula activity
  - Active: T2 hyperintense, enhancing
  - Chronic: T1 and T2 hypointense, no enhancement
- Presence of ischiorectal fossa abscess

REFERENCES

de Miguel Criado, J., del Salto, L. G., Rivas, P. F., Aguilera del Hoyo, L. F., Velasco, L. G., ... Diez Pérez de las Vacas, M. I. (2012). MR imaging evaluation of perianal fistulas: Spectrum of imaging features. *Radiographics, 32*(1), 175–194.

Morris, J., Spencer, J. A., & Ambrose, N. S. (2000). MR imaging classification of perianal fistulas and its implications for patient management. *Radiographics, 20*(3), 623–635.

CASE 165

MRI in Pregnancy: Acute Appendicitis

1. C. The provided images demonstrate a fluid-filled dilated tubular structure with adjacent inflammatory fat stranding in the right lower quadrant, representing findings of acute appendicitis.
2. D. These are all features of acute appendicitis on MRI.
3. E. According to the 2013 ACR guidance document on MR safe practices, data have not conclusively documented deleterious effects of MRI exposure on the developing fetus, and pregnant patients can undergo MR scans in any trimester of pregnancy, following risk-benefit analysis by a qualified radiologist.
4. B. Gadolinium is a pregnancy class C drug, indicating that safety in humans has not been proven. According to the 2013 ACR guidance document on MR safe practices, gadolinium-based MR contrast agents pass through the placental-fetal barrier, and there are no documented fetal indications for the use of MRI contrast.

Comment

Abdominal Pain in Pregnancy

- Diagnosis in pregnant women may be confounded by a number of factors:
  - Nonspecific leukocytosis
  - Displacement of abdominal organs from their typical locations
  - Difficult abdominal physical examination
  - Nonspecific nausea and vomiting

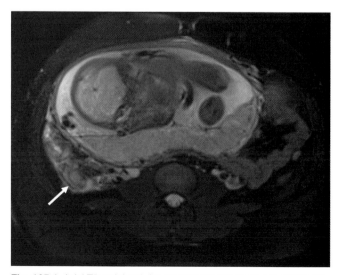

Fig. 165.1 Axial T2 weighted, fat-suppressed image demonstrates T2 hyperintense signal surrounding a tubular structure in the right lower quadrant *(arrow).*

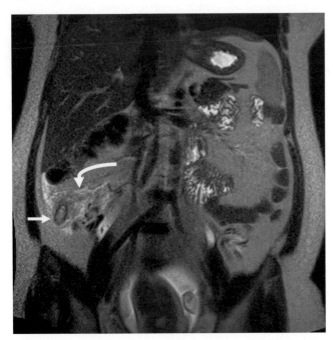

Fig. 165.2 Coronal T2 weighted image demonstrates a dilated tubular structure *(arrow)* with surrounding mesenteric stranding and edema *(curved arrow).*

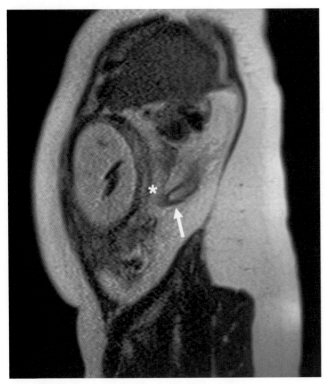

Fig. 165.3 Sagittal T2 weighted image demonstrates the dilated tubular structure *(arrow)* to arise from the cecum *(asterisk),* representing acute appendicitis.

- Imaging techniques
  - US evaluation of the abdomen of a pregnant patient may be obscured by the gravid uterus
  - CT poses risk of ionizing radiation
  - MRI allows for cross-sectional imaging with excellent soft tissue contrast resolution, without ionizing radiation

MRI in Pregnancy

- According to the 2013 ACR guidance document on MR safe practices:
  - Data have not conclusively documented deleterious effects of MRI exposure on the developing fetus
  - Pregnant patients can undergo MR scans in any trimester of pregnancy, following risk-benefit analysis by a qualified radiologist
- Gadolinium contrast in pregnancy
  - Pregnancy class C drug: safety in humans has not been proven
  - Gadolinium-based MR contrast agents pass through the placental-fetal barrier, are filtered by fetal kidneys, and excreted into amniotic fluid
  - No documented fetal indications for the use of gadolinium contrast
  - In rare instances where contrast may be helpful in assessing maternal anatomy or pathology, a rigorous risk-benefit analysis is advised

MR Diagnosis of Acute Appendicitis

- Appendicitis is the most common nonobstetric cause of abdominal pain resulting in surgery among pregnant patients
- MR reported to have 100% sensitivity and 94% specificity for acute appendicitis
- Imaging features:
  - Appendiceal diameter >7 mm
  - Appendiceal wall thickness >2 mm
  - Luminal contents with T2 weighted signal hyperintensity
  - Hyperintense perappendiceal fat stranding and fluid
  - Borderline features may be considered indeterminate and warrant follow-up
- Alternative (nongynecologic) diagnoses
  - Inflammatory bowel disease
  - Diverticulitis
  - Small bowel obstruction
  - Cholelithiasis/acute cholecystitis
  - Pancreatitis
  - Hydronephrosis

REFERENCES

American College of Radiology, Society for Pediatric Radiology. (2015). ACR-SPR practice parameter for the safe and optimal performance of fetal magnetic resonance imaging (MRI). Available at https://www.acr.org/-/media/ACR/Files/Practice-Parameters/MR-Fetal.pdf?la=en. Accessed March 29, 2020.

Expert Panel on MR Safety. (2013). ACR guidance document on MR safe practices: 2013. *Journal of Magnetic Resonance Imaging, 37,* 501–530.

Spalluto, L. B., Woodfield, C. A., DeBenedectis, C. M., & Lazarus, E. (2012). MR imaging evaluation of abdominal pain during pregnancy: Appendicitis and other nonobstetric causes. *Radiographics, 32,* 317–334.

Index of Cases